HISTORY OF INDIAN MEDICINE

HISTORY OF INDIAN MEDICINE

Containing Notices, Biographical and Bibliographical, of the Ayurvedic Physicians and their Works on Medicine

From the Earliest Ages to the Present Time

by

Girindranath Mukhopadhyaya, Bhisagacarya
B.A., M.D., F.A.S.B.

Volume II

Munshiram Manoharlal
Publishers Pvt Ltd

ISBN 81-215-0660-3
This edition 1994

Originally published in 1922-29
by University of Calcutta, Calcutta

Printed and published by Munshiram Manoharlal Publishers Pvt. Ltd.,
Post Box 5715, 54 Rani Jhansi Road,
New Delhi 110 055.

DEDICATED

TO

THE MEMORY OF MY BROTHER

MR. SATYENDRANĀTH MUKERJEE

MEDICAL PRACTITIONER

WHOSE UNSELFISH DEVOTION TO SCIENCE AND
TO THE NEEDS OF THE POOR AND HELP-
LESS CAUSED HIS UNTIMELY DEATH
IN THE DISCHARGE OF HIS
DUTIES TO A POOR
PATIENT

WORKS BY THE AUTHOR

1. The Surgical Instruments of the Hindus, With a Comparative Study of the Surgical Instruments of the Greek, Roman, Arab and the Modern European Surgeons. Griffith Prize Essay for 1909. Published by the Calcutta University, in two volumes. Vol. I: Text. Vol. II: contains about 400 illustrations

2. Tropical Abscess of the Liver
   Thesis approved for the Degree of Doctorate in Medicine, Madras University. Published by the Calcutta University

3. Muscles of the Human Body, arranged in tabular forms. Fourth Edition

4. The History of Indian Medicine containing Notices, Biographical and Bibliographical, of the Āyurvedic Physicians and their Works on Medicine. Griffith Prize Essay for 1911. In six volumes Calcutta University Publications. With a Foreward by Sir Asutosh Mookerjee, Kt., C.S.I., M.A., D.L., D.Sc., etc., Vice-Chanceller, Calcutta University.

   Vol. I
   Vol. II
   Vol. III.

5. Glossary of Indigenous Medicinal Plants.

6. Medicine in the Atharva Veda.

7. Medicine in the Vedic Times.

8. Lathyrism or the Kheśāridāl Poisoning

9. Some Human Parasites as mentioned in the Atharvaveda.

10. Treatment of Syphilis

11. The Bengali Scientific Glossary of the Terms of Medicine

PREFACE

A considerable lapse of time has occurred since the publication of the first volume and the second volume of History of Indian Medicine is now submitted to the public. In arranging the scheme and determining the scope of this work, certain points demanded consideration and it has by no means been easy to arrive at a decision regarding them. A History of Medicine would not be complete if the account of the Sages who promulgated the science did not find a place here. Medical science in ancient times was a subject of study which all learned men, sages, and kings learnt for the benefit of the human race.

In this volume the consideration of the pre-historic period—the account of the gods and sages who took part in the development of the healing art in India, has been dealt with. To know the History of Medicine in Ancient India is to know the entire domain of Indology as the teachers of medicine were sages who were seers of the Vedic hymns, elaborated the philosophical systems, speculated on the existence of God, and were, in fact, concerned in the intellectual history of Ancient India. To deal with such a vast field of study is impossible for any man and many shortcomings would be found in the book. It is restricted to the collection of data which are not even logically and classically arranged. Genealogical tables have been inserted wherever they were needed to elucidate the text.

The article on Śālihotra appeared in part in the *Historical Quarterly*, Vol. I and Vol. II. The introduction appeared in the *Journal of Āyurveda*, Vol. II and Vol. III.

The life of Atri has been described twice through oversight.

My thanks are due to authors for quotations from their books and much of the best in this treatise is due to others. I am under a pleasing obligation to my son Jitendranāth Mukerjee for valuable assistance in the correction of proofs.

156, Haris Mukerjee Road,
Bhowanipur, Calcutta.
1st September, 1926.

G. N. MUKERJEE

As regards the transliteration of Sanskrit words, we have employed the method adopted in the Congress of Orientalists and circulated in the Journal of the Royal Asiatic Society, ignoring in fact, the unpleasant characters of the Sacred Books of the East.

1

SANSKRIT AND ALLIED ALPHABETS.

अ	*a*	ओ	*o*	ट	*ṭ*	ब	*b*
आ	*ā*	औ	*au*	ठ	*ṭh*	भ	*bh*
इ	*i*	क	*k*	ड	*ḍ*	म	*m*
ई	*ī*	ख	*kh*	ढ	*ḍh*	य	*y*
उ	*u*	ग	*g*	ण	*ṇ*	र	*r*
ऊ	*ū*	घ	*gh*	त	*t*	ल	*l*
ऋ	*ṛ*	ङ	*ṅ*	थ	*th*	व	*v*
ॠ	*ṝ*	च	*c*	द	*d*	श	*ś*
ऌ	*ḷ*	छ	*ch*	ध	*dh*	ष	*ṣ*
ॡ	*ḹ*	ज	*j*	न	*n*	स	*s*
ए	*e*	झ	*jh*	प	*p*	ह	*n*
ऐ	*ai*	ञ	*ñ*	फ	*ph*	ळ	*l*

ं (*Anusvāra*) . . . *ṁ*	ऽ (*Avagraha*) . . . ’
ँ (*Anunāsika*) . . *m̐*	(*Udātta*) . . . . . _
: (*Visarga*) . . . . *ḥ*	*Svarita* . . . . . . ^
× (*Jihvāmūlīya*) . *ẖ*	*Anudātta* . . . . . ‿
≍ (*Upadhmānīya*) *ḫ*	

CONTENTS.

CHAPTER VIII.

CHAPTER IX.

CHAPTER X.

CHAPTER XI.

CHAPTER XII.

CHAPTER XIII.

INTRODUCTION

INTRODUCTION

It is no doubt interesting to find that the public has at last been awakened by a sense of responsibility as to their duty to help in the regeneration and development of Indian medical science. The Hindu physicians themselves have felt the necessity of an organisation among their professional brethren for the consideration of the ways and means for the proper study and improvement of the science of medicine and for propaganda work to train public opinion and enlist public sympathy in its favour. The All-India Ayurvedic Conference was thus ushered into existence. It has been doing useful work in this direction and holds its sittings in different provinces year after year. Important discussions relating to some department of medical science are held there amongst the physicians of various parts of India and Ceylon, irrespective of caste or creed. Such deliberations have not only enriched science but cemented the friendship of delegates who represented the different sections of the population of India. The Head Office of All-India Standing Committee—The Āyurveda Mahāmaṇḍala and Vidyāpīṭha—is located at Cawnpur for the present. About two dozen centres have been opened in the various parts of India to conduct examination of students in Āyurveda. Such centres of examination exist in Bengal, Behar, Oudh, Central India, Delhi, United Provinces, Rajputana, Central Provinces, Punjab, Sindh, Orissa, Drāviḍa, Andhra Deśa, Bombay, Karnatic, Berar, and Ceylon.

Our Government could not sleep over this consciousness of the people to regenerate their own system of medical practice. Colleges for systematic study and research have been established by the philanthropic and public-spirited citizens which have not failed to attract a due share of sympathy and patronage, however insufficient in comparison to the universal good, the object of such institutions,—from the Government. The municipal and other corporate bodies have realised their duty towards the development of the indigenous system of cure which alone can reach the teeming millions of poor inhabitants through a network of charitable dispensaries and hospitals which will distribute remedial agents at a comparatively cheaper cost. Madras has got its Government School of Indian Medicine, besides the Channa Purai Āyurveda Kalāśālā, established by its public-spirited citizens. Āyurvedic Department has been opened in the Hindu University of Benares with a hospital attached. In this sacred city of the Hindus, and the ancient seat of Hindu learning and culture, the Āyurveda Vidyāprobodhini Pāṭhśālā has been founded. In Rishikul, Hardwar, the Āyurveda Vidyāpīṭha; in Rishikesh, the Bawa Kali Kamblewaleka Āyurveda Vidyālaya; in Pilibhit, the Lalit Hari Āyurveda College; in the Presidency of Bombay, the Prabhurām College;—all bear testimony to the self-sacrifice and energy of the founders and promoters of these centres of education. The Āyurvedic College of Gurukul, Kangri; the D. A. V. College of Lahore; and the Āyurvedic and Unani Tibbi College of Delhi, are now recognised institutions for the cultivation and advancement in the science of Āyurveda.

The Indian chiefs were not slow to manifest their sympathy towards this renaissance of Āyurvedic treatment. Jaipur had been the seat of a college of Āyurveda—the Jaipur Rāj Āyurvedic Vidyālaya—financed and maintained by the State from a long time. The Mahārājā of Alwar is well-known for his encouragement towards

Āyurvedic studies. The Gawalior Rāj Āyurveda Vidyālaya, the Mysore Government Āyurveda College, the Patiala Rāj Āyurveda Vidyālaya, the Trivandrum Government Āyurveda College, and the Baroda Rāj Sanskrit Parikṣā Samiti and the Āyurveda Mahāvidyālaya, Patan, Baroda State, are unmistakable proofs of the faith of the noble Princes who are at the helm of these principalities. The Thakore Saheb of Gondal is well-known for his interest in the Āyurvedic science. Bharatpore spends a good sum for the treatment of its subjects according to the Āyurvedic method, and other States are helping in this regeneration of Ayurveda.

Besides the Madras Government College of Āyurveda, there are other colleges founded by our Government: The Behar Government Āyurveda Vidyālaya at Jagganathpore; the Muzzaffarpore Government Āyurveda Vidyālaya; and the Āyurvedic and Unani College at Delhi. The U. P. Government has the intention to appoint a committee to enquire about the indigenous system of medicine. The Government of the United Provinces has sanctioned the annual recurring grants-in-aid of Rs. 30,000 for the benefit of the Āyurvedic institutions under its jurisdiction and for the sanction of a donation of Rs. 50,000 and an annual recurring grant of Rs. 5,000 in aid of the Rishikul Āyurvedic College.

In Bengal an Āyurvedic Committee was appointed by the Government of Bengal in August 1921. In 1925 the Committee submitted a Report for the consideration of the Government. The decision of the Government of Bengal is being anxiously expected by the people but we do not know when it will be made public. Three Āyurvedic Colleges have been started in Bengal; the Aṣṭāṅga Āyurveda Vidyālaya, the Vaidya Śāstra Pīṭha, and the Āyurveda Vidyālaya named after Govinda Sundarī the mother of Mahārājā of Cossimbazar. Of these the Aṣṭāṅga Vidyālaya is better equipped with library, laboratories, etc., and is likely to have its buildings completed soon. The Corporation of Calcutta appointed a Committee to find out means for the amalgamation of the three colleges, but notwithstanding the best efforts of the committee the amalgamated College of Āyurveda could not be established. I was a member of the committee, and the report we submitted is annexed herewith for the information of the public. The Corporation has sanctioned grants-in-aid for the three schools. The Corporation has opened Āyurvedic charitable dispensaries in the different quarters of the town. Four charitable dispensaries have already been started in its four districts,—an example which has stimulated other provinces and even villages. The Municipalities, District Boards, Union Boards and benevolent citizens have thus recognised the claims of Āyurveda as a system of medicine which requires improvement and help.

In Ceylon, the Laṅkā Āyurvedic Medical College with a Hospital attached has been opened at Jaffna. The Karnataka Āyurvedic College of the Andhra Research University has been established at Vizianagram. Even institutions established to teach Western system of medicine have incorporated Āyurveda as one of its subjects in the final examination. The Jātīya Āyurjībana Vidyālaya or the National Medical Institute of Calcutta teaches Āyurveda in its fifth year as a subject in the curriculum of studies.

Associations for the cultivation and improvement of the science have been founded. Two associations— the Āyurveda Sabhā and the Brāhman Āyurveda Sabhā have been established in Calcutta, and are doing useful work.

A Journal of Āyurveda has been started in Calcutta.

Contribution from renowned physicians of Calcutta and eminent Vaids in the domain of Āyurveda and kindred science are being published month after month. Similar journals are being published from other provinces, though the scientific value of such publications requires better management as regards choice of articles and contributions. When I began to study Āyurveda contributions from the Graduates of the Medical Colleges of India were few and far between, but now well-read and experienced physicians are coming forward with their excellent articles on some aspect of Āyurvedic studies. Thus an attempt is being made to resuscitate the knowledge embodied in the Āyurvedic literature, not only by the practitioners of the art but also by the learned men from a love of scientific investigation.

The original works on Āyurveda are written in Sanskrit language. Many of the works have been translated in the vernaculars of the different provinces. The works of Caraka and Suśruta have been translated in the English language, and it is available to all in its European garb.

Attempts are being made to write original treatises in Sanskrit and to edit and revise well-known text books, incorporating modern scientific knowledge in the light of Āyurvedic theory and practice. Some of the original productions of the Ṛiṣis have been edited with original commentaries written by the editors.

Publications of Āyurvedic books are being taken in hand by the enterprising proprietors of the Nirnayasāgar Press, Bombay, Śrī Venkateśwar Press, Lakśmī Venkateśwar Press, Jñānsāgar Press; Benimādhab Dey, Jīvānanda Vidyāsāgar, Baṅgabasī Press and C. K. Sen and Co. of Calcutta. The University of Calcutta has given me every facility in the publication of my contributions towards the study of Hindu Medicine, and has published the highly original treatise of Bhela which was not available to scholars. It is no doubt highly gratifying to me that Bhela Saṁhitā has been edited and published as I pointed out the desirability of the publication of its manuscript from the Tanjore Library in the Introduction to Vol. I, p. 34, of this book. The example thus set forth by the University of Calcutta should be followed by the other Universities of India.

The Śāstric medicines are being tested scientifically at the School of Tropical Medicine and the Āyurvedic Conference has recommended the necessity of inclusion of effective and useful medicaments of other systems of medical practice in the science of Āyurveda. Consequently we may entertain the hope that in the near future the system would be thoroughly renovated to be of practical use to the people for whom it is intended.

As I was requested to express my opinion on the desirability of the restoration and development of the Āyurvedic medical science and to give evidence before the Āyurvedic Committee appointed by the Government of Bengal, I submitted my report for the consideration of the committee. The scope of my inquiry is described in the following letter, dated the 1st of September, 1923. After the submission of my report I received the questionnaire prepared by the Committee as to the points on which information was required. The oral evidence before the Committee was taken on the 6th November, 1923, and an abridged copy of it is also attached with the report.

The Committee referred to in the letter consisted of learned members, official and non-official. Dr. M. N. Banerji, B.A., M.R.C.S. (Eng.), L.S.A. (Lond.), was the President of the Board; and Major R. N. Chopra, M.A., M.D., B. Ch. (Cantab.), I.M.S., was its Secretary.

I received the following letter from the Secretary :

AYURVEDIC COMMITTEE,
BENGAL.
School of Tropical Medicine.
Calcutta, 1st September, 1923.

To

Dr. Girindra Nath Mukerjee,
B.A., M.D., F.A.S.B.

SIR,

The Government of Bengal appointed a committee to consider and report, after taking such evidence as may be thought necessary, what practical steps can be taken for the restoration and development of the Ayurvedic system of treatment, with special attention to the question of teaching of that system, with any necessary modifications, under proper supervision and control.

The committee so appointed circulated a questionnaire last year to nearly 400 distinguished Kavirajas and other gentlemen interested in this subject, but received replies from sixty only. A large majority, whose views could be of great value and help to the committee, refrained from replying or expressing their opinion.

It has been urged that the question of restoring and developing the Ayurvedic system of medicine is very important to the country not only from economic considerations but also from the point of view of bringing medical relief within easy reach of the great masses of suffering humanity especially in the rural areas.

Western medicine has done and is doing a lot towards this end, but inspite of all efforts a large majority of the population are without adequate medical relief.

It has also been urged that even in Calcutta where

there are so many Government and other hospitals and dispensaries, a great number of people resort to Ayurvedic and other institutions of the indigenous systems, either for preference or for low cost of treatment. From the evidence already obtained it appears that the Ayurvedic system for various reasons has not made much progress for many centuries and in some instances has actually lost ground. The question before the committee now is in what way can this system be restored and developed, and also how it can be taught to suit modern requirements.

In consideration of the very important issues involved, may we appeal to you to please give us your views on this subject with special reference to-

(1) Need for restoring and developing the system on scientific lines to suit present-day requirements and the way in which it can be accomplished.

(2) Teaching institutions and hospitals required with a scheme of their working.

(3) General qualification of students before commencing Ayurvedic study Medium of instructions suited for Bengal. Period of study and course of instruction. Diplomas which may be granted.

(4) Present condition of the literature and the steps which can be taken for making it available to the students and practitioners in suitable form.

(5) Present status of Ayurvedic practitioners, its disadvantages and the remedies for the same. Whether registration is necessary.

(6) Steps to ensure proper production, collection and sale of drugs. Standardisation of preparations in common use.

(7) How the Government, local bodies (such as Municipalities and District Boards), Universities and private enterprise can help in developing the system.

The Committee will consider it a great favour if you would kindly give your opinion on all or any of the above points in a written statement or make it convenient to meet the Committee at any time or place that may suit you so that they may have an opportunity of discussing various important points with you.

As the Government are pressing for a report the committee solicits a reply to the undersigned before the 20th of September.

Yours faithfully,

(Sd.) R. N. CHOPRA,

Major, I.M.S.,

Secretary, Ayurvedic Committee, Bengal,

School of Tropical Medicine, Calcutta.

I submitted my views on the 25th of September, 1923. Then the Secretary sent me the questionnaire with the following letter :—

AYURVEDIC COMMITTEE, BENGAL.

School of Tropical Medicine.

Central Avenue, Calcutta.

DEAR SIR,

I am in receipt of your very interesting memorandum in reply to my circular letter dated 1st September, 1923 and I thank you for the very valuable information you have conveyed.

I am herewith sending you a copy of the questionnaire and if you can throw any more light on any points mentioned therein the Committee will feel very grateful.

I hope the Committee will have the opportunity of meeting you soon. They particularly wish to discuss with you the full working details of the Central Ayurvedic College and Hospital you have suggested. If you can give any further information in writing before we meet it will help the discussion considerably.

Yours faithfully,
(Sd.) R. N. CHOPRA,
Major I.M.S.,
Secretary.

Questions to Witnesses.

1. What sections of the Indian public take advantage of the Ayurvedic system of medicine?

Please give figures from charitable institutions or from your personal experience if possible.

Will adoption of the system facilitate medical aid in general to the section of the population who are not getting it at present?

2. How would you revise the system and restore it?

Would you do it in all eight divisions (Ashtanga)?

If so, what methods would you suggest?

Are you in favour of scientific investigation and of incorporating new discoveries into the system?

3. What is the special field, if any, of Ayurvedic medicines as practised at the present day?

Please specify any line of treatment of drugs which in your opinion are specially efficacious and superior to those in other systems.

4. To what extent was the Ayurvedic literature developed at the time of the original exponents of the system?

What is its present condition and what are the causes which led to it?

Have attempts been made to bring the system up to date?

How can such attempts be encouraged?

5. With a view to more efficient teaching of the system to meet present-day requirements, would you please state the position of existing literature in :—

Human Anatomy and Physiology; Materia Medica; Medicine and Surgery (including Pathology); Gynæcology and Obstetrics; Hygiene and Preventive Medicine.

Please give a list of important works in these subjects. Have these been printed, if so are they suitable for students and probationers?

If there are any deficiencies, how can they be made good?

6. What steps can be taken for collecting and publishing standard editions of Ayurvedic works so as to make them available in sufficiently easy form for average class of students and practitioners?

7. What is the present method of obtaining crude drugs and making preparations?

Have any attempts been made,

(*a*) To standardise and to find out therapeutic and lethal doses of drugs and preparations in use?

(*b*) To ensure proper production, collection and sale of drugs?

Please give your suggestions as to how this can be carried out effectively so as to have a uniform standard for the guidance of all concerned.

8. How does the cost of treatment by this system compare with Allopathic systems? If possible please quote figures from records of existing institutions or your own cases?

Is it true that the cost of some of the drugs is prohibitive?

9. What are the present arrangements for teaching of this system in India generally?

Is there any central organisation controlling the students? If so what are its methods?

Please give suggestions as to how these can be improved.

10. If an Ayurvedic school recognised by the Government is established, would there be

(*a*) Sufficient number of students forthcoming?

(*b*) Possibility of getting requisite number of qualified teachers in different branches?

(*c*) Sufficient clinical material available in the hospitals attached for training of students?

Would such a school improve the status of Kavirajes passing out? What in your opinion would be the cost of a well equipped teaching institution?

11. What should be the general qualifications and preliminary training of students before starting the study?

What should be the period of study and medium of instruction?

12. Do you consider the study of modern scientific methods as illustrated by the study of Physics, Chemistry, Biology, Human Anatomy and Physiology, in the early part of training, and Pathology and Bacteriology in the latter part essential or not?

With a view to economy, would it be possible for the lectures and practical training in these subjects to be attended in any of the recognised medical schools?

Can any other subject such as Surgery be treated in this way? If not what would you suggest?

13. Should the course for the students be prepared with special reference to progressive standards (*e.g.*, L.M.P. of Medical Schools as in cases of Sub-Assistant Surgeons and M.B.,B.S., and M.D., of Universities as in cases of Assistant Surgeons) or otherwise?

14. What are the disadvantages from which Ayurvedic practitioners suffer and what remedies can you suggest?

15. Do you consider registration on the same lines as medical registration desirable?

If so, how would you constitute the Registration Board and what safeguards would you propose for existing practitioners ?

If not, how will it be possible to distinguish real Vaidyas from quacks ?

16. How in your opinion can, the Government, local bodies such as Municipalities, Universities and private enterprise help in restoring, developing and fostering the system ?

17. Can you give an idea as to cost of restoration and development of the system, to suit modern requirements, on the lines indicated by you ?

I sent the following reply on the 25th September 1923 :

Reply

To

MAJOR R. N. CHOPRA, M.A., M.D. (Cantab.), I.M.S.,
Secretary, Ayurvedic Commitee, Bengal.
School of Tropical Medicine, Calcutta.

SIR,

I beg to acknowledge the receipt of your letter dated the 1st September, requesting me to supply you with information on the question of restoration and devolopment of the Ayurvedic system of treatment, and, in reply, I have the honour of submitting for the consideration of the Committee the results of my inquiry and my individual experienee on the subject.

2. Before we enter into details of the various questions mentioned in your letters it may not be amiss at the outset of an inquiry, to set out with a short description of the work done by our Government to resuscitate knowledge in the Ayurveda.

3. Dr. Buchanan, as quoted by Mr. Montgomery in his work "*The History, Antiquities, Topography, and*

Statistics of Eastern India" 1807, states as regards the province of Behar: "Medicine is taught by several of the Pandits, some of whom also, although they are grammarians, practise the art." "Besides the Professors of Medicine, about 700 families of Brahmins, almost all of Sakadwipa, practise the art, and are the only Hindu physicians who possess anything like science, except three of the Medical tribes from Bengal, who have settled at Patna." The traditional system of training of Kabirajes which has lasted for many centuries in Bengal, has always been exclusively literary in character. The Vaidyas learn their medical science mainly from books and from oral tradition from the *Gurus*—the learned physicians of the time, who generally taught a number of students without fees. Similar practice still exists in the '*Tols*.'

4. In 1811 Lord Minto recommended the establishment of Colleges at Nadia and Trihut with a view to the restoration of indigenous learning in Bengal under the management and control of the Government. The East India Act of 1813 authorised the Governor-General in Council to set apart a sum not less than one lac of rupees from the public revenue and spend it for the revival and improvement of Sanskrit literature and to the introduction and promotion of knowledge of European sciences amongst the people of the country. The Court of Directors pointed out that the Sanskrit language contained many excellent treatises on ethics, medicinal plants and drugs, astronomy and mathematics; and they ordered that steps should be taken to induce the people to adopt modern improvements in sciences. The Court directed the Governor-General to submit proposals to give effect to the principles laid down.

5. The Sanskrit College was opened on the first day of January 1824. This year forms a landmark in the history

of education in India. The Calcutta Madrassa (1781) and the Hindu College (1817) had already been founded but at the personal expense of Warren Hastings and by public subscriptions respectively. The establishment of this College marked the first definite recognition by the East India Company of its responsibility for the education of the people. The purpose of the Institution was laid down in the famous Resolution of Government dated 21st August, 1821 : "The Committee will bear in mind that the immediate object of the institution is the cultivation of Hindu literature. Yet it is in the judgment of His Lordship in Council a purpose of deeper interest to seek every practicable means of effecting the gradual diffusion of European knowledge." In this college, the "General Committee" decided to impart knowledge of medical science—European and Indian—to the students of Sanskrit College. In 1826, Dr. Tytler began his lecture on Medicine according to Western method, and Professors were appointed to teach Caraka, Suśruta, Bhāva Prakasa, etc. Classes for the Āyurvedic students were opened in 1827. The classes were well attended. The justly celebrated Pandit Madhusudan Gupta was a student of this class and learned the science according to both systems. He became one of the Professors entrusted with the teaching of the science. His students handled bones and dissected animals. We quote the words of Professor Wilson, the Oriental scholar, who examined the students of the medical class : "The triumph gained over native prejudices is nowhere more remarkable than in this class, in which not only are the bones of the human skeleton handled without reluctance but in some instances dissection of the soft parts of animals performed by the students themselves." (See *Minutes of Evidence of the House of Commons on the*

Affairs of the East India Company, 1832, page 994.) In 1831, Dr. J. Grant began his lectures on Anatomy and Physiology, Diagnosis and Surgery.

6. In 1833 Lord William Bentinck, the then Governor General of India, appointed a Committee for the revision of the whole question of medical education in Bengal. The Committee comprised the following gentlemen :

Surgeon J. Grant, Apothecary General.

J. C. C. Sutherland, Esq., Secretary to the Education Committee.

C. G. Trevelyan, Esq., Deputy Secretary, Political Department.

Assistant Spens, Body Guard.

Assistant Surgeon Bramley, Marine Surgeon.

Baboo Ramcomal Sen.

In 1834, the Secretary to the General Commitee requested Dr. Tytler about his opinion as to the advisability of adopting English as the medium of instruction, of teaching the students books on European medical science only, and of abolishing the Āyurvedic classes, as many doctors were of opinion that the studends should be taught according to a definite system of medical study. Dr. Tytler was for the continuance of the system in vogue, *i. e.*, European and Ayurvedic systems. The Committee worked for twelve months. Rev. Dr. Grant was its President. It was decided that English should be the medium of instruction, and medical classes in Sanskrit College and the Madrassa should be abolished. The final decision of the Committee was submitted to the Government in an elaborate Report on the 20th October, 1834.

Dr. Tytler is better known to the public for his correspondence with Rājā Rām Mohan Roy, occasioned by a passage in a letter of the Doctor, published in the *Bengal Hurkara* of the 30th May, 1823, regarding the doctrine of Divine Incarnation. It appears that the Doctor was completely silenced by the renowned Rājā, under the pseudonym of Rām Dāss.

By the famous Minute of the 2nd February, 1835, Lord Macaulay won the definite victory of the Western School over the Orientalists. Rev. Dr. Duff and his Anglicist party decided that English should be the medium of instruction, against Dr. Tytler, the Superintendent of the 'Native Medical Institution,' which was founded by Government in 1822, and in which it was found practicable to teach Bengali students the modern science of medicine through the medium of the Bengali language.

The Committee prefaced their recommadations thus :—

"The scheme of reform, too, we would especially submit to your Lordship, ought to be ample, comprehensive, and worthy of a great Government, not intended merely to supply the wants of the State, but of the people, and to become, what it may confidently be expected it will, a moral engine of great utility and power."

7. The Medical College of Bengal was established on the 20th February, 1835, with Dr. Bramley as the Superintendent and H. Goodeve as his assistant. The Government ordered on the 28th January, 1835, abolition of the Native Medical Institution and the medical classes in the Sanskrit College and the Madrassa. Pandit Madhusudan was transferred to the new College and had two assistants assigned to him. The question of dissection of the human body was found to be a stumbling-block to the progress of the students in Anatomy, and the Pandit showed his manly courage in defying the time-honoured prejudices of his countrymen by his dissection of the cadaver on the 10th January 1836. This date marks a new era in the history of Western education in India. Opinions differ as regards the exact date,

Some say that on the 28th October, 1835, four young Hindus (Madhusudan being leader of them) dissected a cadaver.

The study of the Āyurveda gradually came to an end by the establishment of the Medical College, where European medicine began to be studied with enthusiasm. No attempt has been made by the Government since then to revive the study of the Indian medical science, although the science is still studied by many in Bengal and elsewhere:—the torch of light has been kept burning by the zeal and the scientific spirit of the poor physicians without any help from the State which has done so much in educating the Indian youths in other branches of learning. The scientific men in the Indian Medical Service, trained in the most up-to-date methods of the West, naturally thought the study of the medical science of the Hindus mere waste of time, and the Kabirajes, confident of getting no encouragement from a foreign Government, kept themselves aloof from the modern scientific world; even they looked with a suspicious eye towards any interference by the State in shape of improvement in the various branches of the science It is for this reason that you have received so scanty response to your very important Questions which you circulated amongst many distinguished Kabirajes of Bengal.

8. As regards the need for restoring and developing the system on scientific lines to suit modern requirements, I take the liberty of referring you to the *Introduction, pp. 67-157,* in *Vol. I* of my work on the '*History of Indian Medicine*,' recently published by the Calcutta University. Apart from questions of academic and historical interest which the study of the Āyurveda may solve, there is a practical side of the study which we cannot ignore. It can be said without fear of contradiction

that medical aid, as at present available, does not meet the requirement of the rural population in Bengal. There is a steady and increasing demand for medical men, of somewhat lower standard than that of the Sub-Assistant Surgeon,—medical men of a type similar to the old type of the Native Doctor, as the income of a doctor in a village is not attractive to the highly trained Assistant- and Sub-Assistant Surgeons. The spread of education will increase the urgency for more trained men, and as the Medical Colleges and the Medical Schools are full, rather over-crowded, it is the duty of the civilised Government to provide for this increasing demand of the population. Medical Schools may multiply but the Medical Colleges take time to develop; and the cost of establishing such institutions is almost prohibitive. The need for qualified physicians for rural districts may be met with in three ways:

(1). The establishment of Vernacular Medical Schools. A similar institution once existed in Bengal. In 1832 an additional Urdu class, and in 1852, a Bengali class were opened for instruction of the students. The qualified students from such schools were called H.A., or V.L.M.S., or "Native Doctors." Such doctors would have to compete in the practical field with the Graduates of the Medical Colleges, the Licenciates of the State Faculty and the Hospital Assistants from Medical Schools maintained by Government. The older class of Native Doctors died a natural death long before, and the repetition of the same experiment would give us the same result.

(2). By an increase in the number of students in the existing Medical Schools we may increase the number of the Hospital Assistants. The Medical Schools are at present over-crowded, and new institutions must be established to cope with the increasing demand. Apart from the cost of maintaining such schools by the State, the poor villagers in the rural areas would not be able to satisfy these trained doctors who consider their services too valuable for the poor.

(3). We may avail of the services of the Āyurvedic physicians trained in a scientific way. With the establishment of the Āyurvedic College, knowledge of such physicians may be improved by modern methods of teaching medical sciences. It is useless to deny that still the Āyurvedic system of treatment has much influence over educated Indians who are fully aware of the immense benefit of the Western methods of cure. I need not enter here as to the cause of this strange mentality of the Hindus. But so far I am sure that the people of the rural areas would consider it a blessing if they can secure the services of scientifically trained Kabirajes whose charges for treatment would be deemed reasonable by the public and who will be satisfied with their comparatively smaller earnings.

9. *The importance of the Āyurveda.*—The methods of treatment according to the Āyurveda are called empirical. But the so-called empirical methods of treatment were founded on experiments, observations and experience which extended over many centuries. Even some of these observations have been declared by competent authorities to be reliable. About the importance of the subject, I have dealt with it in '*The Conclusion*,' *Chap. IX* of *Vol. I* of my contribution on "*The Surgical Instruments of the Hindus*," published by the Calcutta University in 1913, and I again take the liberty of referring you to its pages 329-362. Here I may mention a few examples of our indebtedness to the indigenous system :—the use of the salt-free diet in the treatment of the dropsical affections, the use of salt in the treatment cholera, liquid food in typhoid

fever, in which even milk is withheld, cooling regimen in small-pox and measles as advocated by Sydenham, the importance of bael and kurchi in dysentery, the use of preparations of mercury, iron and arsenic internally, use of neem and chalmugra oil in leprosy, musk and makaradhwaja as stimulant, and other medicaments too numerous to mention. In the fields of surgery, obstetrics, pathology, and hygiene, we come across observations which, if known earlier, would have saved the labour of scientific men to an appreciable extent. The use of various cooling oils in the treatment of nervous disorders should be scientifically investigated, as there is a deep-rooted belief in the Indian minds that we scarcely possess any curative agents which are equally efficacious.

10. I may here point out that all sections of the Hindu community take advantage of the Āyurvedic system of treatment. The Hindu widows, as a rule, prefer the indigenous medicines and object to taking medicines imported from the West. The old men and patients suffering from chronic diseases show a decided bias towards the medicines prepared by the Vaids. The Bengali Musalmans also use medicines prescribed by the Kabirajes. The educated Indians firmly believe that the indigenous medicines which are generally freshly prepared act better on the constitution of the native population than the medicaments of the British Pharmacopœia imported from Europe.

As regards the methods for restoring and developing the system of medical treatment opinions differ. But the majority of those learned men who have bestowed any thought on the subject consider the following items as the principal methods of popularising the study of the Āyurveda :

(1). The establishment of a Central College of Āyurveda, managed under Government control or under a

Board of Āyurvedic Study under Government supervision. The subjects must be taught according to modern scientific method

(2). Establishment of hospitals for the treatment of patients according to Āyurvedic system.

(3). Foundation of charitable dispensaries in rural areas for the treatment of the poor people.

(4). Foundation of a scientific Library for the use of the students, professors, and practitioners of the healing art. In such a Library not only books on the Āyurvedic system should be collected and catalogued, but also books dealing with the cognate sciences of medicine and other methods of treatment should be available.

(5). Translations of Sanskrit books and manuscripts into English should be encouraged, for then only can we expect healthy criticism from the savants of the world.

(6). The text books as read by the students of Āyurveda require to be recast and re-edited to suit our modern conditions of life. The Ayurvedic system suffered many vicissitudes, and text books were compiled and edited to suit the changed conditions of life. During the Vedic period the vegetable simples only were used and its literature is scattered in the *Atharva Veda* and in the *Āyurveda* which is lost to us. In the Pre-Buddhist period Agniveśa and Suśruta wrote their treatises which were recast by Caraka and Nāgārjuna respectively. Caraka's edition was again improved and enlarged by Dṛḍhvala during the Paurānic period. The *Caraka Saṁhitā*, as we find it in its present form, is a systematic treatise, which has undergone additions and corrections by different physicians in different times. Lastly came the *Rasa Granthas* the chemico-medical texts of the physicians of the Iatro-chemical school, who began to cure diseases by means of mineral drugs of which mercury was the most commonly used. Bhāva Miśra wrote his compilation, a voluminous work, the Encyclopædia of Hindu Medicine, some 350 years ago, in which the author boldly advocated many new drugs of foreign origin and described many new diseases unknown to former authors. This proves that the Kabirajes are not unwilling to improve themselves as regards new innvovations in the methods of treatment and inclusion of new diseases and new drugs not hitherto mentioned in their works.

(7). Exhibitions of drugs, appliances, the actual methods of preparation of medicines requiring technical knowledge, the methods of collecting, sorting and storing medicines, and various articles of interest to the physicians in their daily practice may be held to stimulate curiosity and investigation in a scientific spirit.

(8). Popular lectures dealing with improvements in hygiene and cognate sciences illustrated by lantern slides, pictures and drawings to elucidate the subject.

(9). Therapeutic gardens : *vide infra.*

(10). Museums. The importance of a museum in teaching a scientific subject has been recognised by eminent authorities, and our space forbids any detailed description of a museum for medical studies.

For the rôle played by the library, exhibitions, museums, and popular lectures, I take the liberty of referring you to *Vol. I* of "*History of Indian Medicine,*" *pages 138-169.*

11. *The establishment of teaching institutions.*—It is absolutely essential that a Central College maintained and recognised by the Government for the teaching of the Āyurveda be established in Bengal without further delay. In the College, provisions should be made for the study of the various sub-divisions of the Āyurveda, namely medicine, surgery, midwifery, children's diseases, pathology, materia medica, anatomy, physiology, hygiene, medical jurisprudence, and the elementary sciences, *viz.*, biology.

physics, chemistry, according to the modern scientific methods.

Tols.—The system now in vogue, *viz.*, the students learning the science of medicine from individual teachers or *Gurus* has, no doubt, much to be said in its favour. Such a system has all the advantages of a residential university and is well adapted for teaching literary subjects in a poor country. But the teaching of subjects which require manual dexterity from the votaries must fail in its object if learned in theoretical lectures only—no matter how eminent the professor or lecturer may be. The college should be the central institution where the students from these indigenous *tols* should attend to complete their studies. They must attend the practical classes which can only be arranged in a college fitted with laboratories for the different subjects prescribed in the curriculum of studies. At present the *tol* system may be retained, and as in Sanskrit education we have the Sanskrit College and the *Tols*, the dual system of study may be followed for a time. But it must be, however, clearly borne in mind that sooner the *Tol* system of medical education be stopped, the better.

There are, no doubt, considerable difficulties to surmount. Instruction is to be delivered in a foreign tongue in the college to students full of prejudices and of inactive habits. The lecturer shall have to teach, and translate. He shall have to create a demand for medical and surgical skill, where there was felt no want for them. The pupils, on the other hand, cannot be very enthusiastic—their prospect in life distant and somewhat indefinite. In private practice, they shall have to fear ridicule and opposition from the Graduates of the Medical Colleges and Licenciates from the Medical Schools who may vaunt for their superior knowledge. There are no text books suited to modern times : such books must be written in English and vernacular. The preliminary education acquired by the students who intend to prosecute their studies is far from satisfactory ; the level of their general knowledge is too low for the superstructure of medical science. But by zeal, energy and devotion to work progress can be made, and ultimately success may be achieved.

12. *Hospitals.*—No medical institution is complete without hospitals. A complete knowledge of diseases can only be acquired in the wards of a hospital. It is, at the bedside of the patient, and not from books, that the practical application of medical studies can be mastered, clinical knowledge gained, observations on diseases made and the methods of cure studied. As the system of teaching now stands, students attend to the preparation of medicines and thus learn pharmacy and materia medica practically. They attend to the patients who come in number to the dispensary of their teacher and thus learn diagnosis and treatment. But surgery cannot be learned without a hospital, and we have evidence that in ancient times and even at comparatively recent times the Āyurvedic surgeons practised their art in hospitals. I may mention here that the Chāndsi doctors, who still carry a lucrative trade in Calcutta, are in the habit of keeping patients in their own house in a room called by them 'hospital' at their own cost and thus acquire skill in performing certain surgical operations, *e.g.*, piles and fistula-in-ano. The Māls learn reclination of cataract in a similar way, and the Madrasi doctors become, as they say, experts in fistula operations.

13. *The location of the college and the hospital.*—To establish college and hospital, ample space must be acquired for class rooms, laboratories, and libraries. The problem of students' residence must be solved ; residential

hostels, houses for the staff and playing ground for the students must be provided. The Principal requires a separate house to live in, and the Resident Surgeon and Physician must have quarters assigned to them. The acquisition of land in the centre of Calcutta is very costly. But it is not desirable, on many grounds, that the college is established in any rural area at a very great distance from the town. The college may conveniently be established in a suburban site, preferably towards Tollygunge, or Chetla, or Alipore, where land is still available to any extent required by Government for the purpose. A college located in these places would be easily accessible to students who reside in Calcutta and its neighbourhood.

14. *The scheme of the proposed college and hospitals and their working.*—The college should have a four-year course, and the different subjects may be studied as follows:

First-year—Physics, Chemistry, Biology and Anatomy. Dissection and Practical training in scientific subjects.

Second-year—Anatomy, Physiology, Materia Medica, Pathology, Dissection, Practical classes, and Hospital duty.

Third-year—Medicine, Surgery, Midwifery, Hygiene, Clinical Medicine and Surgery, Labour cases, Hospital duty—medical and surgical, and Operative Surgery.

Fourth-year—Same as in the third year, Medical Jurisprudence and History of Medicine.

After a few years, it would be found that a five-year course would cover the subjects better than a course of four years. The preliminary scientific studies should be taught in a very elementary manner, and only with special reference to the subjects required for proper elucidation of the medical science.

To run such an institution efficiently, the services of the following professors are absolutely necessary :

1. Professor of Biology.
2. „ Physics and Chemistry.
3. „ Anatomy and Physiology.
4. „ Materia Medica and Clinical Medicine.
5. „ Medicine including Mental diseases, and Hygiene. He is to act as Principal of the College.
6. „ Surgery including Dentistry, and Diseases of the Eyes, and Clinical Surgery.
7. „ Midwifery, Diseases of Women and Children.

The salary of the professors should be from Rs. 150 to Rs. 300, and the salary of the Principal should be Rs. 500 per month.

There would be required Demonstrators for Biology, Physics and Chemistry, Anatomy and Physiology, on a salary of Rs. 75 to 150 per month. All the professors and demonstrators must have medical qualifications.

The State must encourage original researches in the medical and allied sciences by special grants from the public treasury. Endowments or establishment of Fellowships, Lectureships, and Readership for researches in the Āyurvedic studies should be sanctioned. There should be scholarships, prizes or rewards for the meritorious students.

The Hospital must contain wards for medical, surgical and gynæcological cases and should have provision for out-door patients. It is not necessary to enter here into detail of the hospital work.

The capital outlay necessary for starting the college and the hospital on the basis of my recommendation could not be put below two lacs of rupees. Considering the present financial difficulties of the State, a start may be made in some existing Government buildings, where accommodation for laboratories, lectures and hospitals is available. A library with seminar rooms, offices and Principal's quarters will be located in the same buildings. I am not aware of any such Government building being available, except the premises known as the "*Hastings* House" situated in Alipore. This house may serve our purpose admirably for the present and may be used permanently if the authorities so desire. The house with a historic fame has ample accommodation for a college, is situated in the southern division of the town and is easily accessible to students from all parts of Calcutta. In this building an educational institution was started a few years ago, but as it exists no longer, the authorities are free to sanction its use for a more useful institution which will prove highly beneficial to the public at large, and will redound to the glory of the benign administration under whose care we all live.

The amount of the recurring annual grant from the State for the college, necessary to run it efficiently,—though we cannot name a figure offhand,—cannot be less than Rs. 25,000 per year for the present. It is possible that a successful administration may be able to achieve the result desired at a comparatively less cost; but as the details are to be worked out afterwards we need not consider about the exact figure. We must make attempts,—and we believe such attempts would meet with favourable response,—to tap new sources of revenue as from Municipalities, District Boards, and to obtain benefactions from the public.

15. *Qualifications of students who intend to study Āyurveda.*—There is difference of opinion as regards the minimum qualification of the students who would be eligible to prosecute studies in the college. I have referred to what Suśruta says about this question in page 37 of "*History of Medicine,*" *Vol. 1,* and I need not dilate it here. There can be no doubt on the dictum that "a physician should be a man of science trained after the best manner and according to the discipline of the science of the age." There is a vast number of students who have passed the Matriculation and I. Sc. Examinations of the University. They do not find any accommodation in colleges of science or arts to prosecute further studies. Admission the Medical Colleges is difficult for them as the number of applicants far exceeds the maximum number of students who can possibly receive adequate facilities to learn the subjects of study in the colleges. The result is that the students sit idly at home as they find no work for them. I would not be astonished if these educated young men without any work and hope in this world, were easily led astray by designing men and ultimately became criminals. These students would like to study the science of Āyurveda, and I hope they will come in number and will welcome this new field of activity open to them. What they want is that they should be regularly taught and that they should be recognised by Government if they can pass their examinations creditably. Under these circumstances, I am of opinion that the minimum qualification should be the Matriculation of the University, but the I. Sc.'s should be given the preference, and I fear that within a very few years the classes would be filled up with I. Sc. and B. Sc. students.

For the *Tols,* the minimum qualifications should be fixed to the *Ādya* and *Madhya* examinations of the

Sanskrit Board. Then they will be able to follow the Āyurvedic Texts which are, as a rule, written in classical Sanskrit.

16. *Accommodation for students in medical institutions.*—I have stated above that the medical institutions are overcrowded. To support this statement I cannot refrain from quoting the Questions and Answers in the local Legislative Council:

Question 10. Mr. J. N. Maitra wanted to know

(*a*) whether large numbers of candidates for admission into the Calcutta Medical College, Carmichael Medical College and Campbell Medical School were annually refused admission owing to want of accommodation.

Ans. (*a*) Yes.

(*b*) Whether many candidates for admission into the Campbell Medical School possessed the qualifications necessary for admission into the Medical College.

Ans. (*b*) No, it is not strictly correct. At the last admission out of 237 I. Sc.'s admitted only 15 were First Division and 22 were Second Division men. The Medical College could fill their admission list with B. Sc.'s alone and Second Division I. Sc.'s have very little chance. The Campbell admits I. A.'s. The figures at the last admission were 9 First Division, 19 Second Division, and 4 Third Division—total 32. The Medical College does not admit I. A. candidates.

(*c*) If so whether the Government would raise the status of the Campbell Medical School to that of a Medical College at an early date.

Ans. (*c*) No.

17. *The medium of instruction in Bengal.*—The difficulty about the medium of instruction in Bengal cannot be solved easily. It is no doubt true that students will appreciate the lecturers if they impart instruction in

their mother tongue. It is undoubtedly a sad waste of time and energy in learning sciences in a foreign garb. All educationists now agree that the mother tongue of the students should be placed over foreign languages. The learner's attention would not then be diverted from the study of science to that of foreign languages.

We know with what good results the mother tongue has been employed for the moral and religious development of children. The Venerable Buddha delivered his sermons to his nation in its own speech,—Pali,—not even in Sanskrit. To learn a foreign language is difficult and certainly it is very inconvenient to express our ideas in another language which has little or no affinity with our mother tongue. But whether we like it or not, the Bengali students begin to learn English even from a very tender age, and when they grow older, I am sorry to remark, they like to express themselves in a foreign tongue. Considering all these facts, I hold that for the present, it is desirable that English language should be the medium of study in the college. It will bring the education of the students up to modern standard of method and efficiency, and will keep them in touch with European learning and progress. The lecturers, however, ought to be prepared to explain difficult questions in the vernacular.

I quote here the remarks of the Committee in their Report of 1834 as regards the medium of instruction and believe that the reasons set forth therein still hold good for the present time. "A knowledge of the English language we consider as a *sine quă non*, because that language combines within itself the circle of all the sciences, and an incalculable wealth of printed works and illustrations; circumstances that give it obvious advantages over the oriental languages, in which are only to be found the crudest elements of science or the most irrational substitutes for it."

But to bring the means of medical instruction within the reach of the masses, who are still for the most part ignorant of the English language, vernacular should be adopted as the medium of instruction. And it was for similar reasons that a Hindusthani class was opened for the education of the native doctors in 1838, with Urdu as the medium of teaching, and a Bengali class, in which the students were taught in Bengali, was added in 1851-52. The students who passed their final examinations from these institutions were known as native doctors who were employed for military and civil duties respectively. Thus there were opened Bengali classes in the Medical College of Bengal in 1852, and in the Medical School at Agra, vernacular was the medium of instruction which was imparted in accordance with European methods. Similar schools were opened at Lahore, Dacca, Hyderabad, Patna, Cuttack and many other places; but in most of these schools the medium of instruction has changed;—the vernacular has gradually yielded its place to English which is liked by the teachers and students alike. It may be laid down as a general rule that vernacular should be retained for the lower standard and the *Tols*, and English for higher examinations in the college. In the examinations, however, the students should be allowed to have the option of writing their answers either in the vernacular or in English, and this mixed system would be found to be educationally economical.

18. *Diplomas.*—The University Commission of 1917-19, it is true, did not deem it correct to establish degrees and diplomas in ancient systems of medicine with a view to authorise the recipients to undertake the practice of their profession. But it was admitted that careful

investigation of the science would throw light on its origin and growth. The report continues,—"If adequate provision is made for this purpose in the reconstituted University, it is not unreasonable to hope that the exponents of the indigenous system of medicine will gradually become linked with students trained according to the most approved Western method."

Practically, there is scarcely any very marked difference between the Āyurveda and the modern scientific medicine. The Āyurveda is not a conservative system of medicine; we can distinctly trace its growth through the different strata of thought. We have abundant testimony,—the internal evidence of the medical books themselves,—that the Āyurvedic system often utilized new methods of treatment, but in a manner peculiar to itself. The treatment advocated in the *Vedas* differs from the treatment recommended by the Ātreya School of physicians; the system of Caraka and Dṛḍhavala is not identical with the teaching of Agniveśa; the treatment of Caraka has undergone a complete change, and the treatment of diseases by mineral medicines is an advance introduced by the physicians of the Iatro-chemical School. Nāgārjuna redacted the *Suśruta Saṁhitā*. But the science of surgery finds no place in the hands of the learned kabirajes of the present time. Bhāva Miśra described some new diseases, *e.g.*, the Firanga roga or Syphylis in his work, but he referred for the treatment of the disease to the ancient Seers (Ṛṣis) although the disease was not even mentioned by his predecessors. Opium, mercury, and arsenic were unknown, to the ancient physicians, or if known, were not commonly used by them; but the modern kavirajes can hardly treat cases without these remedies. It will come to you as a surprise that many Āyurvedic physicians now use quinine in malaria but though they do not admit it, we should not be astonished to find in some tantras or purānas later on, the properties of the drug described in the form of a dialogue between Śiva and Pārvatī. It would be done so, not to cheat the public, but to create a faith in the minds of the patients; and we know that similar devices had been adopted in recent times by Europeans, when, in order to stimulate faith in vaccination, some Sanskrit poems were composed to show that vaccination was sanctioned by the religious books of the Hindus. In the system as practised now-a-days, many medicines from the Unani system have found a permanent place in the Āyurvedic materia medica. We should always bear in mind the famous couplet of Caraka:

"That alone is the right medicine which can remove disease;
He alone is the true physician who can restore health."

In a note on the Sanskrit College, Jeypore, dated the 28th October, 1894, which appeared as an appendix to Dr. Hendley's article on "*The Indian System of Medicine and the Lesson that may learned from them*" (*vide Transactions of the First Indian Medical Congress*, 1894). Mr. Kalipada Banerjee, the then Principal of the Jeypore College writes: "The titles conferred here in the medical examinations are Bhisak at the Upadhaya, Bhisagvara at the Sastri, and Bhisagacharya at the final examination. But the titles conferred in Bengal are Kaviraja, Kavirajan (kaviranjana ?), Kanthabharana, and Dhvanantari; and in the N. W. Provinces Vaidya, Vaidyaraja, and Vaidyachuramani. I must mention in this connection that nowhere besides Jeypore Hindu medicine is systematically taught in the College; and everywhere the science is taught privately by distinguished native vaids." "The medicine is nowhere taught in India in the vernacular, medical education being everywhere given entirely in Sanskrit." In the Punjab University, the titles of Vaidya Vachaspati and Kaviraja are conferred. Any of these titles may be selected for the students who pass their examinations from the *Tols.*

But the students who successfully pass the final examinations of the Colleges should get titles which may indicate that they are qualified medical men entitled to practice Medicine, Surgery and Midwifery. They may be designated Indian Physicians or Surgeons, or Āyurvedic Doctor or similar titles. The Homeopaths without any pretensions to medical education often add such titles as M. B. and M. D. Any title similar to M. B., B. S. or L. R. C. P. might be granted to these trained medical men.

19. *The present condition of the Āyurvadic literature*: For the present state of the Sanskrit literature of Āyurvedic medicine, I would refer you to *Chapter I, Introduction.* on the "*Ancient Medical authors and their works*" in *Vol.* I of my thesis on the *Surgical Instruments of the Hindus,* and also to the *History of Indian Medicine.* which is in course of publication by the University. The literature is poor in scientific subjects. Many books still exist as manuscripts, and only a few have been edited and printed. But it is not difficult to edit books which may serve as suitable text books for the students of the proposed college. New books can be written in easy Sanskrit, Vernacular or English. There are books on materia medica and medicine which may serve as text books for students if brought up to date by new editions in which descriptions of new diseases and their scientific treatment are incorporated.

Memorandum of Sanskrit medical works generally studied by an educated Kabiraj of the present days :

At Jeydur Sanskrit College the following books form the curriculum of studies :

" At the Upadhyaya (Proficiency) Examination in Ayurveda (Medical science) the following are the text books :

Nidan, the great work on the diagnosis of diseases, by Madhava Acharya (?), better known as Madhava Kara.

Narivijnan, a tract on feeling pulse, by Ram Chandra Das.

Bhavaprakas, a later compilation of medical works, by Bhava Misra.

Paribhasapradipa, a book on Hindu Materia Medica, by Govinda Sen.

Chikitsa Sara Sangraha, an ancient compilation from Charaka and Susruta, by Chakradatta.

Rasamanjari, an elementary treatise on Chemistry, by Basli Nath.

At the Sastri (Honours) Examination the text books are :

Bhavaprakas, as at the Upadhyaya Examination.

Astangahridaya, a work on the diseases of the heart and the whole body (*lit.*, the heart of the Octopartrite Science), by Bagbhata.

Susruta Sanhita, Chapter on the body.

Charaka Sanhita, Chapters on treatment.

Rasendra Sara Sangraha, a work on Chemistry, by Gopalkrishna.

At the Acharyya (Final) Examination, the text books are :

Susruta Sanhita.

Charaka Sanhita.

Astangahridaya of Bagbhata.

Bhaisajya Ratnavali, a modern Hindu pharmacopœia.

Rasendra Chintamani, the best work on the chemical or mineral drugs, by Ram Chandra.

I may add here that these are the Sanskrit medical works generally studied at Calcutta, Benares, and other parts of India. There are besides these many other famous works, but they are not in much use at present."

Manuscripts of Sanskrit works on medicine still lie scattered in the country. These MSS. may be collected, edited and published by the learned editors under the auspices of the Government, Societies and also private enterprise. Many such works are being printed in the Āyurvedīya Granthamālā, in the Anandasram Series, and other publications from Bombay, Poona and Calcutta. There are also signs of an awakening amongst our countrymen, and we find a few graduates of our Medical College writing books on the science and have devoted themselves in the improvement of the Āyurveda.

20. *The present status of the Āyurvedic practitioners*: The vaids are still honoured in this country. The learned Kabirajes demand fees for their visits like the doctors of the modern schools, and the public do not grudge to pay them. This method of receiving fees is certainly an innovation for it was the practice in former times to receive gifts from patients after they were cured, especially on the day when the patient was allowed to eat his normal diet. The sale of medicines by means of advertisements, which they often do, is certainly not to be encouraged, if not prohibited.

There are certain disadvantages from which they suffer. But these disadvantages are the result of their inactivity and ignorance: as for instance, their attitude towards Surgery. At present there are many Kabirajes in affluent circumstances but they take little or no interest in the improvement of their science. They never think of the debt they owe to the science they practise. Recently some colleges have been started, but these institutions are more or less of a proprietary nature and there is scarcely any certainty that any of them would last long after the death of their Founders. Already there are signs, not of healthy rivalry, but of obstructive hostility between them. Anyhow there is no likelihood in the near future of imparting knowledge in Surgery to the students of Āyurveda, and the vaids of the present day may justly be compared with "a bird with but one wing." Suśruta says: "Only the association of medicine with surgery forms the perfect physician. The Physician who is deficient in the knowledge of one of these branches resembles a bird with but one wing."

Certificates:—Many Kabirajes, for whose learning and skill as a practitioner of the healing art, I entertain profound respect, have expressed their sorrow at the attitude of our Government in not rocognising the certificates issued by them to their patients who had been under their treatment. Such an attitude of the Government has caused results which are far from desirable. The public have been forced to resort to uncanny practices in which even the qualified practitioners are known to have taken part. To take a concrete example: a clerk in an office becomes ill. Perhaps he lives in a village where qualified practitioners are not available, or if available their services cannot be secured on financial grounds. A kaviraj practices in the village, and the clerk naturally calls him for treatment. He appplies for leave on medical grounds. As usual a certificate from a registered practitioner is wanted by the officer in charge of the office. The clerk informs him about the true state of things. The officer demands from him in reply that under the rules, a certificate from a qualified practioner is absolutely necessary to procure leave on medical grounds. What the clerk does next is well known to all. The dignity of the profession of medicine suffers in the end. There is no law in India to prosecute a quack, and it is necessary to protect the public by training these kabirajes and recognise them, if they pass the test, as qualified medical men.

Registration : There should be a list of qualified kabirajes in Bengal. When trained according to scientific methods, their certificates to patients should be recognised. For the present, the learned physicians should be entrusted with the power of granting certificates, for amongst them we find men whom the Government have bestowed the highest Honours for their professional attainments, such as Mahāmahopādhyāya, Vaidyaratna, etc.

21. *Proper protection, collection and sale of drugs* : The Government should establish a Therapeutic Garden where the medicinal plants should be grown, and where the students should be taken to study the plants and recognise them. A trained Botanist should be in charge of such a garden, and a learned Kabiraj should take charge of the drug store, the main object of which would be to take proper protection, collection, supply, and sale of the certified drugs to different centres, to be established in the different districts of the Province. A Garden of Medicinal Plants and a Materia Medica Museum should be started for the proper identification of all medicaments of vegetable origin. A Chemist should be appointed for the preparation of mineral medicines. At present, it is difficult to secure reliable medicines, and it is highly desirable that medicinal agents should be supplied from a well organised drug store under Government control or supervision.

22. *Standardisation of drugs* : For the present crude drugs may be used as the kabirajes do it now;

but standardisation must be gradually introduced in the preparation of medicinal products. The kabirajes are not hostile to improvements; they are now selling their medicines in tablet forms.

23. *The sale of drugs*: The cost of medicines in the Āyurvedic system is decidedly less than that of medicines used by the doctors. And the cost may be reduced if a central organisation be started for supplying crude vegetable and mineral drugs to the medical men under State supervision. The cost of maintaining such an establishment would be satisfactorily met from the profit realised from the sale of drugs, if manufactured on a commercial scale. As examples of succesful business in the shape of a druggist's store, I may mention the Sakti Pharmacy of Dacca, Jhandu Pharmaceutical Works, Kalpataru Ayurveda Bhavan, Messrs. C. K. Sen and Co., Ltd., and other firms dealing with Āyurvedic medicines.

The recent world-war has taught us a lesson. We have been reminded of our utter helplessness in getting a supply of medicines from Europe. The cry for imported drugs has abolished the trade in indigenous medicine, the well-tried and efficacious drugs of our country. The formation of a Drug Manufacturing Committee to investigate the possibilities of cultivation of medicinal plants in India and manufacture of drugs from them on a commercial scale is a move in the right direction; and if it be successful, there will be no lack of private enterprise to undertake its manufacture. The Cinchona plantation and the manufacture of Quinine tablets in the Reformatory Jail, Alipore, are instances of successful enterprise that has enriched the State, and at the same time benefitted the poor inhabitants of the country.

24. *The duties of the Local bodies,—University, Municipality, District Boards.*—It is the duty of the University to do something to stimulate the proper study of the indigenous system of Āyurvedic medicine. There is scope for study and research by medical students, in the investigation of the empirical truths which have proved beneficial for centuries, by scientific methods. But in the University of Calcutta nothing has been done to stimulate such researches. In the list of endowments, there is no donor for the Āyurvedic studies. There have been Lecturerships, Readerships and Professorships in the varied branches of learning. I am the last person to minimise their importance; but I am sorry to remark that, besides what the Government have done for the western medical science, the University has taken no active interest for cultivation of knowledge in medicine, far less in the medical studies of the indigenous system;—a system which is still believed, and followed by the innumerable inhabitants of the country, and is still doing an amount of good to the suffering humanity. That the teaching of Āyurveda is not incompatible with the ideals of University, has been shown by the University of Punjab which has an Āyurvedic Board and which grants diplomas to the successful students. If the premier university failed to take the initiative, let a Board of Studies in Āyurveda be formed in the Calcutta University without further delay and there are many Fellows of the Senate who are eligible to be its members. I do not think that the study of the Āyurveda is less interesting to, or has less claim on, the Senators than any other study which has a board for it.

The Municipalities and the District Boards should open Āyurvedic dispensaries for the treatment of the poor people. The cost incurred would be less than that of similar institutions under Government control. In the dispensaries should be employed one or two apprentices who will help the Kabiraja in his pharmaceutical preparations and in serving his prescriptions. These dispensaries will not only be the means of affording relief to the sick, but will be instrumental in disseminating medical knowledge among the masses. It must be clearly remembered that I would not for a moment think of transplanting the indigenous system in the place of the Western science which has done so much good in the past and which is destined to do more in the future. My object is to give the Āyurvedic physicians a scientific training. Allow me to quote the words of Suśruta: "The ignorant physicians are allowed to exist and practise their profession from carelessness of the King."

156, Haris Mukerjee Road,
Bhowanipur, Calcutta.
Dated the 25th Sept. 1923.

I remain, yours faithfully,
(Sd.) GIRINDRA NATH MUKERJEE.

Āyurvedic Committee, Bengal.

Oral evidence by Dr. G. N. Mukerjee, B.A., M.D., F.A.S.B, dated the 6th November, 1923.

Answers to the questions put by Dr. M. N. Banerjee, M.R.C.S. (Eng.). L.S.A. (Lond.), C.I.E., the President.

Q.—What do you mean by the word 'literary' in the sentence "The traditional system of training of Kavirājes which has lasted for many centuries in Bengal has always been exclusively literary in character" (para. 3, p. 14)?

A.—They learn the science of medicine from the text books, and the teachers explain those subjects in detail. The students do not get much of practical training. Only in the preparation of mineral medicines they have to do practical work. These text books contain scientific facts

Examples :—(1) *The development of the fœtus* has been described by months and these statements have been recorded since the Vedic times (*Garbha-upaniṣad*). But all along the same story is repeated in all the books, and the teachers teach the students according to these books. But these facts are never shown practically to the pupils nor do they corroborate the truth of these statements by observation.

(2) *Surgical operations.*—It is distinctly laid down in the *Suśruta Saṁhitā* that in case of boils, it must be opened by the knife, or cautery, or fire; and it is mentioned that if a doctor does not open a boil if there be pus in it, then he is considered as 'caṇḍāla.' Also there are mentions about application of ointments, etc., prior to

operations. But the students are taught the local applications only and not the practice of surgical operation.

Q.—Do you think that they are accurate descriptions?

A.—With the knowledge of the Western science, I think, we may find them to be fairly accurate and to contain many true facts and observations.

The barbarians who burned the famous library of Alexandria are called by us fanatics, but I think they were sincere; they believed the Koran to be the only book that contained truth, and as they had it, it was useless, they argued, to allow the library to stand as the books in it, as they were not Korans, contained no truth and so must be destroyed. If the Āyurvedic books are rubbish it is better to burn them for there is no truth in it, but if there is any Koran it should be allowed to live and be studied.

Q.—What is the history of medical education in Bengal?

A.—*Vide* Dr. Mukerjee's paper, para. 4-7, pp. 14-18.

Q.—How was the Āyurvedic system taught in those days?—when was it taught in the Sanskrit College?

A.—The following information has been received from the grandson of Pandit Madhusūdan Gupta. Madhusūdan was a student of the Sanskrit College. His teacher, Pandit Kṣudirām Biśārad had an abscess in the ear and took leave. Then Madhusūdan became the teacher. He used to dissect small animals. It is not a fact that Madhusūdan did the first dissection. Dissection of animals used to be done in the Sanskrit College. The Āyurvedic teaching was a part of the Sanskrit study; the course was for two years. Pandit Naba Kumur Gupta was another teacher of Madhusūdan in Āyurveda.

Q.—What is 'Native Medical Institution'?

A.—The Government first started a separate institution in 1822 long before the Medical College was established. They used to train ordinary apothecaries in Urdu or Bengali for state emergencies. In 1835 Government ordered abolition of the school (see Dr. Mukerjee's paper). They had it from 1822 to 1835.

Q.—What did Madhusūdan do when he was transferred to the Medical College?

A.—The information is not complete whether he taught the Āyurveda or began to learn the Western science. He learned English from David Hare. Hare, Bethune and Madhusūdan were friends. His son was one of the first ten students of the Medical College. His name was Gopal. The students had a superficial knowledge of English; scholarship was awarded to each, and books and dissecting cases were provided. Bethune presented the Pandit's portrait to the Medical College.

Q.—Were there two classes in the Medical College?

A.—When Madhusūdan came to the Medical College, the students of the Āyurvedic class in the Sanskrit College divided themselves into two groups—one came with Madhusūdan and the other did not. When he entered the dissection hall, most of his students fled. I think that the first batch of students in the Medical College got a mixed training,—training in the Āyurvedic and Western science. Anatomy was studied with the help of dry human bones and dissection of goats. Then gradually the Western system was introduced.

Q.—What is the origin of the Military Assistant Surgeons?

A.—At first in the Native Medical Institution the Indians (especially Mahomedans and Hindusthanees) used to get the training. With the establishment of the

Medical College the Anglo-Indians began to get their training in the Medical College and formed the Military Assistant Surgeons.

Q.—What is the utility of the Ayurvedic study ?

A.—Summary of pages 67 to 157 of Mukerjee's book *History of Indian Medicine, Introduction*—about the utility, restoration and development; I have dealt there with the origin of medicine, some obsolete customs, about therapeutic measures, *e.g.*, massage, hypnotism, exercise, and diseases, such as identity of cholera, small-pox since the old days.

Some of the facts mentioned in the original works are not so popularly taught and spoken of because the teachers in these day, lecture on the subjects which they like best (pharmacy, materia medica, medicine). and not all the subjects (surgery, midwifery) which are in the Āyurveda.

Q.—Who were the Native Doctors? Why did the native doctor die long ago ?

A.—Because the graduates of the Medical College came out, and it is a fact that the better qualified seniors always try to oust the juniors and less qualified medical men in practice.

Native doctors.—Before the establishment of the Medical College and Native Medical Institution, it was customary to employ Indians as subordinates in hospitals superintended by British Surgeons to carry out their instructions. Gradually these subordinates acquired skill and experience in medical science and were called "Native Doctors." They were recognized by the Government as such and were ordered to be attached to regiments and civil stations. They acted as compounders and dressers and had to undergo examinations, before they were entitled to higher status. They formed the 'third class' of native doctors. In 1822, the Calcutta Native Medical Institution was established to carry on a better and uniform system of education in medical sciences. Jameison, Breton and Tytler were Superintendents of this school. An excellent class of native doctors—the second class—was the result. They were employed in the army and civil stations.

In 1835 this Institution was abolished and the Calcutta Medical College was established "for the instruction of native youths in the various branches of medical science, through the medium of the English language. The passed students were to receive certificates allowing them to practise medicine and surgery and were to receive pay as native doctors. In June, 1838, the demand for native doctors in the army was great, and the reply of the Council to the Government demand was "that the college in its present state, is not likely to afford a supply of subordinate medical officers to the native army. That the duties of the native doctor, and his pay, are incommensurate to the education given in the college." It was then resolved by the Government that students of this college should, on passing their examination, receive the title of Sub-Assistant Surgeons. They are now known as Assistant Surgeons.

A secondary or military class was then formed for the instruction of native doctors through the medium of their vernacular. They were required to live in the college precincts and to be amenable to military law.

In 1847-48 regulations were drawn up for the education in the college of pupils for the European subordinate medical department. The students on passing their examinations, used to furnish Apothecaries and Stewards to the hospitals of European troops.

In 1851-52, the establishment of classes for the education of Bengali native doctors was added to the secondary class. The students, after passing their examination, were employed in jails and civil stations of lower Bengal. The students who were successful in their examination were also called native doctors. The Bengali class developed afterwards into a separate school—the Campbell School in 1875. The students, on passing their examination from this school had been known as Hospital Assistants. They are now styled as Sub-Assistant Surgeons.

Q.—Do you think that teaching in Bengali or English would make any difference ?

A.—The students like to study medicine in English. At first training was given in English and Bengali in the medical schools but gradually the English came into use because the students liked it better than the Bengali. Really the students find that the English books are easier to learn and the Bengali synonyms of scientific terms are very difficult sometimes. In the case of the Āyurvedic medical schools they would not have so much difficulty as with the western school for in the first case they will have to deal with one class of students.

Q.—Would you sacrifice the advance of Bengali by imparting training in English ?

A.—No—for the present only ; so long as there are no good books or translations in Bengali. Only up to that time they will be taught in English. When good Bengali books will be available then they will be taught in Bengali. Mādhavakar's *Nidāna* is a good book. It has also been recast. The final medium of training would be Bengali.

In his address to the students of the Medical College of Calcutta, Professor Sir William O'Shanghnessy said "The progress of the principles of Normal and Vernacular Education cannot now be checked. These facts have deprived the Anglo-vernacular party of even a pretext for advocating the exclusive use either of English or of the learned native tongues. Let those who wish well to India, and desire to see its inhabitants flourish in knowledge, visit the secondary schools of the new Medical College, and they will see the first fruits of the Normal system. I have felt it an imperative duty to publish these important facts."

When the Orientalists and the Anglicists were fighting to determine the medium of instruction of Indian youths, the celebrated scholar Mr. Hodgson cherished equal doubts about the fitness of the Sanskrit, the Arabic and the English languages as the medium of studies for the various nationalities and races which inhabit India. Dr. Wilson in 1838 remarked—"Mr. Hodgson's advocacy of the vernaculars is most powerful and convincing. They must be the medium of the regeneration of India, as they have been such of every country on the face of the globe."

Q.—Why do you say that most of the methods of treatment are "empirical"?

A.—This is the idea of the people taught in the western science. All the teachings of the Āyurveda cannot be accidental; they must have been founded on facts, experiments and experience. But nowhere are given reasons for the facts, *e.g.*, salt-free diet in ascites and liquid diet in typhoid. They have only described the facts in *sutras* and the commentators and teachers only dilate these facts to the students.

Q.—What is your idea about the text books?

Paragraph 10 (6), page 22—"the text books require to be recast, etc." (*vide* Dr. Mukerjee's paper).

A.—The teachings of the modern sciences must be incorporated with the teachings of the Āyurveda; If there is anything in the Āyurveda that does not corroborate scientific facts, it must be discarded.

Q.—Are there any Botany, Biology, Physics, Chemistry in the Āyurveda?

A.—From the following it will be seen that biology was taught in the Āyurveda in the olden times:

Jīvaka was a student in the University of Taxila. When he finished his studies he wanted a certificate from his teacher. His teacher ordered him to go and examine the plants which were within a few miles of that University and to note all the plants that were of any medicinal importance. After inspection he reported that there was not a single plant which had not had some medicinal property.

In the *Atharva Veda*—there are mentions about various worms. The description of the worms given by the Ṛṣis are exactly the same as given by the writers of the present age. Strange it is that the Ṛṣis in their description made the same sort of mistakes, as were done at first, by the early writers of the western science. I would refer you to my book "*Human Parasites in the Atharbaveda.*" There are no separate text books of Biology, Physics, Chemistry, etc.

Q.—What are the subjects which have distinctive characters in the Āyurveda?

A.—Medicine and Materia Medica. The text books on Biology, Physics, Chemistry, Anatomy and Physiology may be written on the model of the Āyurveda with the addition of facts from other sciences.

Q.—You say that there ought to be a Central College, etc. (*vide* Mr. Mukherjee's paper, paras 11-15)—Why?

A.—If an Āyurvedic College be established and recognised by the Government then the old Kavirajes who had a different training in the *Tols* shall have great difficulty in their practice. So there ought to be a separate system of teachings for those Kavirajes to give them some idea about modern advancements.

Q.—The scheme that you have given is too expensive. Can you curtail it ?

A.—Yes, the scheme is expensive but you cannot get good men for anything less than the amount. But you can get some good men who will be glad to do honorary work.

Q.—What is the nature of the Āyurvedic teaching that is given by the Punjab University.

A.—See Calendar of the Punjab University.

Q.—How will the District Board be a source of teaching to the mass ?

A.—They will get training as apprentice—and only practical training like that of the compounders.

Question asked by Mahāmahopādhyāya Gananāth Sen.

Q.—In case the Government is unable to start a Government Central Āyurvedic College, under the present financial condition, do you think that a suitable subsidy to an existing Āyurvedic College would suffice for the proper teaching of the Āyurveda ?

A.—I want a thoroughly equipped model institution maintained by the Government. But if the Government is unable to start such an institution immediately, then any of the existing institutions may be subsidised, provided the subsidy is sufficient to bring it to the standard of a model institution.

Q.—What would be proper control that Government would exercise ?

(*a*) If the College be a Government one—there should be a board to manage the working of the College. In the Board members will be nominated by the Government from Government officials, from Āyurvedic practitioners, from doctors and from laymen. It should not be maintained and managed like the Calcutta Medical College.

(*b*) If it be a subsidised College—the College must be a public institution—there should be one Government official, the other members will be from the doctors, kavirajes and laymen.

The internal management of the College will be in the hands of the Principal.

Q.—If proper arrangements are made for the teaching of the Āyurvedic medicine up to the required standard, should the University grant degrees and diplomas for Āyurveda to the regularly trained students ?

A.—Yes. I think it is the duty of the University.

Report of Ayurvedic Colleges Amalgamation Special Committee.

Preface.

In April, 1924, the Principal of the Baidyasastrapith applied to the Corporation for (1) a capital grant of Rs. 25,000, (2) a recurring annual grant of Rs. 10,000 and (3) a plot of rent-free land measuring not less than 3 bighas for the erection of a College and Hospital. The Public Health Standing Committee of the Corporation on the 23rd May, 1924, referred the matter to a Sub-Committee. The Sub-Committee inspected the various Ayurvedic Institutions, and the first question that struck them was whether it was not desirable and necessary to start a really efficient Ayurvedic College in Calcutta for the promotion of Ayurvedic learning. They were further prompted to raise this question by the fact that there were such institutions in other parts of India and they particularly referred to the Ayurvedic College in Madras. They communicated with the Principal of the Ayurvedic College, Madras, the Madras Corporation, the Bombay Corporation, the Poona Municipality and the Principal of the Delhi Tibbi College of Science with a view to ascertain their views. They consulted the authorities of the existing three Ayurvedic Colleges in Calcutta, *viz.*, the Astanga Ayurvedic College, Baidyasastrapith and the Govinda Sundari Ayurvedic College and invited them to attend their meetings with a view to help them in their deliberations and to consider whether the different Ayurvedic Institutions could be amalgamated into a first-class Ayurvedic College. From the discussions the Sub-Committee had with the authorities of these institutions, they gathered that they were all willing to amalgamate provided the Corporation took the necessary steps in the matter. The Public Health Standing

Committee discussed the matter threadbare at two of their meetings, agreed with the Sub-Committee in their views and strongly recommended as follows :—

(1) That the support of the Corporation be extended to the Ayurvedic, Unani and other indigenous system of medicine and treatment.

(2) That the question of grant to a new Ayurvedic College having regard to the views expressed by the authorities of the three existing Ayurvedic Colleges and other eminent gentlemen interested in the promotion of the Ayurvedic system of medicine and treatment, the Committee are of opinion that in the existing state of things, it is highly desirable that the three existing Ayurvedic Colleges of Calcutta, *viz.*, Astanga Ayurvedic College, Baidyasastra Pith and Govinda Sundari Ayurvedic College should be amalgamated and that a really efficient Ayurvedic College should be started in Calcutta with a well-equipped Ayurvedic Hospital and Outdoor Dispensary and a Herbarium under the management of a representative Ayurvedic Board to be registered.

Appointment of the Special Committee and their ·ecommendations.

The Corporation at their meeting held on the 4th September, 1924, accepted the recommendations of the Public Health Standing Committee and with a view to give effect to the proposal appointed a Special Committee constituted as shown in the margin to frame a detailed scheme for an amalgamated Ayurvedic College and a constitution

(1) Dr. Sundari Mohan Das.
(2) Dr. B. C. Ghose.
(3) Babn Jogesh Chunder Sen.
(4) Babu Sukumar Ranjan Das.
(5) Babu Ramaprosad Mukhopadhyaya.
(6) Kaviraj Shamadas Bachaspati, Principal, Baidyasastrapith.
(7) Kaviraj Shib Nath Sen.
(8) Dr. Amiya Madhab Mallik.
(9) Dr. Pramatha Nath Banerjea.
(10) Dr. Grindra Nath Mukerjee.
(11) Dr. K. S. Roy.
(12) Mahamahopadhyaya Gananath Sen, President, Ayurvedic Sabha.

(13) Kaviraj Jamini Bhusan Roy, Principal, Astanga Ayurvedic College.
(14) Kaviraj Ram Chandra Mullick, Principal, Govinda Sundari College.

for the said Ayurvedic Board. The Special Committee have held 12 meetings. At the 1st meeting held on the 13th November, 1924, Dr. Pramatha Nath Banerjea, M.L.C., was elected President of the Committee. Mahamohopadhyaya Gananath Sen, President Ayurvedic Shabha, Kaviraj Shamadas Bachaspati, Principal, Baidyasastrapith, Kaviraj Ram Chandra Mullick, Principal, Govinda Sundari College and Kaviraj Jamini Bhushan Roy, Principal, Astanga Ayurvedic College were requested to send their suggestions for a scheme for an amalgamated Ayurvedic College and a constitution for an Ayurvedic Board with a special reference to the following points :—

(1) Constitution, (2) Location, (3) Name of institution, (4) Equipment including, (*a*) College, (*b*) Hospital, (*c*) Herbarium and (*d*) Miscellaneous, (5) Scope of studies, (6) Funds, and (7) Existing arrangements of each of the institutions.

The Committee further agreed that they would consider any scheme submitted by any other member of the Committee in this connection.

Mahamohopadhyaya Gananath Sen and Kaviraj Jamini Bhushan Roy submitted a joint scheme and Kaviraj Ramchandra Mullick and Kaviraj Shamadas Bachaspati submitted their schemes separately touching on all the points referred to above. No other scheme was submitted by any other member of the Committee. It would appear from the schemes submitted that the authorities of the three institutions are sincerely in favour of an amalgamation. They have also assured the Committee that they would abide by their decision in every matter in this connection. The Committee have carefully gone into the schemes submitted, have discussed the various points raised therein and have considered all matters ancillery thereto. They beg to submit the following recommendations to the Corporation :—

(1) *Amalgamation.*—The three Ayurvedic Colleges, *viz.*, the Astanga Ayurvedic College, the Baidyasastrapith and the Govinda Sundari Ayurvedic College be amalgamated.

(2) *Name of the Institution.*—The amalgamated College be named "The Ayurveda Mahavidyalaya."

(3) *General Society.*—The Committee agreed that there should be a Society and that any person having sympathy with the objects of the society should be eligible to be a member of the Society.

That for the purpose of amalgamation, all members of the Institutions namely Baidyasastrapith, Astanga Ayurvedic College and Gobinda Sundari College, should be eligible to become members of the Society in accordance with the Rules and Regulations.

(4) *Governing Body.*—That there should be a governing body for the purpose of carrying on the work of the amalgamated college and hospital according to the rules and regulations for the time being in force and the resolutions of the Society.

(5) *Provisional Ayurvedic Board.*—That for the first year there should be a Provisional Ayurvedic Board for the purpose of organising the amalgamated college and hospital and conducting the affairs of the institution. The Provisional Board should be constituted as follows :—

(*a*) Each of the existing three colleges should elect 3 members	9
(*b*) The Special Committee should elect—	
(*i*) 3 eminent Kavirajes not connected with any of the existiug colleges ...	3
(*ii*) 6 members from the general public ...	6
(*c*) The Corporation to nominate 3 members ...	3
Total	21

(6) *Office Bearer.*—For the present there should be the following principal office-bearers :—

(*i*) The President of the Board.
(*ii*) The Rector of the College.
(*iii*) The Principal of the College.
(*iv*) The Secretary or Secretaries to the Board.
(*v*) The Superintendent of Hospital.

That the Principal of the amalgamated college should be a paid officer and should devote his whole time in the work of the college.

That the Principal should be appointed by the Provisional Ayurvedic Board.

That Kaviraj Shamadas Bachaspati should be President of the Provisional Board.

That Mahamahopadhyaya Kaviraj Gananath Sen should be Rector of the College.

That Kaviraj Jamini Bhushan Roy and Ram Chandra Mullick should be the Joint Secretaries of the College.

That Kaviraj Shibnath Sen should be the Superintendent of the Hospital and that the post should be honorary for the present.

(7) *The Corporation Contribution.*—Having regard to the schemes submitted by Kaviraj Shamadas Bachaspati, Mahamahopadhyaya Gananath Sen and Kaviraj Jamini Bhusan Roy, the Committee are of opinion that about 5 bighas of land would be required for the amalgamated College and Hospital. The capital expenditure for buildings and equipment would be about Rs. 3 lakhs and annual recurring expenditure would be in the neighbourhood of Rs. 60,000. They recommend that the Corporation should give a plot of land measuring about 5 bighas in a suitable locality in Calcutta for the amalgamated College and Hospital, contribute a lakh of rupees towards the cost of

the buildings and equipment and make an annual grant of Rs. 30,000 for maintenance.

(8) *Memorandum of Association and the Rules.*—The Memorandum Association of the Society and the Rules are appended hereto.

(9) *Representatives on the Provisional Board elected by the existing Ayurvedic Colleges.*—The authorities of the existing three Ayurvedic Colleges have selected the following representatives on the Provisional Board :—

(*i*) The Baidyasastrapith.

1. Kaviraj Shyamadas Bachaspati.
2. Kaviraj Sarat Chandra Kabya-Byakaran-Sankhya-Vedantatirtha.
3. Kaviraj Bimalananda Tarkatirtha.

(*ii*) The Astanga Ayurvedic College.

1. Mahamahopadhyaya Kaviraj Gananath Sen, Saraswati, M.A., L.M.S.
2. Kaviraj Jamini Bhusan Roy Kaviratna, M.A., M.B.
3. Kaviraj Hem Chandra Sen, Bhisagratna.

(*iii*) The Govinda Sundari Ayurvedic College.

1. Maharaja Sir Manindra Chandra Nandy, K.C.I.E.
2. Maharaj Kumar Srish Chandra Nandy, M.A.
3. Kaviraj Ram Chandra Mallik, Kavya-Vyakaran-Sankhyatirtha. Sathdarsanacharya, Bhisakshastri.

NOTE OF DISSENT.

4th April, 1925.

To

The SECRETARY,

Corporation of Calcutta.

DEAR SIR,

I beg to acknowledge receipt of a copy of the Minutes of the Proceedings of the last meeting of the Special Committee appointed to frame a detailed Scheme for an amalgamated Ayurvedic College and a Constitution for an Ayurvedic Board, containing the Report as adopted by the Committee. As the Report is going to be placed before the Corporation soon, I would request you to place my note of dissent along with it before the Corporation.

1. We began our work as members of the Special Committee with the object that the proposed Ayurvedic College would be formed by the amalgamation of the three existing Ayurvedic Colleges, *viz.*, Astanga Ayurveda Vidyalaya, Govinda Sundari Free Ayurvedic College, and the Vaidya Sastrapitha. We tried our best for the desired amalgamation and we framed a detailed scheme for the amalgamated college. But for some reasons which would be apparent from the Extracts of the Proceedings of the Governing Bodies of the colleges concerned, amalgamation was not found possible. I do not blame anybody for their decision to which they arrived after mature deliberation ; but as the amalgamation failed, the scheme formulated in our Report could no longer be called a detailed scheme for the amalgamated Ayurvedic College.

2. In the formation of a Provisional Ayurvedic Board, item No. 5 in the report, it was unanimously adopted that (*b*) the Special Committee should elect (*i*) 3 eminent Kabirages not connected with any of the existing colleges, (*ii*) 6 members from the general public. But no such election of the members took place, and we were obliged to send our Report incomplete. We were told that the Special Committee had not been entrusted with the power of election of the members by the Corporation, and consequently the 9 members were elected by the Corporation. Personally I do not think that any gentleman who is sympathetic to a particular college should be debarred from being appointed a member; but as we provided that the 3 colleges should select 3 representatives each, it was settled that members under 5 (*b*) should be selected from gentlemen not connected with the 3 existing colleges. But some of the gentlemen selected by the Corporation are connected with the Colleges mentioned above.

3. In the item No. (6), the principal office-bearers have been selected by the Special Committee, and names of gentlemen had been recommended for the posts. The representatives of the three colleges were also elected by the colleges, and the names of the gentlemen so elected had been accepted by the Special Committee. If the Special Committee had no power of election, the names of gentlemen elected for the principal offices should be deleted from the Report. Then our Report would consist of a scheme and a constitution of the proposed college and the provisional Board, and to be consistent throughout, no name should have been suggested. Either we should have elected the members according to our resolutions, or we ought to have ceased to nominate any. In fact, our recommendations for the

principal office-bearers were made on the basis of the resolution 5. The result of the election (12 by the Corporation and 9 by the three Colleges) wast hat 21 members of the provisional Board had no voice in the election of the principal office-bearers. The office-bearers themselves expressed their doubts about the procedure adopted.

On all other points I fully approve the Report.

Yours faithfully,

(*Sd.*) G. N. MUKERJEE.

Appendix

Memorandum of Association of Ayurveda Mahavidyalaya.

1. The name of the Society shall be the "Ayurveda Maha-Vidyalaya Parishat."

2. The Registered Office of the Society shall be situated in Calcutta.

3. The objects of the Society shall be the imparting of Ayurvedic Education to students in a systematic manner, the advancement of the Ayurvedic science for the benefit of the suffering humanity; and for the attainment of the aforesaid objects the Society may adopt any or all of the following means, namely :—

(*a*) To establish and maintain a College or Colleges and a Dispensary or Dispensaries, Hospital or Hospitals and construct, equip and manage such buildings, Lecture-rooms, Museums, Laboratories, Herbarium and Gardens, Libraries, Hospitals, Dispensaries, Hostels, Boarding Houses and other necessary buildings to be used in connection therewith and as adjuncts or as accessories thereto.

(*b*) Provide for the admission and treatment of in-door and out-door patients in the Hospital or Hospitals or Dispensaries which may be started or may hereafter come under the control of the Society.

(*c*) Provide for the moral training of students of the College in keeping with the best traditions of the country.

(*d*) Make and amend rules and regulations in connection with the management and control of the said College and hospital and other institutions that may be established or taken over by the Society and for the residence for the students and officers and servants and particularly in connection with the admission and conduct of students and regulation of studies.

(*e*) Encourage research in the Ayurveda and allied

sciences by grants from the funds of the Society or by the establishment of Fellowships, Scholarships, Prizes or Rewards and in such other manner as the Society may determine upon.

(*f*) Endow or establish Professorship, Lectureships, Readerships in the Ayurveda or allied sciences.

(*g*) Encourage systematic study of diseases and drugs according to Ayurvedic and if necessary modern methods.

(*h*) Grant Diplomas, Certificates of Proficiency, Medals, Scholarships, Free-studentships or Rewards to students of the College under such terms and conditions as the Society may think fit.

(*i*) Establish farms for the cultivation, distribution and supply to the profession of medicinal plants under such conditions as the Society may determine.

(*j*) Collect manuscripts and compile, edit, translate, print, publish, sell or help in the compiling, editing, publishing, printing and selling of books or journals, for the use of students, practitioners or the general public.

(*k*) Publish, circulate or sell or help in the publication or circulation or sale of a journal of a character specially adapted to the needs of the Ayurvedic science and for purposes of making Ayurveda better known amongst the people of the country and for purposes of creating general interest in Ayurveda.

(*l*) Publish, distribute or sell records of transactions and calendars of the Society and bulletins and reports of the work done in the Hospitals, Dispensaries and Laboratories connected with the Society.

(*m*) Consider the law of India and all questions affecting the Ayurvedic profession and adopt such measures from time to time regarding the same as may be deemed expedient or necessary.

(*n*) Purchase, take on lease or otherwise acquire, hold,

manage, let, sell, exchange, mortgage or otherwise dispose of movable or immovable properties of every description and all rights or privileges necessary or convenient for the purpose of the Society, and in particular any lands, buildings, furniture, household and other effects, utensils, books, newspapers, periodicals, instruments, fittings, apparatus, appliances, conveniences and accommodation and when deemed necessary or desirable in the interest of the Society, sell, demise, let, hire, mortgage, transfer, or dispose of the same.

(*o*) Invest the moneys of the Society not immediately required in promissory notes of the Government of India or any securities which are or may be authorised by any Act of Indian Legislature or by the High Court of Calcutta for the investment of Trust moneys.

(*p*) Assist, incorporate or co-operate with any other Society or Association whether incorporated or registered or not and having altogether or in part objects similar to those of the Society.

(*q*) Accept grants-in-aid from Government, or Indian States or Municipalities or other Corporate Bodies and enter into such arrangements with Government, or Indian States, or Municipalities or Corporate Bodies as the Society may think fit.

(*r*) Accept gifts and endowments on such terms as the Society may consider reasonable.

(*s*) Undertake and carry out the execution of any trusts which the Society may deem to be directly or indirectly conducive to its interests.

(*t*) Borrow or raise money by the issue of or upon bonds, debentures, bills of exchange, promissory notes or other obligations or securities of the Society or by mortgage or charge of all or any part of the property of the Society and collect donations and subscriptions for the purpose of the Society.

(*u*) Establish, endow, contribute to, organise and manage provident or benevolent funds for the benefit or assistance of the staff employed by the Society and their families and dependants.

(*v*) Do all such other things as may be lawful, incidental or conducive to the attainment of the foregoing objects or any of them.

4. If at any time it is found advisable or desirable to discontinue the society, it shall be dissolved in the manner provided by the Societies' Registration Act (Act XXI of 1860) and its property and assets shall be given or transferred to some other institution or institutions having objects similar to the objects of this society in accordance with the provisions of the said Act, subject to the terms and conditions of any agreement which may be subsisting at the time with any donor or lessor.

RULES.

Constitution.

1. The Society shall consist of four classes of Members, namely, Life Members, Ordinary Members, Ex-officio Members and Honorary Members.

2. Any person making a donation of Rs. 500 or more to the Funds of the Society shall be entitled to become a Life Member.

3. Any person paying an annual subscription to the Society of Rs. 12 shall be entitled to become an Ordinary Member.

4. The Trustees, Professors and Lecturers and Visiting Physicians and Surgeons of the Maha-Vidyalaya and the

Members of the Committee nominated by the Calcutta Corporation, shall be Ex-officio Members.

Any person of eminent position and attainments, who is specially interested in the objects of the Society may be elected an Honorary Member at a meeting of the Society on the recommendation of the Executive Committee. Such election may be for life.

6. Any person of eminent position who may take interest in the Institution and give substantial help to it, may, on the recommendation of the Executive Committee be elected a Patron or Vice-Patron at a meeting of the Society. Such election may be for life or for a definite term.

7. Any person above the age of 18 years may be elected a Member. Such person shall be duly proposed, seconded, and elected at a meeting of the Executive Committee.

8. If the whole amount of the Annual subscription of an Ordinary Member be not paid during the year for which it is payable and within six months thereafter, his rights of membership shall *ipso facto* be suspended. Thereafter, the Executive Committee may, after giving him at least one month's notice in writing, remove his name from the list of Members with effect from the 1st Baisak of the following year, or such later date as the Executive Committee may fix.

Meetings of the Society.

9. Meetings of the Society shall be called General Meetings. An Annual General Meeting shall be held every year not later than the last day of Baisak, at which the following business shall be transacted :—

(*a*) To consider the Report of the Provisional Board and the Executive Committee for the previous year ·

(*b*) To consider the audited accounts of the previous year and the balance sheet;

(*c*) To pass the Budget for the new year;

(*d*) To elect the office bearers for the new year;

(*e*) To elect members of the new Executive Committee,

(*f*) To appoint Auditors;

(*g*) To transact any other business that may be brought forward by the Executive Committee or of which a week's notice in writing has been given by any member.

10. A Special General Meeting may be convened at any time by the Honorary Secretary of his own motion, and shall be convened by him at the instance of the President or of the Executive Committee. If the Honorary Secretary shall fail to call such meeting within 7 days after being requested to do so by the President or by the Executive Committee, the President or the Executive Committee, acting through any Member or Members authorized by them in that behalf, may call the meeting.

11. The Honorary Secretary shall call a Special General Meeting on receipt of a requisition signed by not less than 10 Members of the institution. If he shall fail to call such meeting within one week after receipt of such requisition, the requisitionists or any 10 of them may themselves call such meeting.

12. Seven Members shall form a quorum at a General Meeting of the Members.

13. If within half an hour of the time fixed for a meeting, a quorum is not present, the meeting shall, when it has been called by or at the instance of the Executive Committee or the President, or by the Honorary Secretary of his own motion, stand adjourned to another day and hour to be fixed by the Members there present, and the Members present at such adjourned meeting shall form

a quorum whatever their number may be. If, however, the meeting has been called by the Honorary Secretary on the requisition of Members or by the requisitionists themselves, it shall be dissolved.

14. At least 7 days' notice of a General Meeting shall ordinarily be given to each Member. The notice shall specify the place, the day and the hour of such meeting, and the nature of the business to be transacted at such Meeting. In case of an emergency, a General Meeting may be called on shorter notice.

15. The non-receipt or short service of a notice of any General Meeting or of any Meeting of the Executive Committee or of any Sub-Committee shall not invalidate the proceedings of such meeting.

16. Every question arising at a General Meeting shall, unless otherwise provided, be decided by a majority of votes of the Members present and voting on the question. In case of an equality of votes the Chairman of the Meeting shall have a second or casting vote in addition to his ordinary vote.

17. The President of the Society, when present, shall preside at all General Meetings. In his absence, the meeting shall elect its own Chairman.

18. The Society shall have ultimate authority in all matters relating to the institution except such as are expressly provided for in the Rules and Regulations.

Executive Committee.

19. The management and control of the property, business, and affairs of the institution shall be vested in an Executive Committee, who shall have full power to deal with all matters connected with the institution, subject only to the Rules and Regulations for the time being in force and the Resolutions of the Society.

20. The Executive Committee shall consist of not more than 17 members including the officers and they shall be elected or appointed as follows :—

(a) 8 members to be elected by the Society at its Annual General Meeting ; provided that not more than two of such members shall be members of the staff in receipt of salary ;

(b) 3 members to be elected by the Corporation of Calcutta ;

(c) 1 member to be elected by the college staff of the Mahavidyalaya and 1 by the Hospital staff ; and

(d) The Principal, the Rector and the Secretary or Secretaries of the Mahavidyalaya *ex-officio.*

If any vacancy occurs during the interval between any two Annual General Meetings, it shall be filled up by the body concerned.

21. The Executive Committee shall elect its Chairman every year. They shall ordinarily meet once every month to transact all necessary business. A Special Meeting of the Executive Committee may be called by the Honorary Secretary or the Chairman whenever he thinks it necessary and shall be called by the Honorary Secretary on a requisition made by not less than three members of the Executive Committee. Seven shall form a quorum.

22. The Executive Committee may from time to time, appoint Sub-Committees for the convenient transaction of the business of the institution.

The Chairman shall preside at every meeting of the Executive Committee. In his absence, the meeting will elect one of its members as Chairman.

Office Bearers.

23. The Society shall have a President, a Rector, a Treasurer, a Secretary or two Secretaries and a Superintendent of Hospital.

The Rector shall have power to guide the Principal in regard to all academic matters and supervise studies in the college in a general way.

The Principal shall be responsible for carrying on the academic as well as administrative business of the college and in particular shall be responsible for the maintenance of internal discipline in the college.

24. The Honorary Secretary shall have charge of the executive work of the institution. He shall keep the minutes of meetings, carry on correspondence, look over the accounts and records, superintend the collections and be responsible jointly with the Honorary Treasurer, for the due application of the funds of the Society. He shall be responsible for giving effect to the Rules and Regulations of the Society, and the resolutions of the Executive Committee and of General Meetings.

25. The Honorary Treasurer shall be the custodian of the moneys of the institution. He may delegate his powers in respect of the collection and expenditure of small amounts to any other Office-Bearer or to a Subordinate Officer, but such Office-Bearer or Subordinate Officer shall remain duly responsible to the Honorary Treasurer and the Executive Committee. The Honorary Treasurer shall furnish the Honorary Secretary with funds for meeting the current expenses of the institution and such other amounts as may be sanctioned by the Executive Committee. On emergent occasions, any absolute necessary disbursements may be made by the Honorary Treasurer, subject, however, to ratification by the Executive Committee at its next meeting. The Honorary Treasurer shall deposit all funds not required for current expenses in a Bank to be approved by the Executive Committee. All cheques on the Bank shall be signed by the Honorary Treasurer and the Honorary

Secretary jointly. In the absence of the Honorary Treasurer, the Executive Committee may entrust his duties to any other Office-Bearer.

Trustees.

26. The property of the institution shall be vested in Trustees, whose number shall not be less than three not more than five.

27. The first trustee shall be........................

28. The trustees shall hold office for life or until they resign their trusteeship in writing.

29. A new Trustee shall be appointed only at a General Meeting.

30. The Trustees shall have power, in pursuance of a resolution passed at a Meeting of the Executive Committee and confirmed at a General Meeting, to accept any gift, or hold any property, or sell, mortgage, transfer lease, dispose of or deal with in any particular manner whatever, any property movable or immovable of the Society or acquire or take on lease any property.

In case of disagreement between the Society and the Board of Trustees on any matter it shall be referred back to the Society for reconsideration at a special meeting, whose decision shall be final and binding on the Trustees.

31. Any three of the Trustees may exercise all or any of the rights and powers of the Trustees under these Rules.

General.

32. The income and property of the Society, whencesoever derived, shall be applied solely toward the promotion of the objects of the institution as set forth in the Memorandum of Association, and no portion thereof shall be paid or transferred, directly or indirectly, by way of dividend, bonus, or otherwise by way of profit, to the persons who at any time are or have been members

of the Society or to any of them or to any person claiming through any of them. Provided that nothing herein contained shall prevent the gratuitous distribution among or sale at a discount to, Members or Subscribers to the funds of the Society or otherwise, relating to all or any of its objects, nor the payment, in good faith, of remuneration to any officers or servants of the Institution or to any Member thereof or any other person, in return for any services actually rendered to the Society.

33. An Office-Bearer, or a Member may be removed for good and sufficient cause by a resolution passed by a majority of three-fourths of the Members present at a General Meeting and confirmed at a subsequent General Meeting called within a period of not less than a fortnight and not more than two months after the first meeting.

34. The Executive Committee may frame regulations not inconsistent with these Rules, subject to ratification at the next General Meeting.

35. The Executive Committee may make suggestions for additions to or amendments of these Rules. Any individual member shall also have the power to propose any additions or amendments at a General Meeting of the institution, provided that due notice of such additions or amendments shall have been specifically given to the Honorary Secretary at least a fortnight before the meeting and the Honorary Secretary shall have circulated such notice among all the Members.

36. Additions to or amendments of, any of these Rules shall only be made by a majority of two-thirds of the Members present at a General Meeting. The Memorandum of Association shall not be altered or amended except at a Special General Meeting by the votes of three-fifths of the total number of Members on the roll, other than those whose rights have been suspended

under Rule 8, and confirmed by the votes of three-fifths of the Members present at a second Special General Meeting.

Transitory Provisions

1. There shall be a Provisional Ayurvedic Board which shall manage and control the affairs of the Institution for one year from the date of amalgamation. This Board shall be constituted as follows:

(*a*) Each of the existing three Colleges shall elect 3 members ...	9
(*b*) The Special Committee shall elect—	
(*i*) 3 eminent Kavirajes not connected with the existing Colleges ...	3
(*ii*) 6 members from the general public ...	6
(*c*) The Corporation shall nominate 3 members	3
	21

2. The first Trustees shall be elected by the Provisional Board.

N.B.—A copy of the report was sent to each of the Governing Bodies of the three existing Colleges for an expression of opinion. The Governing Bodies of the Baidyasastrapith and the Govinda Sundari Ayurvedic College have approved of the scheme framed by the Special Committee for an amalgamated Ayurvedic College, but the Governing Body and the Board of Trustee of the Astanga Ayurvedic College are of opinion that at present it is not desirable that the Ashtanga Ayurvedic College be amalgamated with the other two existing Colleges.

EXTRACTS FROM THE PROCEEDINGS OF THE MEETINGS OF THE GOVERNING BODIES OF THE THREE COLLEGES.

Letter from the Secretary, Gobinda Sundari Free Ayurvedic College, dated the 13th March, 1925.

With reference to your letter No. S-7025, dated the 7th March, 1925, forwarding, for an expression of opinion, a copy of the report of the Special Committee appointed by the Corporation to frame a detailed scheme for an amalgamated Ayurvedic College, I have the honour to state that the report was duly laid before the Governing Body of this College at their meeting held on 11th March, 1925, and an extract from the proceedings of the meeting is appended.

Extract from the Proceedings of the meeting of Governing Body of the M. C. G. S. Free Ayurvedic College held on 11th March, 1925.

Read letter No. S-7025, dated 7th March, 1925, from the Secretary to the Corportion of Calcutta with enclosures.

Resolved—

That the Corporation be informed that the Governing Body fully concur with the scheme framed by the Special Committee of the Corporation for the management of the amalgamated Ayurvedic College. Resolved further that their sincere thanks be conveyed to the Corporation for what they have done so far for the amalgamation of the three existing Ayurvedic Colleges.

Letter from the Secretary, Baidya Sastra Pith (National Ayurvedic College), dated the 14th March, 1925.

Re AYURVEDIC COLLEGE AMALGAMATION.

With reference to your letter No. S.-7027, dated the 7th March, I have the pleasure to inform you that the report of the Special Committee forwarded with the letter was placed before our College Council (Governing Body) on 12th instant for consideration and that the Council unanimously passed the following resolutions supporting amalgamation and the final report of the Committee and heartily thanked the Special Committee for their effort.

Resolved—

(1) That considering the present state of "Ayurveda" this Council is of opinion that all Kavirajes should leave aside all personal and sectarian interests and devote their energies for the uplift of Ayurveda.

This Council has already intimated its desire for the amalgamation of the three existing Colleges and it reiterates the same agaih and conveys its sincere eagerness for amalgamation and also tenders thanks for the efforts of the Committee for the last six months to bring about amalgamation.

(2) This Council while recognising that the proposed grant is not adequate, considers that there are one or two points in the report of the Special Committee which needs looking into but in view of the loss of time and resultant delay in starting work that will take place, requests that the report of the Special Committee be adopted.

(3) The Council understands that Mahamahopadhyaya Gananath Sen has informed the Special Committee at their last meeting that the three eminent Kavirajes nominated by the Corporation were connected with the Baidyasastra Pith and this action of the Corporation was contrary to the constitution of the Provisional Board.

The Council of the Biadyasastra Pith considers it necessary to inform the Special Committee that the three Kavirajes elected by the Corporation have no connection whatever with the Baidyasastra Pith and their names were put in on the assurance being given by one of the members of the Council that they would help the Baidyasastra Pith by teaching the students of the College but as they did not agree to the suggestion, this fact was recorded in the letter of resignation submitted by them.

Letter dated the 14th March, 1925, from the President, Executive Council, Astanga Ayurveda Vidyalaya, Calcutta.

With reference to your letter No. S-7026, dated 7th instant, addressed to the Secretary of the Astagna Ayurveda Vidyalaya, I beg to state that I placed before the Governing Body and the Board of Trustees of my College a copy of the Report of the Special Committee appointed by the Corporation "to frame a detailed scheme for an amalgamated Ayurvedic College" for favour of their opinion and guidance.

The Governing Body and the Board of Trustees in a combined meeting held on 13th instant have expressed their opinion as follows :—

I. That this meeting of the Governing Body and the Board of Trustees of the Astanga Ayurveda Vidyalaya offers its heart-felt thanks to the Corporation of Calcutta for recognising that support of the Corporation should be extended to the Ayurvedic system of medicine.

II. That the Astanga Ayurveda Vidyalaya has been attempting the resurrection and growth of Ayurveda in all its eight branches, *piz.*—

(1) Shalya or Surgery and Midwifery (together).

(2) Shalakya or Surgery of the Eye, Ear, Nose, and Throat, etc.

(3) Kayachikitsa or Practice of Medicine.

(4) Bhutavidya or Treatment of mental diseases (including the so-called obsessions).

(5) Kaumara-bhritya or Hygiene and Treatment of children.

(6) Agada-tantra or Diagnosis and Treatment of Poisons, vegetable, mineral and animal, including Snake-bite, Rabies, etc.

(7) Rasayana or Hygienic and Preventive Medicine for the attainment of longevity and rejuvenation in old age.

(8) Vajeekaran-tantra or Sexual Science inclnding sexual Hygiene and Treatment of Sexual diseases, and has adopted modern scientific methods where necessary for the said purpose and is not based on blind orthodoxy; but it appears that the two other Ayurvedic Colleges do not attach the same importance to the modern methods of scientific investigation; and in consequence, an amalgamation of Colleges which might hold fundamentally different ideas and ideals would not increase their efficiency.

III. That the proposed amalgamation of the existing Colleges although conceived in the best interests of the Ayurvedic Science, is not in the present circumstances likely to be conducive to its healthy growth.

IV. That this meeting is of opinion that at present it is not desirable that the Astanga Ayurveda Vidyalaya should be amalgamated with the Vaidya-Shastra Pith and Govinda-Sundari Free Ayurvedic College.

Appendix.

The Committee appointed by the Government of Madras on the indigenous medicines drew up the following Questionnaire :—

1. What is the division or divisions of the indigenous systems of medicine,—Ayurveda, Unani or Siddha—that you propose to deal with ?

2. (*a*) What are the theory or theories of causation of disease according to your system ? Please favour the committee with your views as to how far your theory or theories stand the tests of modern scientific criticism. (*b*) What are the principles and methods of diagnosis and treatment followed in your system ? Please favour the committee with your views as to the general efficacy of treatment adopted in your system, supporting your statements by facts and figures wherever possible. (*c*) Do you hold that the view that indigenous systems of treatment are more efficacious in certian conditions than other systems ? If you do, please adduce evidence in support of your statement.

3. (*a*) Are you connected directly with any institution on indigenous lines ? (*b*) Do you consider that the existing institutions of indigenous systems are satisfactory from the standpoint of (1) adequacy of medical relief provided : (2) suitability as centres of medical education. If your answer is in the negative, please state in what respect you consider the existing arrangements deficient and how you propose to remedy them. (*c*) Do you consider that there exists at present sufficient provision for medical relief and medical education on indigenous lines ? If your answer is in the negative, please state what measures you would propose to remedy the insufficiency.

4. (*a*) Do you consider that the ideal medical training

of indigenous systems of medicine requires (1) That the students should be placed under personal guidance of teachers of first-rate ability and of recognised standing in their subjects; (2) that the teachers and students alike should have access to well appointed hospitals, laboratories, libraries and museums; (3) that the teachers should have sufficient leisure to be able to pursue independent investigations in their own subjects? If you share in this view as to the essentials of medical training, do you consider that this ideal is attained or attainable in the near future in any institution in this Presidency or elsewhere where there is provision for medical training on indigenous lines? (*b*) If you consider that this ideal is too high for the present, what would you substitute in its stead, as (1) the ideal to be ultimately achieved, (2) the idea to be worked out in the immediate present.

5. Do you agree with the view of the Calcutta University Commission that "There is an obvious and promising desire at the present moment among the numerous adherents of these (indigenous) systems for closer touch with modern scientific methods. In time, no doubt they will be able to make available for the practitioners of western medicine the traditional knowledge which is of real value and will reject, as western medicine continually rejects, those theories which are mere survivals, and cannot stand the test of experiments. The distinction between Indian and western systems of medicine will then disappear." If you agree that a unified system of medicine as indicated in the above passage is the ideal to be aimed at, what steps would you suggest for the fulfilment of such an ideal?

6. Do you agree with the view that the curriculum of studies of indigenous medicine should include a study of modern scientific methods as illustrated by such subjects

of study as modern physics, chemistry, and biology, as also a study on modern lines of anatomy, physiology, pathology, bacteriology, and surgery in all its branches? If you agree with the above view, in whole or in part, please favour the committee with a precis of the course of studies you would propose for students of indigenous medicine, with special reference to (*a*) the progressive standard corresponding for example, to the existing allopathic qualifications of Licentiate (L. M. P. of our allopathic Medical Schools), Graduate, Masterate and Doctorate (L.M.S., M.B., M.S., M.D., of our Universities). (*b*) The preliminary qualifications and periods of study for each of the standards proposed. (*c*) The medium or media of instruction proposed.

7. What are your views on the question of extending Medical Registration to Indigenous Systems of Medicine? If you hold that such extension is necessary and desirable, please favour the Committee with your views regarding (*a*) the formation of a suitable Registration Board for admitting competent practitioners into the medical register, (*b*) any changes in, or additions to, the existing legislation on Medical Registration.

8. What is your opinion regarding the comparative cost of treatment, according to allopathic and indigenous systems? Please give reasons for your opinion.

9. What, in your opinion, are the causes of decay of the indigenous systems of medicine? Kindly favour the committee with your suggestions for revival?

10. Please state your views as to how the indigenous systems of medicine can be fostered and prompted by (*a*) the State, (*b*) the local boards, (*c*) the Universities, (*d*) Private agencies (individuals or association).

BIBLIOGRAPHY OF WORKS ON INDIAN MEDICAL SCIENCE.

General Medicine.

1. Wilson : On the Medical and Surgical Sciences of the Hindus (*Oriental Magazine, 1823*). Works 3, 269-76, 380-93. London, 1864.

Indian Physicians at Bagdad. J.R.A.S.

2. Royle : An Essay on the Antiquity of Hindu Medicine. London, 1837, Cassel 1839, 200s.

3. Wise : Commentary on the Hindu System of Medicine. Calcutta, 1845; London, 1860 and 1900.

Review of the History of Medicine. London, 1867.

Medical Knowledge of the Hindus, Lancet, Vol. II, 1846.

4 Stenzler : Zur Geschichte de Ind. Medicin, Janus 1, 411-54. Breslau, 1846.

5. Lassen : IAlt. 2, 511-13. 1849.

6. Weber : ILit. (1) Aufl. 1852, (2) Aufl. 1876, 283-90.

History of Sanskrit Lit., Trubner and Co., English trans., pp. 265-70.

7. Brian : Coup d'oeil sur la Médicine des Anciens Indiens. Paris, 1858, 15s.

8. Daremberg : Recherches sur l'etat de la médecine. Ann. méd., Paris, 1867, S. A. 24*s*.

Fragments d'histoire et de bibliographie. Gaz. hebd. de méd. 1883 f.

Resume de l'histoire de la médecine. Paris, 1897, 25-36.

Le Médecine Charaka, etc., in Bull. de l'Ac. de méd., May 11, 1897.

" Suçruta." Dict. Encyclop. des sciences medicales.

9. Liétard : Lettres historiques sur l'etat de la Médecine chez les Hindous. Paris, 1863, 76s.

10. Mrs. Manning : Ancient and Mediæval India. London, 1869, 1. 334-58.

11. Häser : Lehrbuch der Geschichte der Medicin. 3 Aufl. Jena, 1875, 4-38, mit Beitrogen von Stenzler.

12. Hessler : Allgemeine übersicht der Heilkunde dei altern Inder. Sitzungsberg Math.-phys. Cl., Munchen, 1887, 1, 137-49.

Der Ayurveda des Sushruta. Erlangæ. I 1844, II. 1847.

13. Schroeder : Indiens Literatur und Cultur. Leipzig 1887, 729-33.

14. Dutt : History of Civilization in Ancient India. Vol. II, Ch. IX. Calcutta, 1890, 3, 382-95.

15. Brendes : Die Pharmacie bei den alten culturvolkern. Halle. 1891, 1, 1-30.

16. Kuhn : KZ. XIII. 49.

17. Jolly : Early medical literature of India. Trasac, 9, Cong. of Orient. London, 1903, 454-61.

Médicin von Julius Jolly. Grundriss De Indo-Arischen Philologie und Altertumskunde. Encyclopædia of Indo Aryan Research, 111 Brand, 10 Heft. Strassburg, 1901.

Knoblauch, Festgruss an Roth, p. 18.
Fur Quellen Kunde der Indischen Medizin. Zt.d. Deutsch. Morgent-Geschichte, 1904.
Medicine and Divination, Bower MS., JASB. 1891.
IA. XXI. 29, 129.
WZKM. V. 103.
Indian Medicine.

18. Sir B. Sinh Jee : A Short History of Indian Medical Science. London, 1896.
19. Pagel : Geschichte der Medicin. Berlin, 1898, 32-7.
20. Macdonnel : History of Sanskrit Lit., London, 1900, 426f., 435f.
21. Cordier : Origine, evolution, et décadence dela Méd. Indienne. Annales d'Hygiene, 1901, 77-89.
Vāgbhaṭa et l'Aṣṭāṅgahṛidayasaṃhitā. Besançon, 1896.
Études sur la Médecine Hindoue temps Védiques et héroiques. Paris, 1894.
Bibliographie Medicale de l'Inde.
Nāgārjuna et l'Uttaratantra de la Suçruta Saṃhitā. Anantarivo, 1896.
22. Dietz : Annalecta Medica.
23. Elphinstone : History of India, 5th Ed. pp. 159-60.
24. Ward : Hist., Lit., Mytho. of the Hindoos, Vol. II. Serampore, 1815-18.
25. Coats : Transactions of the Literary Society of Bombay, Vol. III, p. 232.
26. Grohmann : Medicinisches aus dem Atharva-Veda mit besonderem Bezug auf den Takman in I. st. ix. 381 ff. 1865.
IS. IX. 381.

27. Böthlingk : St. Petersburg Dict. Supplement, Vol. VII—Medical Authors. 1879.

28. Roth : Z. D. M. G. xxvi, 441 and 448, 1872. Monograph on Caraka.

Article critique sur l'edition. Aṣṭāṅgahṛidaya by Pandit Jîbānanda Vidyâsâgâra in Zeitschrift der D. M. G. : T. XLIX. pp. 184 *et seq.* et Litteraturblatt für orientalische Bibliographie. l. n., pp. 48-50.

29. Gildemeister : Script Arab. de rebus Indicis, pp. 94-97. [Flugel, following in the Fihrist-al-ulum in Z. D. M. G. xi, 148 ff, 325 ff. 1857.]

30. Webb : The Historical relations of Ancient Hindu with Greek Medicine. Calcutta, 1850.

31. Hoernle : Commentaries of Suśruta, J.R.A.S. 1906-7.

Bower Manuscript with English translation. Calcutta, 1895.

Studies in the Medicine of Ancient India, Part I, Osteology. Oxford, 1907.

The Authorship of Caraka Samhita. A. F. Gesch. d. Medizin, 1908.

32. Ray : History of Hindu Chemistry, Vol. I, Calcutta, 1902; Vol. II, Calcutta, 1909.

33. Colebrooke : Transactions of the Royal Asiatic Society, Vol. I.

34. Haas : Die Heiratsbrauche der Altin Inder Webers Indische Studien. 1862.

In Volumes XXX, XXXI of J. Germ. Or. Soc. Z.D.M.G. 1876, p. 617 sq., 1877, p. 647 sq.

35. A. Müller : In Volume XXXIV of J. Germ. Or. Soc. Z.D.M.G. 1880, p. 465.

36. Goldstucker : In Mrs. Manning's Ancient and Mediæval India. London, 1869.

37. Bergaigne : Inscr. Sanscrites de Campa et du Cambodge. Paris, 1893.

38. Derselbe : Hippocrates und die Indische Medizin Z. D. M. G., 31, 647-66.

39. Buck : Growth of Medicine from the earliest times to the end of the 18th Century.

40. Heyne : Tracts on India. London, 1814.

41. Csoma de Koros : J. A. S. B., 1835, Jan. No. 37.

42. Eatwell : On the Rise and Progress of Rational Medical Education in Bengal. Indian Annals of Med. Sc. No. xiii, Art. x.

43. Muhammad Mirza : Memorandum on Mahomedan Medicine in India, *ibid*, Art. xi.

44. Neuberger (translated by Playfair) : History of Medicine : "Medicine of the Indians," Vol. I, pp. 43-60. London, 1910.

45. Chakraberty : An Interpretation of Ancient Hindu Medicine. Calcutta, 1923.

A Comparative Hindu Materia Medica. Calcutta.

46. Mazumdar : Medicinal Science in Ancient India. Calcutta Review, February, 1925.

47. Laufer : Beitrage Zur Kenntnis der Tibetischen Medicin. I and II Teil. Von. Heinrich Laufer, Dr. Med. Berlin, Druck Von Gebr. Unger, Bernburger, Str. 30, 1900

48. Ghose : Sphygmology in Ayurveda, Journal of Ayurveda. Calcutta, 1924.

49. Roy : On the Past and Present State of Medicine in India : Printed as Appendix of Burdwan Fever by Dr. Gopal Chunder Roy. Calcutta, 1876.

50. Bloomfield : Contributions, AJP. vii, xi, xii.
51. Pictet : KZ. U. 24, 321.
52. Gupta : The Ātreya School of Medicine. Calcutta, 1917.
53. Articles in the Āyurveda Journal. Calcutta, 1924-26.
54. Sen, G. : The Medical Science in Ancient India. Calcutta, 1908.
Hindu Medicine, an Address delivered at the Benares Hindu University. Calcutta, 1916.
The Science of Ayurveda. Calcutta, 1925.
55. Sham Shastry : Kautilya's Arthaśāstra, done into English.
56. Kaviratna, A. C. : Caraka Samhita. Eng. trans. Calcutta, 1899.
57. Bhisagratna K. L. : Sushruta Samhita, Eng. trans. Calcutta, 1907-1916. Introduction.
58. Sarkar, J. : Sushruta Samhitā.
59. Vullers : Alt Indische Geburtschülfe. Janus, 1846.
60. Winternitz : Folk Medicine in Ancient India, Nature, 1898, lviii.
61. Zimmer : Alt indisches Leben. Berlin, 1879.
62. I'Tsing : Records of Buddhist Religion (Takakusu's Ed.)
63. Kunte : Astangahṛidaya of Vagbbaṭa. Introduction.
64. Sanskrit Language and Literature in Encyclo. Brit., Vol. XXI, p. 294, 9th Ed.
65. Webb-Johnson : Medicine in India. A lecture delivered at a meeting of East India Association, London, on 24th January 1921.
66. Ghosh, H. N. : Ayurvedic system of Medicine and the Question of its Adaptability. A. B. Patrika, Sept. 1923. C.M.J.
67. Reinaud : Memoire sur L'Inde.

68. Mukerjee, G. N. : Mādhava Kara. J. A., Vol, I. pp. 124-129; 208-217, 1924.
Comparative Medicine, *ibid*, 237-244.
Vṛnda Madhava, *ibid*, 256-259.
Madhavācārya and others, *ibid*, 307-313.
Kārtika Kundu, J. A. Vol. II, 184-187.
Bhāskara, *ibid*, 342-344.
Ravi Gupta and Viṣṇu Gupta, *ibid*, 373-376.
Śālihotra. Historical Quarterly. 1925-1926.

69. Bodding : The Santals and Diseases. Mem, Asiatic Soc. Bengal, Vol. X, no. i.
Santal Medicine, *ibid*, no. ii.

70. Moberly : Amulets as Agents in the Prevention of Disease in Bengal, *ibid*, Vol. I, no. xi.

71. Gupta, U. C. : Introduction to Vaidyaka Savdasindhu. Calcutta.

72. Watanbe : A Chinese Text Corresponding to a part of Bower MS., J. R. A. S., April, 1907.

73. Wustendeld : Geschichte der Arab Aerzte.

74. Cureton : A collection of such passages relative to India, as may occur in Arabic writers. Wilson's note to the above. J. R. A. S., Old Series, vi, 105-115.

75. Heudley : The Indian Systems of Medicine and the lesson that may be learnt from them Transac. First Ind. Med. Cong. 1894.

Botany, Materia Medica and Pharmacology

1. Ainslie : Materia Medica of the Hindustan. Madras, 1813. 48, 301 s. 4, 2 Aufl. London 1826

2. Roxburgh : Flora Indica, 3 Bde, Calcutta, 1832.

3. Watson : Index to the names of Indian plants, London, 1868, 637 s. folio.

4. Waring : Pharmacopœia of India. 1868.
Bazzar medicines of India.

5. Dutta : Materia Medica of the Hindus. Calcutta, 1877.

6. Garbe : Die Indischen Mineralien. Leipzig, 1882, 10, 104s.

7. Dymock : Vegetable Materia Medica of Western India. Bombay. 1883 f.; 2 Aufl, 1886, 1012 s.

8. Dymock, Warden, Hooper : Pharmacographia Indica. 3 Bde, London, 1889-1893, 599, 641, 643, 205 s.

9. Watt : Dictionary of Indian Economic Products. 6 vols. in 9, London 1889-93, 5326 s, Index, 1896.
First Presidential Address, Section Pharmacology and Indian Drugs, First Indian Medical Congress, 1894.
The Commercial Products of India. London, 1908.

10. Irvine : Materia Medica of Patna, 1847.

11. Steuart : Punjab Plants.

12. Arjuna : Bombay Drugs (Catalogue), 1879.

13. Drury : Useful Plants of India, 1872. London. 1873, 2nd Ed.

14. O'Shaughnessy : Bengal Dispensatory, 1841.
Bengal Pharmacopœia, 1844.

15. Pal, N. C. : Indian Herbalist, 1873.

16. Khori and Katrak : Materia Medica of India and their Therapeutics, 1903.

17. Dey : Indigenus Drugs of India, 1867.
Indian Pharmacology—A Review. Second Presidential Address. First Ind. Med. Cong. Calcutta, 1894.

18. Mohideen Sheriff : Supplement to the Pharmacopœia of India, 1869.

Materia Medica of Madras, Vol. I, 1891.

19. Lisboa : Useful Plants of Bombay.

20. Bentley and Trimen : Medicinal Plants. London 1877.

21. Baden-Powel : Economic Products of Punjab. Lahore, 1868-72.

22. Graham : Catalogue of Bombay Plants.

23. Haunigberger : Thirty-five Years in the East.

24. Murray : Plants and Drugs of Sind. London, 1881.

25. Fleming : Catalogue of Indian Medicinal Plants and Drugs. Calcutta, 1810.

26. Pyres or Peris : Letter about Indian Drugs to Manuel, King of Portugal, written from Cochin, 1516. Journ. de Soc. Pharm. Lusit. II (1838), 36. Abel Remusat : None. Melanges Asiatiques II (1829), 203.

Pedro Josse da Silva : Elogio Historico noticia completa de Thome Pires, pharmaceutico e primeiro naturalista da India. Lisboa, 1866. Library of the Pharm. Soc. London, Phamphlets No. 30.

27. Christoval Acosta : Tractado de las Drogas y Medicinas de las Indias Orientales. Burges, 1578.

Aromatum Historia, 1574.

28. Garcin de Orta : Colloquios dos Simples, etc. Goa, 1563.

29. Shirazy : Ulfaz Udwigeh. (1630) Trans. by Gladwin. 1793. No. 543, 551s.

30. Beva bin Khas Khan : Madan-us-Shifa-i-Shikandar. 1512.

31. Mahomed Momin : Tupfat-ul-Muminin.

32. Mahomed Akbar Arzani : Karabadine Kaderi. 1658.

33. Boissier : Flora Orientalis. 1867.

34. Wallich : Trans. of Med. and Phys. Soc. of Calcutta VIII, 1836. Reprinted in Pereira's Mat. Med. Vol. II, Part 2, 1857, 699. Subject : Coptis Teeta.

35. MacIssac : T. M. P. S. (Cal.), 1827, Coptis Teeta.

36. Royle : Illustrations of the Botany of the Himalayan Mountains and of the Flora of Cashmere, 1839.

The Commercial Products of India and the East. 1854.

The Productive Resources of India. 1840.

A Manual of Materia Medica. 1845.

37. Ramkamal Shen : T. M. P. S. (Cal.), 1827. Subject : Gulancha.

38. Banerjee : Indigenous Drugs of India, Transac. First Ind. Med. Congress, p. 533. 1894.

39. Mukharji : Anti-Malarious Drugs. *Ibid*, p. 535.

40. Bagchi : Hæmostatic Plants. *Ibid*, p. 536.

41. Ganga Sing : *Tinospora Cordifolia, Ibid*, p. 536.

42. Morton : Therapeutics of Calatropis Gigantea. *Ibid*, p. 537. I.M.R. 1898, p. 267.

43. Chaitan Mal : Effects of Tribulus Terrestris in Health and Disease. *Ibid*, p. 537.

44. Sen, H. C. : Treatment of Pathological Hæmorrhages. C. M. J. 1906, Vol. I, pp. 233-234.

Spondias Mangifera in the treatment of diabetes and dysentery. *Ibid*, p. 301.

Treatment of Ascites. *Ibid*, Vol. II, p. 109. 1907.

Original Researches in the treatment of Tropical Diseases with Indigenous Drugs.

45. Spencer : Neem Oil in Fever in " A record of Indian Fervers," p. 15. Calcutta, 1899.

46. Birdwood: Practical Bazar Medicines. Calcutta, 1920.
47. Nadkarni: Indian Plants and Drugs. Madras, 1910.
48. Prain: Bengal Plants, 2 Vols. Calcutta, 1903.
49. Indian and Colonial Addendum to the British Pharmacopœia. 1900.
50. Sanyal: Vegetable Drugs of India. Calcutta.
51. Voigt: Hortus Suburbanus Calcuttensis. Calcutta, 1825.
52. Hamilton: Prodromus Floræ Nepalensis. Londini, 1825.
53. Boissier: Flora Orientalis, 1867.
54. Gupta: Vanauṣadhidarpaṇa in Bengali. Calcutta, 1908.
55. Pratt: Flowering Plants.
56. Warden, Bose: False Bikh or Bikhma (*Aconitum palmatum*), Ph. J., 1892.
Note on the presence of Cholesterol in the Roots of *Hygrophila spinosa*. Pharmacographia Indica. Index and App., p. 191.
57. Bose, C. L.: Analysis of East Indian Plantains. *Ibid*, Vol. III, pp. 446-447.
On the Chemistry and Toxicology of *Nerium odorum*, Trans. Chem. Soc. 1901, I. M. G. 1901, Coates Memo. Prize Essay. C. U., 1900.
On the Toxic properties of the fruits of *Luffa Aegyptiaca*, bitter variety (Teeta Dhoondul), C. M. J., 1906.
58. Dutta, R. C.: Kurchicine, the new alkaloid of *Wrightia antidysenterica*, Calcutta Medical News. February, 1880.
59. Ghose, R. D.: The Bark of *Wrightia Antidysenterica*. Transac. Cal. Med. Soc. Vol. I, pp. 175-186. 1880.

60. Ghose, H. N. : A Report on *Ixora Coccinea.* C. M. J., Vol. III, pp. 419-427. 1908-1909.

61. Chopra : The Pharmacology and Thearapeutics of *Boerhavia diffusa* (Punarnava). I. M. G. 1923.

Investigations into the Santonine obtained from *Artemesia brevifolia,* I.M.G. 1924.

Some Medicinal Plants from the Himalayas.

62. Chopra, Bose : Observations on the Anti-diabetic properties of *Cephalandra Indica.* I.M.G. 1925.

Cephalandra Indica in Diabetes. I. J. M. R., 1925.

Note on the Pharmacology and Therapeutics of *Adhatoda vasica.* I. M. G. 1925.

Some Observations on the Pharmacology, Action and Therapeutic properties of *Adhatoda vasica.* I. J. M. R. 1925.

63. Ghosh : Chemistry of Indigenous Drugs : 1. *Adhatoda vasica* (Vāsaka) 2. *Terminalia Arjuna,* (Arjun) 3. *Saussurea Lappa* (Kuṣṭha) Ann. Rep. of C. S. T. M., 1923, p. 48.

64. Ghose, Ghose, Dutt : Chemistry of Silajatu, *Tribulus terrestris* (Gokhura), *Butea froadosa* (Palasa), *Saussurea Lappa* (Kut), *Terminalia Arjuna* (Arjun), *Seraluta anthelmentica* (Somraja), *Holarrhena antidysenterica* (Kurchi). Abhrak Bhasma (calcined mica), Vanga bhasma (calcined tin). Ann. Rep. of C. S. T. M, 1925.

65. Kirtikar, Bose, B. D. ; Indian Medicinal Plants. 2 Vols.

66. Kirtikar : The Poisonous Plants of Bombay, 1903.
Botanical Characters of Indian Poisonous Plants, in Lyon's Medical Jurisprudence for India, 2nd 3d. 1890, pp. 520-30.

67. Birdwod : Catalogue of Matheran and Mahabaleswar Plants.

68. Ghosal : *Terminalia Arjuna.* Coate's Memorial Prize Essay. C. U. 1908.

69. Kurz : Forest Flora of British Burma. Calcutta, 1877.

70. Cooke : The Flora of the Presidency of Bombay. London, 1901.

71. Stewart : Illustrations of the Forest Flora of N. W. and Central India. London, 1874.

72. Haines : A Forest Flora of Chota-Nagpur. Calcutta, 1910.

73. The Second Report of the Indigenous Drugs Committee. Simla, 1909.

74. Strachey : Catalogue of the Plants of Kumaon, Garhwal and Tibet. 1852. Revised by Duthia. London, 1906.

75. Beddome : Ferns of British India. Madras, 1869, 1876.
Ferns of S. India, 2 vols. and Supplt. 1863-70.
Flora Sylvatica of S. India, 2 vols. Madras, 1869-73.
Icones Plantarum Indiæ Orientalis, Madras, 1868-74.

Surgery and Midwifery.

1. Jivanram Vaidya : Forceps used by the Ancients of India. Bombay, 1892.

2. Mukhopādhāya : The Surgical Instruments of the Hindus with a comparative study of

the surgical instruments of the Greek, Roman, Arab and the Modern European Surgeons. Calcutta, 1912.

Midwifery in India : Indian Medical Record. 1925.

The Science and Art of Midwifery as known to the Hindus. 1926.

Restoration and Development of Āyurveda. Journal of Āyurveda, 1926.

3. Holwell : Account of the manner of inoculating for Small-Pox in the East Indies. London, 1767.

4. Das, S. M. : History of Midwifery in Bengal, C. J. M., Vol. II., pp. 140-145. 1907-8.

5. Ghosh : Difficult Labour and its Treatment according to the Ancient Hindu Physicians. Proc. and Transac. of the Second Or. Confer. 1922.

6. Dass, K. N. : Midwifery in India. Indian Medical Record. February, 1924. Am. Jour. Obs. Gynæ., 1923.

7. Banerjee : A note on the Illustrations of the Surgical Instruments of Tibet (Journ. and Text, Budhist Text Society, Part III, 1894, Proceedings IX ; Surgical Instruments and Appliances in Ancient India and Tibet. Plates I, II, III. *Ibid*, Appendix.

8. Mullick : Hindu Midwifery, C. M. J. April, 1916.

9. Walsh : Tibetan System of Anatomy, JRAS.

10. Ray, S. K. : Surgery of the Ancient Hindus, C.M.J. 1925.

11. Mitra : Die Geschichte der Gyn. u. Geburtschilfe des Alt Indiens. Innsbruck Kongress, 1924.

Development of Midwifery and Gynæcology with special reference to that of Ancient India. C.M.J. 1926.

12. Sen, G. : The Practice of Surgery in Ancient India. Indian Med. Record. Oct., 1914. Nov., 1915.

Indian Medicine and Surgery.—a Sketch.—Forward, Nov. 15, 1925.

13. Goswami : Āryadhātrīvidyā and Puṁsavana in Bengali. Calcutta.

HISTORY OF MATERIA MEDICA AND OTHER COGNATE SUBJECTS.

1. Flückiger and Hanbury : Pharmacographia : A History of Drugs, 2nd Ed. 1879.
2. Guibourt : Hist. des Drogues, 1849.
3. Hill : History of the Materia Medica.

A T ALOGUES.

The following catalogues should be consulted for notices of Āyurvedic books:—

Abbreviations. — **Names of Catalogues.**

Z. d. D. M. G. = Zeitschrift der Deutschen Morgenläudischen Gesoelschaft.

B. C. = Sūcipustakam. Cat. of Sanskrit MSS. in the Library of the Asiatic Society of Bengal.

Cat. Cat. = Catalogus Catalogorum. (Leipsic, 1891, Supplement 1896.) It gives a list of Sanskrit MSS. in the alphabetical order of works and authors.

I. O. Cat. = India Office Catalogue.

Oxf. Cat. = Catalogi Codicum Manuscriptorum bibliothecæ Bodlianae codices Sanscritcos, by Aufrecht. Oxford, 1869.

B. M. C. = British Museum Catalogue. By P. C. Bendal. London, 1902.

Bkr: Bhandarkar's Report on the search of Sanskrit MSS. in the Bombay Presidency. Bombay, 1893.

Bkr. 2 Rāj: Bhandarkar's Report of a Second Tour 1904-6 in search of Sanskrit MSS. in Rājputana and Central India.

S. B. L. (Nepal): The Sanskrit Buddhist Literature of Nepal. By R. L. Mitra. Calcutta, 1882.

Tanjore Cat.: A classified Index to the Sanskrit MSS. in the Palace at Tanjore. By Burnell. London. 1880.

L = Notices of Sanskrit MSS. in the Asiatic Society of Bengal. By Dr. R. L. Mitra,

Vol. I-IX. Calcutta, 1880. By H. P. Śāstrī, Vol. X and XI.

Bik. Cat. = Sanskrit MSS. in the Library of H. H. the Maharaja of Bikaner.—A Catalogue of, by Dr. R. L. Mitra. Calcutta, 1880.

Notices (2nd Series): By H. P. Śāstrī. Vol. I; II-III.

Nepal Cat.: Catalogue of MSS. in the Durbar Library in Nepal. By H. P. Śāstrī.

Peterson: Report in the Search of Sanskrit MSS.

Rep.: Report on the Search of Sanskrit MSS. 1895-1900. By H. P. Śāstrī.

Ulwar: Catalogue of Sanskrit MSS. in the Library of H. H. the Maharaj of Ulwar. By Peterson. Bombay, 1892.

Stein: Cat. of Sanskrit MSS. in the Raghunath Temple Library of H. H. the Maharaja of Kāshmir and Yammu. By M. A. Stein.

C. S. (Cat.): Catalogue, Sanskrit College Library, Calcutta.

W.: Weber's Berlin Catalogue.

B. N.: Buniyon Nanjies.

Ep. Ind.: Epigraphia Indica.

C. B. T.: Cat. of the Chinese Transcript of the Buddhist Tripitaka.

G. O. M. L.: Cat. of Government Oriental MSS. Library, Madras, XXIII—Medicine.

Taylor: A catalogue raisonne of Oriental MSS. in the Library of College, Fort St. Ceorge, 3 vols. Madras, 1851-62.

Kielhorn: Classified Alphabetical Catalogue of Sanskrit MSS. in the South Division of the Bombay Presidency, Bombay, 1869.

Report on the search for Sanskrit MSS. in the Bombay Presidency. Bombay, 1880-81.

ABBREVIATIONS.

In these volumes the following abbreviations have been used for the names of authors and their books :

Abbreviations.		Names of Authors and Books.
C. S.	=	Caraka Saṁhitā
S. S.	=	Suśruta „
A. S.	=	Aṣṭāṅga Saṁgraha
A. H. S.	=	Aṣṭāṅga Hṛdaya Saṁhitā
M. N.	=	Mādhava Nidāna
V. M.	=	Vṛinḍa Mādhava
C. P. D.	=	Cakrapāṇi Datta
Bhā	=	Bhānumati
B. P.	=	Bhāva Prakāśa
Śā. S.	=	Sāraṅgadhara Saṁgraha
V. K. V.	=	Vyākhyā Kusumavalī
V. M. K.	=	Vyākhyā Madhu Koṣa
G. N.	=	Gada Nigraha
R. R. S.	=	Rasaratna Samuccaya
R. C.	=	Rasendra Cintāmaṇi
R. H.	=	Rasa Hṛdaya
R.	=	Rasārṇava
A. T.	=	Agniveśa Tantra
B. S.	=	Bhela Saṁhitā
J. S.	=	Jatukārṇa „
P. S.	=	Parāśara „
H. S.	=	Hārīta „
K. S.	=	Kṣārapāṇi „
V. S.	=	Vṛddha Suśruta
V. H.	=	„ Hārīta
V. B.	=	„ Bhoja
A. V.	=	Aśva Vaidyaka
AV.	=	Atharvaveda

RV.	=	Ṛgveda
YV.	=	Yayur Veda
SV.	=	Sāma Veda
Ni. S.	=	Nivandha Saṁgraha
T. C.	=	Tattva Candrikā
K. K.	=	Kartika Kuṇḍu
D.	=	Dallvaṇācārya
G.	=	Gayadāsa
J.	=	Jaijjaṭācārya
H.	=	Haricandra
R. G.	=	Ravi Gupta
A. D.	=	Aruṇa Datta
S. K. D.	=	Śrīkanṭha Datta
V. R.	=	Vijaya Rakṣitā
R. S. S.	=	Rasendra Sāra Saṁgraha
R. K.	=	Rasendra Kalpadruma
Si. S.	=	Sivadāsa Sena
B. M.	=	Bhāva Miśra
V. J.	=	Vaidya Jīvana
Y. R. K.	=	Yogaratnākara
R. N.	=	Rāja Nîghantā
D. N.	=	Dhanvantari Nirghantu
M. P. N.	=	Madana Pāla ,,
Y. T.	=	Yoga Taraṅgini
Ā.	=	Ātreya
A.	=	Agniveśa
R. P.	=	Rasa Pradīpa
V. V. P.	=	Vramha Vaivarta Purāṇa
N.	=	Navanītaka
A. R.	=	Āyurveda Ratnākara

NOTICES, BIOGRAPHICAL AND BIBLIOGRAPHICAL, OF THE ĀYURVEDIC PHYSICIANS AND THEIR WORKS ON MEDICINE

CHAPTER V

AGNI

Agni, to whom next to Indra, are addressed the greatest number of hymns is one of the most important gods in the Ṛgveda. There he is described as the Purohita or Priest (i, 1, 1 ; 44, 10, 12 ; 58, 3 ; 94, 6 ; 127, 2 ; 128, 4 ; iii, 2, 8 ; 3, 2 ; 11, 1 ; 13, 3 ; 21, 3 ; 28, 8 ; v, 11, 2), and as the King and the Superintendent of worship (i, 1, 8 ; 44, 8, 9 ; 65, 10 ; iii, 3, 3 ; 9, 8 ; 27, 2 ; iv, 3, 1 ; viii, 43, 4 ; x, 52). Various functions are ascribed to him : He is Hotri (i, 1, 1 ; 12, 1 ; 13, 4 ; 26, 2, 5 ; 31, 3 ; 44, 7 ; 45, 7 ; 58, 1 ; 67, 2 ; 76, 2 ; 77, 1 ; 94, 6 ; 127, 1, 2, 10 ; 128, 1 ; 141, 12 ; 143, 1 ; 144. 1 ; 149, 5 ; ii, 3, 1 ; 5, 1 ; 6, 6 ; 7, 6 ; 9, 9 ; iii, 1, 22 ; 2, 6, 15 ; 3, 2 ; 4, 4, 5 ; 5, 4 ; 6, 2 ; 7, 9 ; 9, 9 ; 11, 1 ; 14, 1 ; 17, 2, 5 ; 19, 5 ; 21, 1 ; 27, 7 ; iv, 8, 4 ; v, 13, 3, 4 ; 20, 3 ; vii, 16, 5 ; x, 2, 1 ; 91, 8-11), Adhvarju (i, 94, 6 ; iii, 5, 4 ; x, 91, 10), the banner (iii, 3, 3 ; 10, 4 ; 29, 5; vi, 2, 3) and the father of sacrifices (iii, 3, 4), Nestri (ii, 5, 5 ; x, 91, 10), Prasastri (ii, 5, 4 ; x, 91, 10), Potri (i, 94, 6 ; ii, 5, 2 ; iv, 9, 3 ; vii, 16, 5 ; x, 91, 10), Agnidh and Brahmāṇa (x, 91, 10).

He is described as the great (i, 36, 12 ; 79, 5 ; 94, 6 ; 128, 4 ; 145, 2 ; 188, 1 ; ii, 3, 1 ; 6, 7 ; iii, 1, 22 ; 2', 4), the wise (i, 12, 1 ; 31, 2 ; 71, 10 ; 77, 3), and the purifier (i, 12, 9, 10 ; 95, 11 ; 142, 3 ; ii, 3, 1 ; 7, 4 ; iii, 2, 6 ; 5, 7 ; 10, 8 ; 17, 1 ; 21, 2 ; v, 23, 4 ; 26, 1). He is called Tanūnpāt (i, 13, 2 ; 142, 2 ; 188, 2 ; iii, 4, 2 ; 29, 11 ; x, 110, 2), Narāśaṁsa (i, 13, 3 ; 142, 3 ; ii, 3, 2 ; iii, 29, 11 ; v, 5, 2=

Avesta Nairyo-Sanha, *i.e.*, praised by men), Jātāvedas (i, 44, 4 ; 45, 3 ; 49, 5 ; 77, 5; 78, 1 ; 94, 1 ; 99, 1 ; 127, 1 ; ii, 2, 1, 12 ; 4, 1 ; iii, 1, 20, 21 ; 2, 8 ; 3, 8 ; 6, 6 ; 10, 3 ; 11, 4, 8 ; 15, 4 ; 17, 2, 4 ; 20, 3 ; 21, 1 ; 22, 1 ; 23, 1 ; 25, 5 ; 26, 7 ; 28, 1—4 ; 29, 2 ; iv, 1, 20 ; 3, 1 ; 5, 11, 12 ; 12, 1 ; 14, 1 ; v, 4, 4, 10 ; 5, 1 ; 9, 1 ; 22, 2 ; 26, 7), Vaiśvānara (i, 39, 1 ; 49, 5, 6 ; 98, 1—3 ; iii, 2, 3 ; 26, 1 ; iv, 5, 1 ; v, 27, 1) and Vasu (i, 31, 3 ; 44, 3 ; 45, 9 ; 79, 5 ; 94, 13 ; 127, 1 ; 143, 6 ; ii, 3, 4 ; 7, 1 ; 9, 1 ; iii, 4, 1 ; 15, 3 ; 18, 2 ; 19, 3 ; iv, 5,15 ; 12, 6 ; v, 3, 10 ; 6, 1 ; 24, 2). He is Mātāriśvān (i, 96, 4 ; 128, 2 ; 147, 3 ; 148, 1 ; iii, 5, 8 ; 26, 2, 3 ; 29, 11), Jarābodha (i, 27, 10), Uśig (iii, 3, 7, 8 ; 11, 2 ; 15, 3 ; 27, 10 ; iv, 1, 15 ; 6, 11), Aṅgira Ṛṣi. (i, 31, 1, 2 ; 74, 5 ; 75, 2 ; 127, 2 ; iv, 9, 7 ; v, 8, 4 ; 10, 7 ; 21, 1 ; ii, 84, 4 ; 102, 17), Dvaivadāsa (vii, 92, 2 ; viii, 103, 2), and Trāsadasyavam (viii, 19, 22).

His relationship with the other gods.—Agni is identified with the following gods :—Mitra (i, 94, 13 ; ii, 1, 4 ; iii, 5, 4, 8 ; v, 3, 1 ; vii, 12, 3) ; Varuṇa (ii, 1, 4 ; iii, 5, 4 ; v, 3, 1 ; vii 12, 3) ; Tvaṣṭṛi (ii, 1, 5), Indra (ii, 1, 3, 6, 5 ; iii, 9, 2 ; v, 3, 1) ; Indra and Vāyu (Nirūkta, vii, 5) ; Viṣṇu (ii, 1, 3 ; Nir, xii, 19) ; Aryamān (ii, 1, 4 ; v, 3, 2) ; Aniśa (ii, 1, 4) ; Ṛbhus (iii, 5, 6) ; Rudra (i, 27, 10 ; iii, 2, 5 ; v, 3, 3) ; Aditi (i, 94, 15) ; Viśvadeva (i, 3, 4) ; Bhārata (i, 96, 3 ; ii, 7, 1) ; Āditya (ii 3, 4) ; Brahmāṇaspati ; Vidhātṛ (ii, 1, 3) ; Visvāsam (v, 22, 2) ; Asura (iv, 2, 5 ; v, 12, 1 ; 15, 1 ; vii, 2, 3 ; 6, 1 ; 13, 1 ; 30, 3) ; Puṣāna ; Savitṛ ; Bhaga ; Hotrā ; Bhāratī ; Ilā and Sarasvatī (i, 164, 46 ; ii, 1, 3-7 ; iii, 5, 4 ; v, 3, 1-3 ; vii, 12, 3 ; x, 8, 5).

They call him (Sun) Indra, Mitra, Varuṇa, Agni, etc. ; that which is one they call it variously Agni, Yama, Mātāriśvān (Ṛv. i, 164, 46). In v. 3, 1-2, the altar-fire Agni is called Varuṇa and Indra; in him are said to live all the gods. See also x, 114, 5; and iii, 38, 7, where reference to various forms of Agni is given.

Agni becomes Varuṇa in the evening, rising in the morning he is Mitra, becoming Savitṛ he moves through the air, and as Indra he glows in the middle of the sky (Av, xiii, 3, 13). Agni is said to be the mouth of the Ādityas, the tongue of the gods (ii, 1, 13, 14), and the companion of the Ratiṣāk or bounteous gods (ii, 1, 13). Through him, not only the gods, but even the mortals taste their drinks (ii, 1, 14). Agni is said to bring Varuṇa, Indra, and the Maruts to the ceremony (x, 75, 11); he worships them (vii, 11, 3; viii, 91, 16; x, 7, 6), obeys their commands (x, 52, 1) and shares the adoration which they receive (i, 36, 4; ii, 2, 1). He is often prayed for to eat the offerings (iii, 21, 1; 28, 1-6) and drink the Soma juice (i, 14, 10; 19, 9; 21, 1, 3) with Indra (vii, 93, 6; viii, 38, 4, 7-9). He is worshipped by Varuṇa, Mitra, the Maruts and 3,339 gods (iii, 9, 9; 14, 4; x, 69, 9). He helps Varuṇa, Mitra and Aryamān (i, 141, 9).

His Parents.—Agni is said to be the son of Heaven and Earth (i, 140, 7; iii, 2, 2; 3, 11; 25, 1; x, 1, 2; 2, 7; 46, 9), of Tvaṣṭṛ (i, 95, 5; iii, 7, 4; x, 46, 9; see Hillebrandt's Vedische Mythologie i, 522 *seq.*, Bergaigne, Rel. Ved., vii, 26, 6; iii, 47, *seq.*, x, 2, 7), of Ilā (iii, 29, 3), and also as the ghṛta-sprinkling offspring of Manu (i, 45, 1). Agni, the hidden god (i, 95,4; iii, 1, 9, 14; 5, 10; 9, 5; v. 11, 6), is said to be of twofold births,—celestial and terrestrial (i, 47, 4, 5). The terrestrial birth refers to the generation of Agni by means of friction between two kindling sticks, araṇis (i, 68, 2; 127, 4; iii 29, 1, 2, 3; 23, 2, 3; v, 9, 3; vii, 1, 1; viii, 23, 25; x, 5, 3; 7, 5; 49, 15; 24, 4), one the father, the other the mother. Thus his two mothers are described to be the two kindling sticks (i, 31, 2; 128, 3; 141, 4). Sometimes Agni is said to be born with the fingers which twirl the sticks (iii, 26, 3; iv, 6, 8; x, 4, 6) which die when he is born (x, 79, 4). He is also said to have three births;—one in the sea as sun (x, 5, 7), one in the heaven as lightning, and one in the waters (i, 95, 13; x, 45, 3). He is described as the child of water (i, 143, 1; 144, 2; 145, 5; ii, 1, 1; iii, 1, 3; 3, 5; 5, 3; 9, 1, 2, 4; 11, 12; vii, 9, 3; x, 2, 7; 91, 6); or its grandson (x, 8, 5). In x, 51, he is said to have been desired by the gods to come out of water and plants on a promise of his long life and a share in the sacrifice. He is also said to have been born out of heaven, out of the water and the stone, out of the forests and herbs (ii, 1, 1; iii, 1, 13). Indra is said to have generated him between two 'clouds or stones (ii, 12, 3). Bhṛgu discovered (x, 4, 6, 2) and worshipped him in the abode of the waters (ii, 4, 2; iii, 1, 3), appointed him as messenger (i, 71, 4), and placed him among men (i, 58, 6; 143, 4; iv, 7, 1, 4; vi, 15, 2). Aṅgirasa discovered Agni (v, 11, 6), and the Aṅgirasa family introduced and extended the fire worship (i, 71, 2, 3). Another account says that Mātārisvān produced the hidden one (i, 60, 1; 71, 4; 93, 6; 141, 3; 143, 2; iii, 5, 10; 9, 5; vi, 8, 4; x, 46, 9) and brought Agni from the gods (iii, 9, 5) in the sky (x, 5, 7) and gave him as a gift to Bhṛgu who, in his turn, gave him to Manu. In Ṛv. vi, 16, 13, we find that Atharvan Ṛṣi first produced fire निर अमन्थट "Thee, Agni, from out the sky Atharvan twisted." (See x, 21, 5.) This अमन्थ reminds us of the Greek Pramantheus or Prometheus, the son of Titan Iapetus and Clymene. He stole fire from heaven and brought it to men, when Zeus refused mortals the use of fire. This theft displeased Jupiter so much that he sent Pandora to Prometheus with a box that was filled with all sorts of evils. His brother Epimetheos married Pandora, who opened her box and let evils, trouble and diseases hitherto unknown spread over the earth. Hope alone remained in the box.

'No pow'r the pride of mortals can controul:
  Prone to new crimes, by strong presumption driven,
With sacrilegious hands Prometheus stole
  Celestial fire, and bore it down from heaven !
The fatal present brought on mortal race
  An army of diseases; death began
With vigour then to mend his halting pace,
  And found a most compendious way to man."

Horace, Carm, 1, x.

In vi, 16, 14, Dadhici, the son of Athavan is said to have kindled fire. Trita, the son of Vibhuvasa, received Agni on land (x, 46, 3).

The Atharvans were so called as they were appointed to take care of the sacrificial fires : from Atharya = fire. The Persian fire-priests held similar functions as Atharvans. The fire-god of the ancient Iranians was Atar (See Rogozin's Story of Medea, pp. 130-152 ; x, 46, 2, 9.) Some declare that Bhadryāśva first kindled fire, and so he is called Agni Bhadryāśva (x, 69, 1). He is sometimes described as the son of Vala or Strength (iii, 14, 1) or his grandson (ii, 6, 2). He is also said to have been generated by Daus (x, 45, 8), by the Dawn (vii, 78, 3), by Indra and Viṣṇu (vii, 99, 4), by Tvaṣṭā (x, 2, 7), and by the gods (vi, 7, 1 ; vii, 91, 17 ; x, 46, 9) who placed him among men (i, 36, 10 ; ii, 4, 3 ; vi, 16, 1 ; vii, 7, 5 ; viii, 73, 2) as a light to the Aryan people (i, 59, 2). For his three-fold origin see Ṛv., i, 95, 3 ; iii, 26, 7 = Vāj. S, xvii, 66 ; v, 4, 8 ; vii, 39, 8 ; x, 45, 1 = Vāj. S., xii, 18 ; x, 5, 6, = S. V., 1, 65) and for twofold origin, see i, 60, 1 ; 140, 2 ; 149, 2, 3 ; ii, 9, 3 ; vii, 43, 28. Agni's three-fold birth represents " the first triality, which, philosophically, is interpreted as a trinity " (Hopkins) in later times: the sectarian trinity where Viṣṇu is the sun, and Rudra, the lightning.

Varuṇa is described as his brother (iv, 1, 2) and Indra his twin brother (vi, 59, 2). Svāhā is his wife and Uṣā, his daughter (i, 71, 5).

Agni is compared to a delightful new-born infant (i, 69, 4), which like spirits, is difficult to catch (i, 168, 2.............x, 7, 5 ; 49, 15). He consumes his parents after birth (x, 79, 4). He does not suckle her mother's breasts (x, 115, 1) but is nourished by oblations of clarified butter (iii, 21, 1, 3) which is his food (i, 7, 6 ; iii, 17, 1 ; 27, 5 ; v, 11, 3 ; 14, 6 ; vii, 3, 1 ; viii, 39, 3 ; 43, 10, 22 ; x, 69, 1, 2 ; 118, 4, 6 ; 122, 2 ; Av., i, 7, 2), his eyes (iii, 26, 7) and his hairs (viii, 49, 2). He is butter-backed (v, 4, 3 ; 37, 1 ; vii, 2, 4 ; x, 122, 4), shines with butter (iii, 18 ; v, 11, 1 ; x, 21, 7) and issues from butter (ii, 3, 11 ; v, 8, 6). He is all devouring (viii, 44, 26) and is also fed by wood (ii, 7, 6 ; vii, 3, 4 ; x, 45, 8 ; 79, 7). He swallows his food without mastication (x, 79, 1, 2).

His appearance.—He is the never-ageing (i, 27, 9 ; 53, 4 ; 143, 3 ; 144, 4 ; 146, 2, 4 ; iii, 2, 2 ; 6, 4 ; 7, 7), immortal (i, 26, 9 ; 31, 7 ; 44, 6, 11 ; 58, 1 ; 72, 6 ; 77, 1 ; ii, 10, 1, 2 ; iii, 1, 18 ; 2, 11 ; 3, 1 ; 11, 2 ; 17, 4 ; 27, 5, 7 ; iv, 11, 5 ; v, 4, 10 ; 14, 2 ; 18, 5 ; vi, 9, 4 ; vii, 4, 4 ; viii, 60, 11 ; x, 79, 1), young (vi, 7, 7), god (i, 26, 10 ; 31, 8 ; 36, 6, 15 ; 44, 4 ; 145, 3 ; 147, 2 ; 189, 2, 4 ; ii, 7, 1 ; iii, 9, 6 ; 19, 4 ; 23, 1 ; iv. 2, 10 ; 4, 6 ; 12, 4 ; v, 1, 10). He is described as having four eyes (i, 31, 13), or hundred eyes (i, 128, 3), or thousand eyes (i, 79, 12). He is long-tailed (i, 27, 1) with the banner of smoke (i, 23, 11; 44, 3; 94, 10; iii, 10, 4; 11, 3; v, 11, 3; 43, 4; 44, 10; x, 4, 5; 12, 2). His hairs are the terrible (i, 36, 10, 20) blazing (i, 45, 6; iii, 14, 1; 17, 1; 27, 4; v, 8, 2; vi, 41, 10) red flames (i, 36, 9; iii, 14, 1; 17, 1; 27, 4; v, 8, 2)—the grass-consuming sparks (i, 94, 1), with which as the forest—fire, when driven by wind, he shears the hairs of the earth (i, 58, 4, 5; 65, 4, 8; 67, 1) like a barber shaving a beard (x, 142, 4), carves the wood (i, 27, 4) and eats and chews with his sharp jaws the forests (i, 143, 5; ii, 2, 5; 4, 5, 6, which are rendered black by his tongue (i, 143, 5; vi, 41, 10; 60, 10; x, 79, 2). Agni is therefore described as the lord of forests (iii, 8, 1, 3, 6, 11). He is without head and foot (iv, 1, 11) but is sometimes represented as having a burning head (vii, 3, 1), or three heads with seven tongues and seven rays (i, 146, 1; ii, 5, 2). His face is turned everywhere (i, 97, 8). He shakes his thousand horns (i, 79, 2; 140, 6; v, 2, 9). He is gay, beautiful and blameless (i, 31, 9; 94, 7; 143, 3; 144, 7). He is formed of gold (iv, 3, 1; x, 20, 9) and he has golden beard (v, 7, 7). His teeth are sharp (i, 79, 6; 14, 3, 5; iv, 5, 4; 15, 5; viii, 19, 22), burning (i, 58, 5; vii, 23, 4 and brilliant (v, 7, 7),—the golden (v, 2, 3) and iron grinders (x, 87, 2) are set in sharp and consuming jaws (viii, 49, 13; x, 79, 1), the sharp iron (x, 87, 2) teeth (i, 79 6) set in fierce jaws (i, 36, 16; 58, 5). His two teeth (x, 87, 3), strong as iron (x, 87, 2) cut the Rakṣasas, especially the cannibals, and those who steal cow's milk (x, 187, 16).

Forms of Agni.—Agni is the altar-fire. The other fires are verily Agni's branches (i, 59, 1; vii, 1, 14; viii, 19, 33). He has hundred manifestations and shines like the sun (i, 49, 3; vii, 3, 6; 8, 4; x, 91, 4) As sun, he is the bright great splendour of dawn (i, 94, 5;

146, 4; v, 17, 3), the solar hero (ii, 2, 1). He, as moon, determines the season of the dwellers on earth (i, 95, 3). He assumes the fierce appearance which is above, *i.e.*, lightning (i, 95, 8). His triple existence is explained by his three-fold manifestations: Sun in heaven, lightning in the atmosphere and as fire on the earth (x, 88). In this hymn Sun is identified with Agni (v, 6; Yāska in Nirukta, vii, 27, 28).

The Agni in this earth has also three forms. He is caled Kravyād and is besought to burn the body of the dead in such a way as not to destroy it completely (i, 162, 20; x, 16, 4) but to send the soul to the Fathers in the world of the righteous. In x, 16, 9, 10, such a funeral Agni is spoken of as an object to be repelled. In Vāj. S., 1, 17, Agni is prayed to drive away two of his own forms: Krāvyād (=devourer of dead flesh or funeral fire) and Āmād (=devourer of raw flesh or culinary fire) and to bring Yāyā yogyaḥ or sacrificial fire. Compare also Vāj. S., xviii, 51. In Taitt. S., ii, 5, 8, 6, we have three forms of fire mentioned: Hayavāhana for Devas; Kavyavāhana for the Pitṛs (Fathers) and Saharakṣtah for the Asuras.

His power.—He is the divine monarch, strong as Indra (vii, 6, 1), the king of all treasures which dwell in the mountains, in the earth, in the herbs, in the waters, in the sky and among men (i, 59, 3; 72, 1; vii, 6, 7; 9, 3; x, 4, 1; 6, 6; 91, 3). He is the giver of wealth (i, 46, 1, 8; 127, 11), the priest (x, 110, 11; 150, 4) and the swift (x, 6, 4) messenger of the gods (i, 36, 3-5; 44, 7, 11; 72, 7; 183, 1; ii, 6, 6; iii, 3, 2; 5, 2; 6, 5; 11, 2; iv, 2, 2; 8, 1; v, 11, 4; Taitt. Br., ii, 4, 1, 6; Taitt. Sam., ii, 5, 8, the carrier of oblations (i, 36, 10; 72, 7; iii, 9, 6; 11, 2; v, 25, 4) and the law-giver of the gods (i. 31, 2, 10; 15, 3). Agni is the bond of communication between gods and men (i, 12, 1, 2, 4, 8; 27, 4; 36, 3-5; 44, 2, 3, 5, 9, 12; 58, 1; 74, 4, 7; 188, 1; ii, 6, 6, 7; 9, 2; 10, 6; iii, 6, 5; 9, 8; 11, 2; 17, 4; 21, 1, 5; iv, 1, 8; 2, 3; 7, 8; 8, 2, 4; v, 8, 6; 21, 3; vi, 15, 8-10; vii, 11, 4; 16, 4; 17, 6; viii, 19, 21; 23, 18, 19; 39, 1, 9; 44, 3; x, 4, 2; 46, 10; 91, 11; 122, 7). He is god among gods (i, 31, 9; 94, 13), bull among animals (i, 31, 5; 58, 4, 5; 79, 2; 128, 3; 140, 6, 10; 141, 2; 145, 2; ii, 1, 3; 3, 11; 9, 2; iii, 4, 3; 6, 5; 7, 6, 7; 15, 3; v, 2, 12; 12, 1). He kills many enemies in battle with a few companions (i, 31, 6). His weapons are sharp (iv, 4, 4; 5, 3). He slew the Dasyus and Rakṣasas (iii, 15, 1; vii, 13, 1; 15, 10; viii, 23, 3; 43, 26; x, 87, 1, 2, 5; 9, 14) and cut down Śambara. He defeated the Panis (vii, 6, 3; 9, 2) and drove away the Dasyus (i, 59, 2; vii, 5, 6; x, 69, 6). He killed Jarutha, bringing him out of water (x, 80, 3). Like Indra, he is also said to be the slayer of Vṛitra (iii, 20, 4) and destroyer of cities (i, 59, 6; 78, 4; vi, 16, 14, 39, 48; vii, 5, 3; 6, 1, 2; viii, 63, 4; Av., iv, 23, 5; vii, 110, 1). Agni protected Atri, Bharadvāja, Gavisṭhīra, Kaṇva and Tryasdasyu in battlefield (x, 150, 5). He is fearful like an army let loose (i, 66, 8; 142, 4; 143, 5). He roars like thunder (vii, 3, 6; viii, 91, 5; x, 45, 4), like the wind (viii, 91, 5) and like a lion (iii, 2, 11). His flames roar like the waves of the sea (i, 44, 12) and terrify the birds when he devours grasses (i, 94, 10, 11). He resounds as the Maruts and as lightning (i, 143, 5) and is the conqueror of thousands (i, 188, 1).

Divine honours.—He is said to have produced the two worlds and upheld the earth and sky (i, 67, 3, 5; iii, 5, 10) and kept them apart (i, 96, 4; iii, 5, 10; 6, 5; vi, 7, 7; 8, 2, 3; vii, 5, 4, 6). He formed the luminaries of heaven (vi, 7, 7 ; 8, 2) and placed the sun in the sky (x, 56, 4). He adorned the sky with stars (i, 68, 5, 10) and caused the sky to roar (i, 31, 4). He is said to bestow vigour (i, 166, 4) and to grow up with might within the plants, within the children and within the sprouting grass (i, 67, 9 ; 95, 10). He begot Mitra (x, 8, 4) ; and created all creatures that move (x, 88, 4). He is the head of the sky and the centre of the earth (i, 59, 2 ; vi, 7, 1 ; vii, 44, 16 ; x, 88, 5). Before him, the men tremble (ii, 8, 3 ; 9, 1= Vaj. S. xi, 36 ; vi, 7, 5 ; vii, 44, 25 ; 92, 3) and the gods fear him (vi, 9, 7). He sees all creatures (iii, 55, 10 ; x, 187, 4), knows the births of gods and men (i, 70, 1, 3 ; iii, 4, 11 ; vi, 15, 3) and the secrets of mortals (viii, 39, 6). He destroys darkness (i, 94, 7 ; 140, 1 ; x, 88, 2) as he is brilliant (i, 27, 6 ; 140, 1 ; ii, 10, 2 ; v, 2, 3 ; 26, 2 ; vi, 10, 3 ; 15, 2 ; vii, 9, 3 ; 12, 1 ; 15, 10 ; viii, 19, 2 ; 23, 20 ; 4, 3, 31).

Agni's chariot and horses.—His beautiful car (ii, 3, 9 ; iv, 2, 4) is made of gold (iv, 1, 8). As he drives his two ruddy, red, wind-driven horses called Rohita, yoked to his chariot (i, 94, 10 ; ii, 6, 5 ; 10, 2 ; iii, 6, 6) which is variegated (x, 1, 5), and luminous (i, 140, 1 ; 141, 12 ; iii, 5, 3 ; v, 1, 11 ; x, 1, 5) like lightning (iii, 14, 1), he bellows like a bull (1, 94, 10, 11). His path and wheels are marked by blackness (ii, 4, 6 ; vi, 10, 4 ; vii, 8, 2 ; viii, 23, 19). His horses are butter-backed, wind-driven and active, and assume all forms (i, 14, 6, 12 ; 45, 2 ; 94, 10 ; 141, 12 ; ii, 4, 2 ; 10, 2 ; iv, 1, 8 ; 2, 2, 4 ; 6, 9 ; vi, 16, 43 ; vii, 16, 2 ; viii, 43, 16 ; x, 7, 4 ; 70, 2), His horses are said to have seven tongues (iii, 6, 2). He comes, seated in his car (iii, 4, 11 ; vii, 11, 1 ; x, 70, 2), to the sacrificial altar alone (x, 70, 2) or in company with other gods (i, 14, 12 ; iii, 6, 6, 9 ; viii, 64, 1).

Agni and his votaries.—Agni has taken up his abode among men as their guest or Atithi (i, 44, 4; 58, 6; ii, 4, 1; iii, 2, 2; iv, 1, 20; v, 1, 8; 8, 2; 18, 1; vi, 2, 7; 15, 1, 4; vii, 8, 4; viii, 73, 1; x, 10, 5; 91, 2; 92, 1). He is the lord, protector and leader of the people (i, 12, 2; 26, 7; 31, 11; 96, 4; ii, 1, 8; iii, 11, 5). He is their father, mother, brother, son and friend (i, 26, 3; 31, 10; 14, 16; 75, 4; 161, 1; ii, 1, 9; vi, 1, 5; v, 4, 2; viii, 43, 16; 64, 16; x, 7, 3). He is guardian and father, even of the weak (i, 31, 14) and accepts hymns even of the poor (i, 31, 13). He supports men (i, 59, 1 iv, 5, 1) and has 'grouped men in dwelling places' (iii, 1 17). He is their house-priest. He is called "Gṛhapati" or master of the house (i, 12, 6; 36, 5; 60, 4; v, 8, 2 vii, 15, 2), "Viṣpati" or lord of men and rājā or king of men (i, 59, 5; ii, 1, 8; iii, 10, 1; v, 4, 1; vi, 7, 1; vii, 8, 1; viii, 43, 24).

His worshippers turn to him (x, 91, 3) with glad hearts (viii, 43, 31). They prosper and live long (vi, 2, 4, 5; 5, 5; 10, 3; 13, 4; 15, 11; vii, 11, 2; viii, 19, 5, 6; 44, 15; 73, 9). He is protector and friend of the man who serves him (iv, 2, 6; 4, 10; x, 79, 5). He gives him riches (i, 1, 3; 31, 10; 36, 4) and abundant food (i, 27, 7) and makes him unconquerable (viii, 23, 15) in battle. He preserves men from calamities (iii, 20, 4; v, 4, 9; vii, 12, 2). He is the source of all blessings (vi, 13, 1) and is like water in a desert (x, 4, 1). He satisfies his votaries with riches, food, deliverance, sons, etc. (i, 12, 8, 9; 36, 12; 58, 8, 9; ii, 4, 8; 7, 2, 3; 9, 5; iii, 1, 21; 16, 5; iv, 2, 20; 3, 14; 11, 6; v, 3, 11; vi, 1, 12; 4, 8; 5, 7; 6, 7; vii, 5, 13, 19). His worshippers prayed for his protection inside a house having hundred iron walls (i, 189, 2; vi, 48, 8; vii, 3, 7; 15, 14; 16, 10) and forgiveness for folly against Aditi (iv, 12, 4; vii, 93, 7) and Varuṇa (iv, 1, 4).

In vii, 19, 25 and 44, 23, his worshippers assured Agni of every help if they mutually changed their places. ‘Let us be united with thy favour which bestows strength’ is the prayer of the Seers (i, 31, 8) whose invocations the god hears (viii, 143, 23).

He is prayed to strike down the malevolent, the enemy of his worshippers (iv, 4, 4 ; vi, 8, 5 ; Av., iii, 1, 1 ; 2, 1 ; vi, 120, 1) in battle (vii, 43, 21 ; 73, 8 ; viii, 11, 8, 9). He saved Jaratkarṇa (x. 80, 2) and Atri when he fell in a hot well (x, 80, 2).

Agni as a physician.—In the following hymns we find references to the skill of Agni as a physician who cured diseases. In Ṛv., i, 12, 7, Agni is said to be the god who drives away diseases. Agni saved Dīrghatamās, the blind son of Mamatā from distress (i, 141, 3 ; iv, 4, 13 ; MBH. I, 4179 *seq.*, ed. Calc. ; Geldner, Vedische Studien, ii, 145). He is prayed to prolong life (i, 94, 16 ; iv, 12, 6) and he lengthened Praskanva's life that he may reach old age (i, 44, 6). In i, 189, 3, the poet prays : "Agni ! Drive away from us all plagues ;" and in i, 94, 15, he is prayed to grant sinlessness in health and wealth. In Ṛv., vii, 50, 2, Agni is prayed to remedy the poison Vandana which forms at the nodes of trees, and which causes swelling of knees and ankles. Agni is invoked to bestow a renowned son (v, 25, 5). In i, 71, 10, he is prayed to prevent old age. In Av., v, 28, 1 : Agni is thus invoked : "Thou art a physician (bhiṣaj), a maker of remedy (bheṣaja) ; by thee may we gain cow, horse, man (purūṣa)"—Whitney. In 29, 13 : we find a prayer : "Make him, O Agni, exuberant, sacrificial (medhya), free from Yakṣmā ; let him live." In 30, 14 : "With breath, O Agni, with sight unite him ; associate him with body, with strength ; thou understandest immortality (amṛta), let him not now go." The purifying property of Agni is hinted at vi, 62: "Let Vaisvānara (Agni) by his rays purify us, the wind, lively with mists by his breath" (1.) "Take ye hold upon that (f) of Vaisvānara in order to splendour, becoming cleansed, clear and purifying." In Ṛv., iv, 12, 4, fire is said to purify as water purifies a man from dirt and sin. Agni is invoked for relief from insanity (vi, 111) and to put out snake's poison (x, 4, 26).

In vii, 1, 7, Agni is said to cure diseases by reducing high temperature. In vii, 1, 20, 22, he is prayed to purify our food. Prayers are offered to Agni to give his votaries productive virility (vii, 2, 9). He causes the women to deliver many heroic sons (x, 80, 1). Through his kindness Ṛṣi Numedha got a son (x, 80, 3).

In the Mahabhārata Agni is said to have cured indigestion of the gods and the Fathers, caused by eating excessive rice-offerings in Srāddha (Ânuśāsanika Parvādhyāya, Ch. 92).

His character.—He is pure; he is truthful (i, 73, 2; 76, 5; vii, 7, 6). He is kind to his friends; and is always accessible to the poor. He is the upholder of religious order. He lights the earth, gives life and supports men. His deep sympathy for mortals at once destined him to surpass other gods and to become the popular god of the Vedic Hindus.

Agni is also invoked with other gods: especially with Indra as Indrāgni (i, 21; 108; 109; iii, 12, 25, 4; v, 27, 6; 86; vi, 59; 60; vii, 93; 94). They are both described as thunderers, slayers of Vṛttra (viii, 38, 4; i, 108, 3; Bergaigne ii, 295; viii, 8, 9) and shaker of cities (iii, 12, 4, 6; vi, 59, 3; 60, 3; vii, 93, 1-4; viii, 38, 2). In vii, 94, 7, they are prayed for help. They are called "Aśvina" or horse-men (i, 109, 4), the two "ṛtvija" or priests (viii, 38, 1), Indrās or the two Indras and the two Agnis (vi, 60, 1). They are correlative deities and are conceived as one joint deity like the two Asvins.

Agni and Soma : i, 93.

Agni and Maruts : viii, 103.

Agni and Sun : x, 88.

Agni, Sun and Vayu : x, 136.

In the Ṛg-veda the following hymn's are addressed to Agni :—

i, 1 ; 2 ; 13 ; 26 ; 27 ; 31 ; 36 ; 44 ; 45 ; 58-60 ; 65-79 ; 94-99 ; 127 ; 128 ; 140-150 ; 188 ; 189.

ii, 1-10.

iii, 1-29.

iv, 1-15.

v, 1-28.

vi, 1-16 ; 48, 1-10 ; 59 ; 60.

vii. 1-17 ; 50, 3 ; 93 ; 94 ; 104, 10.

viii, 11 ; 19 (except 26, 27, 34, 35) ; 23 ; 38 ; 39 ; 40 ; 43 ; 44 ; 56 ; 58 ; 60 ; 72 ; 75 ; 84 ; 102 ; 103.

x, 1-8 ; 11, 12 ; 15, 11-14 ; 16 ; 20 ; 45 ; 46 ; 53 ; 69 ; 79 ; 80 ; 87 ; 88 ; 91 ; 110 ; 115 ; 118 ; 122 ; 124 ; 125 ; 140 ; 142 ; 150 ; 156 ; 187 ; 188 ; 191, 1.

In a hymn to Agni, in the Mārkaṇḍeya Purāṇa, Sect. 99, vv. 52 ff, the seven tongues of Agni are thus described : (1) Kāli, the final destroyer, (2) Karālī, the cause of the great mundane dissolution, (3) Monojavā, the quality of lightness, (4) Sulohitā, accomplisher of the desire of creatures, (5) Sudhūmravarṇā, the inflictor of diseases on living beings, (6) Sphuliṅgini, the loveliest of all, 7. Viśvā, bestower of blessings on living beings. The seven shafts of Agni are also referred to in the 17th verse of this hymn.

In the Munḍuk Upaniṣad i, 2, 4, the seven flickering tongues of the fire are mentioned : Kālī (the black one),

Karālī (the terrific), Manojava (swift as mind), Sulohitā (the red one), Sudhūmravarṇā (of purple colour), Sphuliṅgini (emitting sparks) and Viśvarūpi (all-shaped). Of these names, Kālī and Karālī are well known to us as the names of Siva's consorts.

In the Gṛhya Saṁgraha, (pp. 782-3), the seven tongues and their functions are described :

1.	Karālī	for eating	Rākṣasas
2.	Dhūmini	,, ,,	Asuras
3.	Svetā	,, ,,	Nāgas
4.	Lohitā	,, ,,	Piśācas
5.	Maha Lolitā	,, ,,	Gandharvas
6.	Suparnā	,, ,,	Yama
7.	Padmarāga	,, ,,	Devas

VĀTA AND VĀYU

The Vāta or Vāyu is the wind-god in the Vedas. He is often invoked with Indra (i, 2, 4; 14, 3; 23, 2; 135, 4). The three daily Soma oblations are made chiefly to Indra and Vāyu. There is some difference between Vāta and Vāyu: Vāta is the wind, and Vāyu is the wind-god. A similar differentiation also occurs in the case of the Sūrya, Sun and Savitā, Sun-girl. The Vāta is the same as the Scandinavian Woden. This deity, as it was known to the Iranians and Teutons, must be one of the primitive gods of the Aryans. The Greek and Latin names, Pan and Pavonius correspond to the Sanskrit word Pavana, another name of Vāyu. Vāyu is one of the god in the Zend Avesta, where he is prayed for by Thrataon (Sanskrit Traitan) for conquering Ajidathak (Ahi, Dahak in Sanskrit). —*Zend Avesta.. Ram Yast* 7. Vāyu is the power or god at the back of the Vāta or wind. The Vāyu is the loftier spiritual conception of Vāta. But the terms used to describe Vāyu are also applied in reference to Vāta, the physical prototype of Vāyu. In i, 142, 12, Vāyu refers to the god, while in V, 19, 5, it represents the wind.

Vāyu is said to have sprung from the breath of Purūṣa (x, 90,13) He is also described to have been generated by the two worlds (vii, 90, 13). The Vāyus are said to be the sons of Rudra (x, 93, 7). He is the son-in-law of Tvaṣṭā (viii, 26, 21, 22). He begets the storm-gods Maruts, (i, 24, 4) from the rivers of heaven. He is attended by Puṣān, Maruts and the Viśva-devas (i, 142, 12).

Most of the hymns simply invite Vāyu and Indra to come to sacrifice on the same chariot (iv. 46, 2; 48, 2; viii, 91, 5). Vāyu alone, or with Indra gets the first drink of the Soma juice (i, 134, 1; 135, 1, 4; 139, 1; ii, 41, 3; iv, 46, 1, 2; 47, 2; v, 43, 3; 51, 4, 6; vii, 90, 5; 91, 4; 92, 2; viii, 8, 26; 26, 23; x, 65, 9; 141, 4). Indra and Vāyu are popular gods. The spiritual exaltation of these gods over the material phenomena is characteristic of the atmospheric and earthly gods. They are invoked together to come quickly to the sacrifice (i, 2, 5, 6) and to drink Soma there (i, 2, 4).

According to Yāska (Nirukta, vii, 5), Agni is the representative of terrestrial gods; Sūrya, of celestial gods; and Indra and Vāyu, of the gods of aerial or intermediate sphere. They had different names according to their functions as Hotā, Adhvaryū, Brahma and Udgātā. In v, 41, 4, the Vedic triad is Fire, Wind, and Indra; (Trita of the sky) and in x, 158. ff. Sun, Wind and Fire form the triad (x, 136).

He is beautiful in appearance (i, 2, 1; vii, 26, 24). He rushes noisily (x, 100, 2). He is described to be swift, wise, and thousand-eyed; and with Indra he is spoken of as touching the sky (i, 23, 2, 3).

His shining car which touches the sky is made of gold (iv, 46, 3, 4). It is drawn by a pair of red or purple horses (i, 134, 3) or by several team of ninety-nine, or hundred, or thousand Niyuta horses (i, 134, 1; 135, 1, 3, 4; iv, 46, 2, 3; 47, 1; 48, 2, 4, 5; ii, 41, 1; vii, 91, 5; 92, 1, 5).

In the family books, the three complete hymns to Wind do not occur, and Indra is always associated with Vāyu in all the hymns (vii, 90-92; iv, 47-48). Similar association also occurs in i, 2, 4, 6; v. 51, 4, 6, 7, 10. In vi, 51, 12, he is associated with Soma.

HYMNS TO VĀYU.

Ṛv., i, 2, 1 : Come, O Vāyu, worthy of sight! and drink Soma juice.

2 : The priests have prepared Soma and are praying for you.

3 : Your words describing the properties of Soma juice go to the worshippers.

4 : O Indra and Vāyu! Come hither. Drops of Soma juice want you.

5 : You know Soma juice. Come soon.

6 : O ye two men! Come near to Soma.

134, 1 : Let the swift Niyuta horses bring you on your car first among the gods to drink Soma. May you approve our hymns.

2 : May the delightful well-made Soma drops please you. Your Nijuta horses are bringing you to the altar. Your votaries are expressing their wishes before you.

3 : Vāyu yokes two red horses to his chariot. As a lover awakes his sleeping sweetheart, you awaken your votaries. You display heaven and earth and brighten Uṣā.

4 : For you the bright Uṣā spread out beautiful garments in their new rays. To you cow pours out her riches. You have brought Maruts from heaven.

5 : From you the Soma rushed to waters. You protect men from fear of evil spirits and robbers.

6 : O Vāyu, you are worthy to drink Soma first. The cows pour out butter and milk for you.

135, 1 : O Vāyu, come on your thousand Niyuta horses and drink Soma. The gods are waiting for you.

2 : The Soma juice, purified and stimulating, men offer you; yoke your horses and go away, being delighted with us.

3 : The priests have prepared pure Soma, which is your due. Come to our sacrifice on your horses.

4 : You two, O Vāyu and Indra, come here with riches and drink Soma.

5 : You are giver of food; you come to drink Soma.

6 : This Soma, purified through a sieve, is for you.

7 : You both go to the house where Soma is being prepared, hymns are chanted, and *ghee* is flowing.

8 : You accept the oblations in this sacrifice. Cows are giving milk. May they not be weak and destroyed.

9 : The young, strong and swift horses are carrying you. It is difficult to stop their motion.

164, 44 : Three hairy beings annually inspect this earth in proper time. One shaves the earth (Agni); a second, acts as her overseer (Sun); and the third, is seen by his motion, his form is never seen (Vāyu).

iv, 46, 1	: Do you drink soma in this sacrifice as you are the first drinker.
2 to 7	: Hymns to Indra and Vāyu.
47	: " " "
48, 1	: Come here on your chariot to drink Soma.
2	: Indra is your charioteer, come to drink Soma.
3	: The Earth and Heaven follow you, come, etc.
4	: May ninety-nine swift horses carry you, come, etc.
5	: Harness hundred or thousand horses to the chariot.
v, 51, 4-7, 10	: Hymns to Indra and Vāyu.
12	: Hymns to Vāyu and Soma

HYMNS TO VĀTA.

Ṛv., i, 186, 10	: Vāta, like Viṣṇu, is free from malice.
viii, 26, 20	: Harness your two horses and then come here to drink Soma.
21	: O Vāyu, the son-in-law of Tvaṣṭā, the lord of sacrifice, may we be maintained by you.
22	: I pray Vāyu, the son-in-law of Tvaṣṭā, for riches.
23	: You bear the goodness of Heaven. Harness the horse to your chariot.
24	: You are beautiful. I pray you to come here

25 : Yon are the chief among the gods; may you graut us food, water and work.

46, 25 : You are giver of riches and strength, I pray you.

26 : Drinker of shining and purified Soma.

27 : You, Pṛthuśravā, wished to give me riches and so ordered your managers Aradva, Akṣa, Nahuṣa, and Sukṛtta.

28 : The pure King, greater than Ucatya and Vapu, has sent us food on the back of horse, camel and dog, through your kindness.

32 : I am a Brahman, I am keeper of of cows and horses. I take a hundred from the slave Valvatha. These creatures belong to you.

101, 9 : You come to our sacrifice. The white Soma in the sieve is for you.

10 : O Vāyu with Niyuta horses, the Adhvaryu is carrying butter and Soma for you.

x, 136, 2 : The Munis of Vātaraśana family became gods and followed Vāta.

3 : We are mad after religious austerities; we raise ourselves upon Vāta. The men see our bodies only.

5 : The Muni is like a horse of Vāta, a companion of Vāyu. He is liked by the Devas.

7 : When Keśī drinks water with Rudra, Vāyu moves the water and breaks the hard snow-balls.

137, 2 : The two Vātas blow even beyond the seas. Let one come to make you strong and let the other flow to destroy your sins.

3 : O Vāta, blow medicine towards this side. What is harmful take away hence. You are medicine in this world You are messenger of the gods.

x, 141, 4 : It is a pleasure to invoke Indra, Vāta and Vṛhaspati ; may they be pleased to grant us riches.

5 : Excite Vāta, Viṣṇu, Indra to generosity.

168, 1 : The chariot of Vāta goes thundering through the sky creating redness, or scattering the dust of the earth.

2 : The gusts of wind go towards the god who accompanies them on the same chariot as the king

3 : He never rests when he moves in the sky. He is friend of waters and is the first-born. Where was he born ?

4 : He is the breath of the gods, the germ of the world. His roars are heard, but his form is not seen. Let us worship him.

186 : 1 : The Vāta wafts as a medicine. May he be propitious and delightful.

2 : You are our father, brother, and friend. Do thou allow us to live!

3 : From the treasure of immortality which is in your house, give us immortality, give us life.

Śat. Br., xi, 2, 3, 1 : Brahma placed Vāyu in the atmesphere.

vi, 1, 2, 1 : Prajāpati connected himself as Agni with the Earth ; from this union sprang an egg, and thence Vāyu ; next through Vāyu he united himself with the Air (Antarikṣa, neuter), and again an egg was produced, and thence Āditya (Sun)—Muir.

Nirukta, vii, 5 : There are only three deities : Agni on earth, Vāyu or Indra in the atmosphere, and Sūrya in the sky. They receive many appellations according to their functions.

Authorship : Vāyu is not known as the author of any medical book. He is said to have narrated the Vāyu Purāṇa consisting 24,000 ślokat :

श्वेतकल्पप्रसङ्गेन धर्म्मान वायुरिहाब्रवीत्।
यत्रैतद्वायवीयं स्याद्रुद्रमाहात्म्यसंयुतम् ॥
चतुर्व्विंशं सहस्राणि पुराणं तदिहोच्यते।

He is also the speaker in the Śiva Purāṇa, which is also said, according to the Bhāgavat Purāṇa, to consist of 24,000 ślokas.

CHAPTER VI.

VṚHAṢPATI.

Vṛhaṣpati is the same god as Brāhmanaṣpati, the lord of Brahma or prayer (i, 40, 5; ii, 23, 1, 2; x, 98, 7). Hillebrandt identifies them with Moon; and Muller, with 'Agni' or Fire as Vṛhaspati is red and golden, and considers the two gods as varieties of Agni. Roth considers them as "Lord of Prayer" or as "impersonation of the power of devotion" as Muir puts it. Hopkins supports Roth with the modification "as the priestly abstraction of Indra," or as a "sacerdotal Indra." Weber holds the same view (Vājpeya Sacrifice, p. 15). Langlois considers Vṛhaṣpati and Brahmanaṣpati as names of Agni (Trans. of Rv., Vol. I, pp. 249, 254, 578, notes, and Index, Vol. IV). Wilson also identifies Brahmanaṣpati with Agni (Intro. Trans. Ṛv., Vol. I, p. xxxvii; ii, 1, 3, 2; iii, 26, 2; v, 43, 12), and Vṛhaṣpati with Indra (Intro., Vol. II, p. ix) as he sends rain and recovers cows, etc. (see also II, 30, 4). Sometimes he is looked upon as a minor god (Ṛv., i, 190).

His parentage.—Vṛhaṣpati is known to us as an ancient Ṛṣi or sage, the son of Aṅgirasa (iv, 40, 1; vi, 73, 1; x, 47, 6; 68, 2) and the preceptor of the Devas. He is the younger brother of Utathya. He is also said to be the offspring of the two worlds (vii, 97, 8), and the son of Tvaṣṭṛ (ii, 23, 17). He composed hymns in the Vedas (Ṛv, 71; 72). "Another Vṛhaṣpati is known as the author of a "Dharmaśāṣtra" or "Law Book" and the founder of the Vārhaṣpatya School (4th century B.C.). There was also an author of some minor "Jyotiṣa" or "Astronomical Tracts"; and other obscure authors of that name are also known. See Aufrecht's Catalogus Catalogorum."

There is no Vṛhaspati known to us as the author of any medical text book, though in the Bower MS. the following formula is distinctly ascribed to him :—

निर्मुसल चक्रहलशब्दाभिहतायाम् भूमौ जातमाश्वगन्धाम् समुलपत्रपुष्पम् सूक्ष्म-चूर्णाणि कुर्य्यात्। ततः सर्पिषा विड़ाल पादकमाहृत्याहनि लेहयेत् पयश्चानुपिवेत् जोर्नान्ते पयसा भोजनमाश्नीयात्॥ एवं एकविंशतिरात्रं बलवान्वृऽच्छवीरश्च भवत्याह वृहष्पतिरिति। वार्हष्पत्यम् वृहत्करणम्।

A Prescription of Vṛhaspati for Promoting Bulkiness[1] :—

" Take Aśvagandhā wine (*Withania Somnifera*) with its roots, leaves and flowers, grown in ground undisturbed by the sound of ploughs, or the din of *battles faught with* clubs and discusses and make it into fine powder. Of this, one may take a Viḍālpada, every day, as a linctus with clarified butter, and follow it up with a drink of milk. When it is digested, one should eat one's food with milk. By *continuing this treatment* for a period of twenty-one nights (or three weeks) *a person* will become strong and stout : so says Vṛhaspati."

In Cakra Datta, Sureśvara Ghṛta is ascribed to Jīvaka ; and by Jīvaka, Śivadāsa, the commentator, means Vṛhaspati, (जीवो वृहस्पति स्वार्थेकः). Jīva is no doubt a synonym of Vṛhaspati, but it seems, however, to be a far-fetched explanation. It really refers to Jīvaka, the well-known Buddhist physician who flourished when the Venerable One preached.

The medical skill of Vṛhaspati, however, is referred to in unmistakable language in the Rāmāyana, Yuddhakāṇḍa, Ch. 50. There Suṣena is reported to have said :

तदा स्म दानवा देवान् शरसंस्पर्शकोविदान्।
निजघ्नुः शस्त्रविदुषश्छादयन्तो मुहुर्मुहुः॥

[1] Bower, MS., p. 149. Prose, 781-785.

तान्नार्त्तान्नष्टसंज्ञांश्च गतासूंश्च वृहष्पतिः ।
विद्याभिर्म्मन्त्रयुक्ताभिरोषधीभिश्चिकित्सति ॥
तान्यौषधान्यानयितुं चीरोदं यान्तु सागरम् ।
जवेन वानराः शीघ्रं सम्पातिपनसादयः ॥
हरयस्तु विजानन्ति पार्व्वती ते महौषधी ।
सञ्जीवकरणीं दिव्यां विशल्यां देवनिर्म्मिताम् ॥
चन्द्रश्च नाम्ना द्रोणश्च चीरोदे सागरोत्तमे ।
अमृतं यत्र मथितं तत्र ते परमौषधी ॥
तौ तत्र विहितौ देवैः पर्व्वतौ तु महोदधौ ।
अयं वायुसुतो राजन् हनूमांस्तत्र गच्छतु ॥

Relationship with other gods.—He is said to be the father of the gods (ii, 26, 3) and to have 'blown forth the births of gods like a blacksmith' (x, 72, 2). With Indra he lead armies in battle. Vṛhaṣpati and Brāhmanṣpati are the names of the same god ; and as such they have been identified with Agni. But Agni is mentioned separately from both these gods in Ṛv., iii, 20, 5 ; iv, 40, 1 ; v, 51, 12 ff ; vii, 10, 4 ; 44, 1 ; ix, 5, 11 ; x, 35, 11 ; 65, 1 ; 68, 9 ; 130, 4 ; 141, 3.

His acts.—To Vṛhaṣpati, 'the lord of strength,' are attributed many deeds of Indra. He breaks the cloud-demon's power with sharp bolt, releases the imprisoned waters of the sky, and so pours water to fertilise the earth ; dispels darkness (x, 68, 5) ; breaks through the caves of, and destroys, Vala, and rescues and carries off the well-formed heavenly kine with milk (x, 68, 3) from the mountains (x, 68, 3, 4), gives offsprings and riches to worshippers, and helps them in battle (vii, 13, 2) ; discovers Uṣā or Dawn and Agni ; and keeps a band of singers like Maruts. He rescued Trita from a well (i, 105, 17), killed Samvara (ii, 24, 2), composed many Ṛks before, and now resides in clouds (x, 68, 12). He is the prototype of the priestly order and is the Purohita of the gods (x, 11, 1, 3).

Relation with the worshippers.—He protects the pious from calamities (ii, 23, 4, 5) and blesses them with wealth and prosperity (*Ibid*, 9 *f*).

His attributes.—He is divine (iii, 62, 4; iv, 50, 6), bright (iii, 62, 5; viii, 97, 7), pure (vii, 97, 7) and omniform (iii, 62, 6). He has hundred wings (vii, 97, 7). He is clear-voiced (vii, 97, 5), opulent and increaser of nutriment (i, 8, 2).

His arms.—He carries a golden spear (vii, 97, 7), has his bow and arrow (ii, 24, 8) and is deseribed as armed with an iron axe which Tvaṣṭṛ sharpens (x, 53, 9). Swift ruddy horses are said to carry him (vii, 97, 6).

His sons.—Bharadvāja was his son. So were Kaca and Saṁyu Ṛṣi who composed many hymns in the Ṛgveda (vi, 44; 45; 48).

In the Ṛgveda the following hymns are addressed to Vṛhaṣpati and Brāhmanaṣpati:

i, 18, 1: Prayer to Brahmanaṣpati to make the worshippers famous like Kakṣivān, the son of Uśija.

2: He is opulent, remover of disease, bounteous, and increaser of nutriment.

3: May you protect us from blasphemy of men.

4: The men whom Indra, Brahmanaṣpati and Soma favour, can never be destroyed.

5: May you, Soma, Indra, and Dakṣiṇā, protect men from sin.

6 : I have prayed for intelligence from Agni (Sadasampati).

7 : He exists in association of our thoughts.

8 : He performs ceremonies successfully and through him our hymns reach the gods.

9 : I have seen the powerful and famous Narasāṁsa.

40, 1 : Rise Brahmanaṣpati, we pray you. O Indra, drink Soma juice with him.

2 : O Son of Strength! Men pray you for riches.

3 : May Brahmanaṣpati, goddess Sunṛti come here. May gods drive away our enemies.

4 : We shall pray Ilā for the man who pays riches to Ṛtvija.

5 : Brahmanaṣpati has uttered a hymn in praise of Indra, Varuṇa, Mitra and other gods.

6 : May we utter it on the festivals.

90, 9 : May Vṛhaṣpati be a source of happiness for us.

190, 1 : I magnify Vṛhaṣpati, the sweet-tongued, the leader of songs.

2 : To him proceed well-ordered words. He is born for ceremonies.

3 : He tries to secure prayers from, and rice and gifts for the worshippers.

4 : He makes all living beings conscious. His arms go towards the enemies.

5 : The sinners who compare Vṛhaṣpati to a decrepit bull must not be given riches.

6 : You are friend of pious worshippers and kings.

7 : All hymns meet with you.

8 : The great Vṛhaṣpati is born for the good of many men. If we pray, he will grant us food, strength and long life.

ii, 23, 1 : Brahmanaṣpati, renowned of sages, monarch of prayers, help us.

2 : Vṛhaṣpati, the generator of all prayers.

3 : He overcomes demons and darkness.

4 : Preserves men from the enemy of devotion.

5 : Preserves them from calamity.

6 : Homage to the wise Vṛhaṣpati, our protector and guide.

7 : Turn away mortals who are hostile to us.

8 : As protector of our bodies, destroy the revilers of gods.

9 : May we acquire riches. Crush our foes.

10 : May we obtain the highest vigour.

11 : You are a real avenger of guilt and subduer of foes in battle.

12 : Preserve us from the shaft of the malicious man.

13 : You are to be invoked in battles and to be worshipped with reverence, you have overturned our enemies.

14 : With your sharp burning bolt, destroy the Rakṣasas.

15 : Prayer for wealth.

16 : Prayer for protection from robbers.

17 : Tvaṣṭṛ generated you, the upholder of ceremonials.

18 : You, Aṅgirasa, opened the cow-pen; with Indra's help, you let loose the stream of water.

19 : May we, blessed with strong men, speak with power at the festivals.

4, 1 : We worship you with a new song. Fulfil our desires.

2 : Brahmanaspati has split open the clouds and the mountains full of riches.

3 : By prayer he split Vala, dispelled darkness and revealed the sky.

4 : He split open the stone-covered fountain of sweet water, which, having been drunk by the rays of the sun, reappears as rain-drops.

5 : He has opened the gates of rain for all time for the worshippers.

6 : The learned Aṅgiras found out the Panis hidden in a fort.

7 : They hurled fire against the mountain.

8: Brahmanaṣpati with his bow and arrows gets his desired objects. Those arrows (*mantra*) are to be seen and heard.

9: He is the priest. All men adore him.

10: His riches are scattered every where and are accessible to all.

11: He protects all men. The bounteous god is the representative of all the gods.

12: O Indra and Brahmanaṣpati, you are opulent. Come to our sacrifices.

13: His swift horses are hearing our hymns as sung by our priests.

14: He rescued the cows.

15: You are the lord over all. May our heroic sons be father of sons

16: You are the lord of this world. May we thus magnify you with our sons and grandsons.

25, 1: The friend of Brahmanaṣp[illegible] lives beyond the age of his grandson.

2: He is famous for the cows. The progeny of his friend become rich.

3: His votary conquers his enemy.

4: His friend gets heavenly water and cows, and conquers his foes by force.

5: His friend becomes happy.

26 : 1 : May his worshipper kill his foes.

2 : O hero, you pray Brahmanaṣpati and start for war against your enemies.

3 : The votary who serves Brahmanaṣpati, the father of the gods, gets food and riches for himself and his sons.

4 : The god rescues his votary from sins, enemy and poverty.

30, 4 : Vṛhaṣpati and Indra are identified and prayed to kill Asura's sons.

9 : Prayer to king Vṛhaṣpati to kill the hidden foes by the thunderbolt.

iii, 62, 4 : May Vṛhaṣpati, the benefactor of the Devas, give us riches.

5 : Worship the pure Vṛhaṣpati with prayers.

6 : I pray him to fulfil my desire.

iv, 49, 1 : I throw Soma on your mouth, O Indra and Vṛhaṣpati.

2 : Soma is given for your drink and pleasure.

3 : Come ye to our house to drink Soma.

4 : Give us riches consisting of a hundred cows and a thousand horses.

5 : We are inviting you to drink Soma.

6 : You drink Soma and be pleased to live in our house.

v, 42, 7 : Pray Vṛhaṣpati the giver of riches ; he makes the worshippers happy.

8 : When you protect men, their enemies become powerless ; and they get riches and sons. May the giver of horse, cow and cloth get riches.

9 : May those, who enjoy happiness but do not make others happy and observe ceremonies, be deprived of the Sun.

43, 12 : Worship the wise, butter-backed, mighty, golden-hued, ruddy god who shines in our house.

v, 50, 1 : The ancient sages placed the pleasant-tongued Vṛhaṣpati in front. He occupies three abodes and holds apart the ends of the world.

2 : You protect the sacrifices of your votaries.

3 : Around you, pravers and Soma are offered.

4 : When first born in the sky, he had seven mouths and he dispelled darkness.

5 : He killed Vala and rescued the cows.

6 : We shall worship our father Vṛhaṣpati. May we be rich and heroic with noble sons.

7 : The king who prays him conquers his enemy.

8 : The king, to whom Brahmanaspati goes first, finds his subjects obedient.

9 : The king who gives riches to Brahmanaspati gets riches from his enemies and subjects.

10 : O Vṛhaspati and Indra, drink Soma and give us riches with progeny.

11 : O gods, ye help us with your kindness. Protect our sacrifice and fight with our enemies.

vi, 45. 31 : Vṛbu sat on the high banks of Gaṅgā among the Panis.

32 : I crave for riches. He gave me thausand cows.

33 : We always magnify Vṛbu.

47, 20 : O Vṛhaspati, guide us in our search for cows.

73, 1 : Vṛhaspati, the breaker of mountain, the first-born, the truthful, Aṅgira, our father, thunders as he rains.

2 : He kills Vṛtra and enemies.

3 : He has secured riches and cows, and has killed the enemy of heaven.

75, 17 : May Brahmanaspati and Aditi make us happy in the battlefield where arrows are falling.

vii, 97, 10 : Vṛhaspati and Indra are the lords of earthly and heavenly riches. May both of you bestow riches on the worshippers.

2 : May we prove innocent before Vṛhaṣpati, the giver of riches.

3 : I magnify Brahmanaṣpati, the eldest of the gods. May the ślokas worship the great king Indra.

4 : May Brahmanaṣpati the adorable, come here.

5 : We shall worship Vṛhaṣpati, with his pure hymns.

6 : May the bright horses bear Vṛhaṣpati.

7 : Vṛhaspati is pure, sweet-tongued and is the giver of food.

8 : He is the son of Earth and Heaven; magnify him. He has made water fluid.

9 : For Brahmanaṣpati and Indra we offer this prayer. Kill the army of our foe.

VII, 98, 7 : Same as above.

X. 67, 3 : Vṛhaspati opened the door of stone. The imprisoned cows loudly bellowed.

4 : He opened three doors of the cave, one below and two above, and rescued the cows.

5 : During night he broke the cave and opened the three doors, and saw the sun and the cows in the morning.

6 : Indra killed Vala by his shouts. He rescued cows from Pani,

7 : He killed Vala, and Brahmanaṣpati took possession of the cows.

8 : They thanked the god presiding over cows. Vṛhaspati brought out the cows.

9 : Let us magnify Vṛhaṣpati when he comes to the sacrifice.

10 : When Vṛhaṣpati gave various foods, the intelligent magnified him.

11 : May my prayer for food be granted; I am your votary; give me shelter and kill my foes.

68, 1 : Prayers were offered to Vṛhaṣpati.

2 : He, the son of Angirā, brought our cows to light.

3 : He brought forth cows from mountain.

4 : He drove away cows which broke the surface of earth.

5 : Dispelled darkness and drove forth cows from Vala.

6 : He clove the defences of Vala and revealed the cows.

7 : He drove out the cows from the mountain.

8 : He found out sweet water covered by rocks.

9 : He discovered the Dawn, the Sky and Agni; dispelled darkness, and killed bull-shaped Vala.

10 : He seized all the cows. The Sun and the Moon again appeared.

11 : The father-like Devas formed the starry heaven and ordained darkness for night and light for day. Vṛhaspati rescued the cows by breaking the mountain.

12 : He composed many hymns. He now resides in heaven. May he grant as cows, horses, servants and food. We salute him.

98, 1 : O Vṛhaṣpati ! For us you go to each god. Whether you be Mitra, or Varuṇa, or Puṣā, or Ādityas, or Indra with the Vasus, you pour rain for Sāntānu.

2 : O Vṛhaspati come to us as messenger from Devāpi.

3 : May we compose a bright hymn for you, so that rains may fall on earth.

4 : Vṛhaspati gave Devāpi a hymn for causing rain.

100, 5 : Vṛhaṣpati is the giver of life.

108, 6 : O Panis ! Vṛhaspati may inflict pain on you.

11 : Vṛhaṣpati, Soma, have found out the hiding place of the cows.

109 : Vṛhaspati divorced his wife Juhu, but being told by the gods and kings that she was a chaste lady, he took her as wife again.

141, 2 :
3 :
4 :
5 : —Vṛhaspati and Brahmanaṣpati are mentioned.

155, 2 : O spirited Brahmanaṣpati ! come here after driving away Alakṣī (misfortune).

164, 4 : O Indra, O Brahmanaṣpati ! may you protect us from sins committed by us.

182, 1 : O Vṛhaṣpati ! destroy our sins, cure the diseases of the worshipper and prevent his fear.

2 : May Narasāṁsa protect us.

3 : May Vṛhaṣpati cause death of the envious Rākṣasas.

In the Atharva Veda we find references to Vṛhaspati as a god of medicine :

Av. v, 25, 11 : Thine embryos let god Vṛhaṣpati place, etc.

v, 26, 12 : He is often invoked at sacrifices.

vii, 53, 1 : "Vṛhaṣpati, thou hast delivered us from dwelling in the realm of Yama, from the curse."

x, 6, 11 : } 12 : } The healthful amulet of Vṛhaṣpati is referrred to. It is said to have yielded the Aśvin twins greatness

UṢANĀ.

Usanā is the name of Śukrācārya, the preceptor of the demons. He was the son of the great Ṛṣi Bhṛgu. He is said to have possessed the mystic power of restoring the dead to life. This power Kaca learned from him (see Kaca). He is said to have become blind of one eye for his objection to the gift of king Valī to Viṣnu.

He had two sons, Ṣanda and Amarka, and one daughter Devayāni. His daughter fell in love with Kaca, the son of Vṛhaṣpati, but her offer was not accepted as Kaca considered her to be his sister, being the daughter of his preceptor. She was afterwards married to King Yayāti, who was cursed by the sage to become old as Devayāni complained to her father against him for having secretly married her maid Sarmiṣthā, the daughter of Dānva King Vṛṣaparva. Yayāti requested his sons to take his old age in exchange of their youth, but the four elder sons refused, and the youngest, born of Sarmiṣthā, consented. His father enjoyed his youth, and after many years, made Puru his heir to the throne.

"Usanas, with the patronymic *Kāvya*, was an ancient Ṛshi or 'Sage' who was the preceptor of the asuras or daityas, the opponents of the dêvas. As such he is always represented, in antagonism to Indra, the chief of the dêvas. It is curious that here the composition of a remedy which was a favourite with Indra is ascribed to him. It is curious also that both he as well as Vṛhaṣpati, the preceptor of the dêvas are named as author of medical formulæ. To both the composition of *mantra* or 'charms' and 'maya' or 'rules of conduct' are ascribed in the Mahābhārata, and there is an antitonic charm, called *Uśanaḥ-stoma* or Uśanas' hymn (see the large Petersburg Dictionary). But there is no Uśanā known as the author of any medical work, though there exists an author, with that name, of a *Smṛiti* or 'law-book' (see Aufrecht's Catalogus Catalogorum)" [1]

Uṣanā in the. Bower Ms., Part II. 846b-847a, p. 65.

Indrapriya Paya.

इन्द्रप्रियः पयः।

पयः पिवेत रात्रिम् यः कृत्स्नाम् जागर्त्ति वेगवान्।
शर्करामधुदुग्धाज्य घृतम् त्रिकटुकम् सरः॥
घृतमेकध्यमेतद्‍वै पिवेदिन्द्रप्रियं पयः।
औशनसो योगः इन्द्रप्रियः॥

The Indrapriya prescription, by Uśanas (846*b* and 847*a*): sugar, honey, milk, clarified butter, the three aorids, and water: all these should be boiled together, and may then be taken as the Indrapriya or potion 'beloved by Indra.'

Indra and Uṣanā are said to have entered the house of Kutsa to kill suṣṇa (Rv., v. 29. 9).

[1] Bower MSS., foot-note 332, p. 157.

CHAPTER VII.

AGASTYA.

In the Ṛgveda, Agastya appears as the author of several hymns and is said to be the son of Mitra and Varuṇa (and so called Maitra-Vāruṇi Aurvaśīya) whose seed fell from them at the sight of Urvaśī. Sāyaṇa says that he was born in a water-jar (therefore called Kalasīsūta, Kumbha-Sambhava and Ghaṭodbhava). He was called Māna as he was only a span in length when he was born, Agastya and Vindhyakūṭa from his having commanded the Vindhya mountains to lower their heads, Pītābdhi and Samudra-chuluka or "ocean-drinker" from his drinking up the ocean. His other namss are Āgneys, Āgnimāruta and Agasti. He is said to have eaten Ātapi and Vātapi asuras, so called Vātapidvit. He is the regent of the star Canopus and is the narrator of Brahma-Purāṇa. His wife was named Lopamūdrā—a girl formed by him out of the distinctive beauties of different animals, as narrated in the Mahābhārata. In the Rāmāyaṇa he appears as the chief of the hermits of the South. He kept the Rākhasas under control and helped Rāma in his exile, by presenting him the Vaiṣnava Bow, two inexhaustible arrow-cases and other weapons of war.

He is "venerated in the South, as the first teacher of science and literature to the primitive Dravidian tribes" and "we shall not greatly err in placing the era of Agastya in the 7th or at least in the 6th century B.C." (Caldwell). Wilson also thinks him to be "instrumental in the introduction of the Hindu religion and literature into the Peninsula."

His works : 1. The Asuras used to conceal themselves in the ocean, and the Devas were unable to kill them. Agastya drank up the ocean and thus exposed the Asuras before the Devas who killed them.

2. He married Lopamudrā who was brought up in the house of King of Vidarbha. To satisfy her he went out in search of money. He went to three kings, but failing to collect the whole amount from them, he next went to Ilvala, King of the Dānavas. To kill his guests, Ilvala gave them flesh of deer to eat. The deer was his brother Vātāpi. The sage in anger ate the flesh and digested Vātāpi. Ilvala then gave him the money.

3. He was the preceptor of the Vindhya mountains. Vindhya requested the sun to turn round him but was refused. The mountain thereupon began to grow higher and higher to obstruct the sun in his daily course from east to west. The devas requested Agastya to interfere. He reached the Vindhya mountain, and as Vindhya lowered his head to salute his preceptor, Agastya ordered him to remain so till he comes back from the South. The sage never came back.

4. King Nahuṣa, son of Āyus, and fifth in descent from Soma, through self-conceit, engaged great sages to bear his vehicle. By his gaze, he could rob any one of his energy. He touched with his foot Muni Agastya who was carrying him. Agastya cursed him : " Fall, thou serpent." He appeased his anger. Agastya told him to wait till Yudhiṣṭhira would free him from the curse. Another account says that Bhṛgu who was concealed in Agastya's hairs, cursed Nahuṣa. (Mahābhārata, Adiparva, 3151 ; Vanaparva, sect. 180 ; Udyogaparva, sect. 10-16 ; Anusāsana Parva 4745-4810).

Books :—

1. Dvaidha-Nirṇaya : As a medical author, Agastya is mentioned in the Brahmavaivartta Purāṇa to have written a treatise on medicine, called " Dvaidha-Nirṇaya " or " Solution of Difficulties." It is not available now.

2. In the Rudantīkalpa, Agastya is said to have prayed the sage Vasiṣṭha to lecture on medicines for the good of men :

Ms. :—GOML 13212. Rudantīkalpah.

On the preparation of a medicine from the leaves of a plant named Rudanti.

Beginning :

कैलासशिखरे रम्ये वेदब्रन्दनिषेविते ।
वसिष्ठं मुनिशार्दूलमगस्त्य: परिपृच्छति ॥
दारिद्र्यदु:खमज्ञानं मृत्युव्याधि: प्रदर्शितम् ।
मनुष्याणां हितार्थाय औषधं कथय प्रभो ॥

ईश्वर उवाच—

साधु साधु महाप्राज्ञ सर्वसत्त्वाहिते रत ।
कथयामि यथातथ्यं मृत्युदारिद्र्यनाशनम् ॥
ओषधीं शृणुष्वेमां चेमां मातेव हितकारिणीम् ।
रुदन्ती नाम विख्यातं(तां) मृत्युदारिद्र्यनाश(नीं)म् ॥

End :

ग्रहनागपिशाचा वा यक्षराक्षसमर्दनात् ।
विषलेपेन सर्वेषां प्रीत्या विषाणि भवन्ति हि ॥
चणककला: खदिरमात्रं विचित्रापत्राणि ।
सितपीतरक्तकृष्णा: भूमिसमो भवति ॥

Colophon :

इति रुदन्तीकल्पस्सम्पूर्ण: ॥

The Formulæ ascribed to Agastya :—

1.	A purgative by Agasti—	Bower Ms. I, vv. 61-67.
2.	Agastya Haritakī Avaleha I.	G. N. Vol. I, p. 145. / Śa. Ś. II, 8, p. 144.
3.	,, ,, ,, II. ...	G. N., pp. 144-5.
4.	Agasti Haritaki ...	... V. K. V., p. 147.
	Agasti Rasāyaṇa	... A. H. S., IV, p. 80.
5.	Agastya Avaleha	S. S., VI, li.
	Agastya Abhayā Avaleha	Śataślokī, p. 26.
6.	Agasti Rasa ...	... R. C., ix, p. 115.
7.	Sūraṇa Vatikā ...	... G. N., pp. 108-9.
8.	Maha Lakṣmī Vilāsa Rasa (used by Kṛṣṇa)	... Saṁkṣiptasāra, p. 33.
9.	Vṛhat Viṣṇu Oil ...	... Do., p. 58.
10.	Bhīma Vaṭaka ...	... H. S. III, xii, p. 205.

1. Agastya's Purgative.

चित्रकार्द्ध' पलम् मूलात्तृब्रृत्‌शातलयोस्तथा ।
+म् दन्तिमूलानाम् कर्षाम् कर्षम् पृथक् पृथक् ॥
पिप्पल्या: सैन्धवाच्चैव तथा हिम्ग्वम्नुबेतसात् ।
विंशतिश्चाभया मुख्या + + विपाचयेत् ॥
गुड़स्याष्टपलात् सम्यक् व्वींत दशमोदकान् ।
फकैकम् भक्षयेत्तस्माद्दशमे दशमेऽहनि ॥
दोषाणामपाचनार्थाय जलमुष्णम् पिबेदनु ।
विरिक्तांते तत: स्नात्वा सात्म्यमन्नं प्रयोजयेत् ॥
नात्र कश्चित् परिहारो वाक्कायमनसाम् सदा ।
सर्व्वर्तुको नरेन्द्राणाम् विरिकोऽगस्ति निर्म्मित: ॥
जरा-मृत्यु प्रमथ्नन: सर्व्वामय विनाशनं: ।
वृष्यो रसायनश्चैव मेधारोग्याभिवर्द्धन: ॥
नापुत्राय प्रदातव्यो नाशिष्याय कथञ्चन ।
राजद्विष्टे न दातव्यो ये चान्येपापचारिण: ॥

Bower MS. (61-67)

"Boil half a pala of the root of Chitraka (Plumbago Zeylanica), likewise of Trivrit (Ipomæa Turpethum) and Sâtalâ (Stereospermum Suaveolens), and one karsha, each of the roots of Danti (Baliospermum Montanum) and ...., and likewise of long pepper, rock-salt, asafætida and Indian sorrel and 20 of the best chebulic Myrobalans,....... From these carefully prepare 10 boluses with 8 pala of treacle, and take one of them on every 10th day. After it one should drink warm water for the purpose of correcting the defects of the humours; and then, after the purgative has taken effect, one should bathe and may then return to one's ordinary diet. There should never be any hesitation with regard to this remedy either in words or deed or thought. It is a purgative composed by *Agasti*, fit for princes, and which can be used in all seasons. It prevents old age and death; it cures all diseases; it also acts as an aphrodisiac and alterative tonic, and increases memory and health. It should never be administered to any one who has no son nor disciple; nor should it be given to an enemy of the king, nor to any other sinful liver." Bower Ms., p. 17.

2. Agastya Haritaki Avaleha I.

अगस्त्यहरीतक्यवलेहः ।

द्विपञ्चमूलीभकणात्मगुप्ताभार्गीशठीपुष्करमूलविश्वाः ।
पाठामृताग्रन्थिक शङ्खपुष्पीरास्नाग्न्यपामार्गबलायवासाः ॥
द्विपालिकास्तत्र यवाढकं च हरीतकीनां च शतं गुरूणाम् ।
द्रोणे जलस्याढकसंयुते तु क्काथीकृते पूतचतुर्थभागे ॥
पचेत्तुलां शुद्धगुडस्य दत्त्वा पृथक्सतैलात्कुडवं घृताच्च ।
चूर्णं च तावन्मगधोद्भवानामनेकरोगौघमथाशु हन्यात् ॥
तद्राजयक्ष्मग्रहणीप्रदोषशोफाग्निमान्द्यस्वरभेदकासान् ।
पाण्ड्वामयश्वासशिरोऽक्षिरोगान्हृद्रोगहिक्काविषमज्वरांश्च ॥
मेधाबलोत्साहमतिप्रदं च चकार चैतद्भगवानगस्त्यः ।

3. Agastya Haritaki Avaleha II.

द्वितीयोऽगस्त्यहरीतक्यवलेहः ।

दशमूलीं स्वयङ्गुप्तां शङ्खपुष्पीं शटीं बलाम् ।
हस्तिपिप्पल्यपामार्गपिप्पलीमूलचित्रकान् ॥
भार्गीं पुष्करमूलं च द्विपलांशान् यवाढकम् ।
हरीतकीशतं चैकं जले पञ्चाढके पचेत् ॥
यवैः स्विन्नैः कषायं तं पूतं तच्चाभयाशतम् ।
पचेद्गुडतुलां दत्त्वा कुडवं च पृथग्घृतात् ॥
तैलाच्च पिप्पलीचूर्णात्सिद्धे शीते च माक्षिकात् ।
कुडवं, पलमानं च चतुर्जातं समावपेत् ॥
लिह्याद्द्वे चाभये नित्यं ततः खादेद्रसायनात् ।
वलीं च पलितं हन्याद्वर्णायुर्बलवर्धनम् ॥
पञ्च कासान् क्षयं श्वासं सहिध्मं विषमज्वरम् ।
गुल्ममेहग्रहण्यर्शोहृद्रोगारुचिपीनसान् ॥
अगस्त्यविहितं धन्यमिदं श्रेष्ठं रसायनम् ।
यथोद्दिष्टान् गुणं कुर्वन्पित्तं चेत्कुरुते यदि ॥
तदा सार्धं गुडो योज्य एष एवाल्पमात्रया ।
पादशेषे कषायेऽव स्विन्ना विद्याद्धरीतकीः
भर्जितास्तिलतैलस्य कुडवे गोघृतस्य वा ।
पचेत्ताम्रमये पात्रे आपाकाल्लोहितोदयात् ॥
शङ्खया फलानां शतशश्चातुर्जातं पृथक्पलम् ।
बद्धा पोटलके पथ्या यवान् स्विन्नांश्च कारयेत् ॥

4. Agasti Haritaki.

अगस्ति हरितकी ।

The same formula as No. 2.

Agasti Rasāyana.

अगस्ति रसायन ।

The same formula as No. 2

AGASTYA HARITAKI.

This formula "Agastya Haritaki" also occurs in another recension in the C. S., vi, 20, 734.

C. D., xi, 37, 219.
Bower Ms., II, vv. 436-440.
V. S., xii, 276.

In the Vaṅgasena, it is found with two additional lines were first of which adds, as a further ingredient, one pala each of the *Chaturjāta* or 'set of four spices.' The other explains the name *Agastya-haritakī* by which the formula is there called, to have been given to it, because it was composed by the great sage Agastya, and because it contains one hundred *haritakī* or 'chebulic mysobalani.'

Bower Ms., p. 119, F. N. 171.

5. AGASTYA AVALEHA.

अगस्त्य अवलेह: ।

द्विपञ्चमूलिभकणात्मगुप्ताभार्गीं शठीपुष्करमूलविश्वान् ।
पाठामृताग्रन्थिक शङ्खपुष्पीरास्नाग्न्यपामार्ग बलायवासान् ।
द्विपालिकान्नस्य यवाढ़कञ्च हरीतकीनाञ्च शतं गुरूणां ॥
द्रोणे जलस्याढ़क संयुते च क्वाथे कृते पूतचतुर्थभागे ।
पचेत्तुलां शुद्धगुड़स्य दत्त्वा पृथक्चतैलात् कुड़वं घृताच्च ।
चूर्णञ्च तावभगधोद्भवाया: देयञ्च तस्मिन्मधु सिद्धशीते ।
रसायनात् कल्कमतो विलिह्याद्द्वेचाभये नित्यमथाशु हन्यात् ॥
तद्राजयक्ष्मग्रहणी प्रदोषशोफाग्नि-मान्द्यस्वरभेदकासान् ।
भाण्डुामय श्वासशिरोविकारान् हृद्रोगहिक्काविषमज्वरांश्च ॥
मेधावलोत्साहमतिप्रदञ्च चकारचैतद्द भगवानगस्त्य: ।

5. Agastya Abhayā Avaleha.

अगस्त्याभयानामावलेह: ।

शङ्खाह्वादशमूलपुष्करशठीयास: स्वगुप्ताबला-
पामार्गेभकणामृतौषधहकी ग्रन्थ्यग्निभार्ङ्गी रसा: ।
द्व्यामा: पथ्यशतं यवाढकमपां पश्चाढकस्वायव-
स्वेदात् पाच्यमिमा: शिवा: सच रसो गौड़ीत्तुलाच्चाञ्जलि: ॥
कृष्णातैलघृतात् पुन: कुड़विकाचौद्रैरगस्त्याभया
कासाऽर्शोग्रहणी-क्षय-ज्वर-जरा-श्वास-प्रतिश्याकृचौ ।

6. Agasti Rasa.

अगस्तिरस: ।

रसोंशुमालीजयपालल्लोहशिलाहरिद्रावलय: समांशा.: ।
व्योषाग्निभृङ्गार्द्रकनिस्वनीरै: निर्गुण्डिकारग्वधमूलकाद्भि: ॥
पृथग्विमर्द्योदरनाशनोऽयमगस्तिसूत: सशिवागुड़ोऽयम ।
सम्पाचनादिक्रमशुद्धदेहे वल्लद्वयोऽथ क्रमसंयुतो वा ॥
कम्पिल्लचूर्णेन समञ्च दत्वा जलोदरादीन् जयतीह रोगान् ॥

7. Suraṇa Vaṭikā.

सूरणवटिका: ।

षोड़श सूरणभागा वह्नेरष्टौ महौषधस्यापि ।
अर्धेन भागयुक्तिर्मरिचस्य ततोऽपि चार्द्धेन ॥
त्रिफला कणा समूला तालीसारुष्करकृमिघ्नानाम् ।
भागा महौषधसमा दहनांशा तालमूली च ॥
भाग: सूरणतुल्यो दातव्यो वृद्धदारुकस्यापि ।
भृङ्गेलि मरिचांशौ चूर्णेऽस्मिन्योजयेन्मतिमान् ।
द्विगुणेन गुडेन युत: सेव्योऽयं मोदक: प्रकामघनै: ।
गुरुवृष्यभोज्यरहितेष्वितरेषूपद्रवान्कुरुते ॥
भस्मकमनेन जनितं पूर्वमगस्त्यस्य योगराजेन ।
भीमस्य मारुतेरपि येन ते महाशना जाता: ॥

अग्निबलवृद्धिहेतुर्न केवलं सूरणो महावीर्य्यः ।
प्रभवति शस्त्रक्षाराग्निभिर्विनाप्यर्शसामेषः ॥
श्वयथुश्लीपदगरजिद्गृहणीं च कफानिलाज्जाताम् ।
नाशयति वलीपलितं मेधां कुरुते वृषत्व च ॥
हिक्कां कासं श्वासं सराजयक्ष्मप्रमेहांश्च ।
प्लीहानमप्यथोग्रं हन्ति च रसायनं पुंसाम् ॥

8. Mahā Laksmībilāsa Rasa.

महालक्ष्मीविलासो रसः ।

पलं वज्राभ्र चर्णस्य तदर्द्धं गन्ध-पारदं ।
वङ्गभस्म तदर्द्धञ्च तदर्द्धं तारकस्य च ॥
तत् समं हरितालस्य तदर्द्धं ताम्रभस्मकं ।
रस तुल्यञ्च कर्पूरं जाती-कोष-फले तथा ॥
वृद्धदारक-वीजञ्च वीजं स्वर्णफलस्य च ।
प्रत्येकं कार्षिकान् भागान् मृत-स्वर्णञ्च शानकं ॥
नागवल्ली रसैः पिष्टा त्रिगुञ्जाफल मानतः ।
वटी कार्य्यानुपानञ्च व्याधिं वीक्ष्य प्रयोजयेत् ।
निहन्ति सन्निपातोत्थान् गदान् घोरान् सुदारुणान ।
प्रोक्तं प्रयोगराजोयं अगस्त्ये न महात्मना ॥
महालक्ष्मीविलासोऽयं वासुदेव जगतगुरुः ।
अस्य प्रसादात् भगवान् लचनारीषु वल्लभः ॥

9. Vṛhat Visṇu Oil.

वृहद्विष्णु तैलं ।

गुहार्काब्दाश्वगन्धाम्बु वृहत्यौ चन्दनं निशे ।
शालपर्णीवर्द्धमाषपूतिकाङ्घ्रिकुरण्टकाः ॥
गवेधकवलाभीरुविसविश्वाकणागुरु ।
लवङ्गं चन्दनं चोचं कक्कोलं वणिता शिवा ॥
जातीकोषफलं दारु पयस्या पुष्करं शटी ।
तालीशकुङ्कुमं धात्री मांसी शैलसमुद्भवं ॥

त्रुटिवल्कलकोशीरग्रान्थिकं कल्क मुत्तमं ।
पृथक् कर्षं समादाय तैलप्रस्थं पचेत् सुधीः ।
चतुर्गुण मज्जाक्षीरं तत्तुल्यं जलमेवच ।
यद्वा चतुर्गुणं गव्यं क्षीरं वारिच तत्र वे ॥
हन्त्यभ्यङ्गात् नभस्वन्तप्रदुष्टं पित्तमुल्वनं ।
वलासं तत् समुद्भूतान् रोगानति सुदारूणान् ॥
वाधिर्य्यं खाञ्ज्य पङ्गुत्वं मूकमिन्मिनगद्गदान् ।
अष्ठीलां ग्रहणीरोगमर्द्दितं कर्णनादकं ॥
सूतिका गर्भिनीरोगमिन्द्रलुप्तं जरां जयेत् ।
वृहद्विष्णुतैलमेतद्गस्त्ये न च भाषितं ॥
सेवनादस्य सर्व्वस्मात् मुच्यते विषमाद्गदात् ॥

10. Bhīma Vaṭikā.

भीमं वटिका ।

त्रिफलमगधजानां मूलतालीशपत्रं
क्रिमिरिपुमगधानां पुष्करं चेत् समांशः ।
मरिचदहनभागश्चैकभागेन शुण्ठी
सकलतुलितुल्यः शूरणस्यैकभागः ।
मदनचपलयुक्तं वृद्धदारैलभङ्ग
कृतमिह परिचूर्णं द्विगुणे जीर्णखण्डं ।
कृतवटकमुखस्तु प्राशते यो मनुष्यो
हरति जठररोगं तस्य चाशु प्रकर्षम्
गदजरुधिरपित्तं कासमन्दाग्निशूलान्
चयतमकहलीमान् कामलांश्च क्रिमींश्च ।
विदधति वलपुष्टिं दापयेच्चाशु मार्गे
प्रवलयति हुताशं योगराजप्रसिद्धः ।
योगराजेन युञ्जीत स्वयमेवाप्यगस्तिना ।
अस्य योगस्य योगेन भीमोऽपि वहुभक्षकः
इति भीमवटको नाम ।

CYAVANA.

The legend of Cyavana and the Aśvins is related in Śatapatha Brāhmaṇa and also in the Mahābhārata. The cure of Cyavana by the heavenly physicians is thus described in the Śatapatha Brāhmaṇa, IV, 1, 5, 1 ff. :—

Cyavana assumed a shrivelled form to perform austerities. Sons of King Saryātas incensed the Ṛṣi by throwing clods against him. Cyavana created discord among them. Saryāta appeased the sage by giving him her daughter Sukanyā in marriage. The Aśvins tried to seduce her pointing out to her husband's appearance. She refused to abandon her husband. Cyavana advised her to tell them that he would make the Aśvins perfect if they make him young again. Cyavana was bathed in a pond and recovered his youth. The gods were then informed that they have been excluded from a sacrifice in Kurukṣetra. The Aśvins remonstrated but were told by the other gods that as they wandered about very familiarly among men performing cures, they have been excluded. The Aśvins pointed out that the sacrifice was headless. The gods invited them. The Aśvins restored the head of sacrifice, became the adhvaryu priests and received the Aśvina draught.

In the Ṭaitt. Saṁ., VI, 4, 9, 1 it has been further added that when the Aśvins restored the head of sacrifice, the gods purified them as they were unclean, for going among men as physicians. Hence no Brāhman must act as a physician as it makes him unclean and unfit to sacrifice.

In the Mahābhārata, Vanaparva, 10, 316 ff. a somewhat different version of the same story is given: Cyavana was covered by an anthill; Sukanyā pierced his eyes, and Cyavana afflicted Saryāta's army with stoppage of urine. The sage was given Sukanyā as wife to appease him. Aśvina restored Cyavana to beauty, on condition that she would be at liberty to choose any one of the Aśvins and Cyavana as her husband. Sukanyā recognised her husband Cyavana. The sage performed a sacrifice for the king and gave the Aśvins a share in the oblation. Indra objected, as Aśvins were physicians, but the sage stayed the arm of Indra when he was about to use his thunder-bolt and compelled him to submit.

He is the famous sage Cyavana, the son of Bhṛgu. When advanced in age he could not give up desires, and married the young and beautiful Sukanyā, the daughter of Śaryāti. He regained his youthful vigour by the judicious medication of the two Aśvins. He repaid the debt of gratitude by compelling Indra to drink with them Soma juice when he refused to do so. The legend is thus related in the Mahābhārata:

"Having given a promise to that effect, Chyavana applied, along with the other gods, to Indra, to allow the Aśvins to partake in the soma juice. Indra answered 'How can they become drinkers of the soma, seeing they are reviled by us, and are not on an equality with the gods? We do not wish to drink soma in their company; but we shall accede to your wishes in any other respect.' Chyavana repeats his request, and urges that the Aśvins also are gods, and the offspring of the sun (7310). He adds that it will be well for the gods if they accede to this demand, and ill if they do not. Indra rejoins that the other gods may drink with the Aśvins if they please, but he cannot bring himself to do it. Chyavana retorts that if he does not, he shall be chastised by the sage, and made to drink soma (with them) at the sacrifice. A ceremony was then instantly begun by Chyavana for the benefit of the Aśvins; and the gods were vanquished by sacred texts. Indra, seeing this rite commenced, became incensed, uplifted a vast mountain (7315) and rushed with his thunderbolt, and with angry eyes, on Chyavana. The sage however sprinkling him with water, arrested him with his mountain and thunderbolt. Chyavana then created a fearful open-mouthed monster, called Mada, formed of the substance of the oblation ** Finding themselves in this predicament, the gods took counsel and said to Indra, 'Make salutation to Chyavana and let us drink soma along with the Aśvins, and so escape from our sufferings.' Indra then, making obeisance, granted the demand of Chyavana, who was thus the cause of the Aśvins becoming drinkers of the soma. He then performed the ceremony, and clove Mada to pieces." [1]

Formulæ ascribed to Cyavana :—

1. The Cyavana Prāśa or the Cyavana Clarified Butter. This formula is ascribed to the sage Cyavana and it is still much used by the Kavirajes of the present days.

The Cyavana Prāśa—See	C. S.,	vi. I.	pp. 312-3.
	C. D.,	X. v. 20.	pp. 95-6.
	A. H. S.,	vol. II, vi. 39	p. 338.
	H. S.,	III. 9.	pp. 180-1.
	Sā. S.,	II. 8.	pp. 142-3.
	Bower Ms.,	II.	p. 98.
	Śataślokī,		p. 32.
	G. N.,	vol. I,	p. 160.
	V. K. V.,		p. 145.

[1] Muir's Sanskrit Texts. Vol. I, pp. 470-71.

In the Hārīta Saṁhitā, the formula is ascribed to Kṛṣṇātreya who is said to have taught it.

क्षयरोगविनाशाय कथितश्चिकित्सा महत् ।
च्यवनप्राशनं नाम कृष्णात्रेयेण भाषितं ॥

2. Laghu Cyavana Prāśa—G. N., I., p. 163.

For the English translation of Cyavana Prāśa, See Bower Ms., p. 98.

1. Cyavana Prāśa.

च्यवनप्राशः ।

बिल्वाग्निमन्थौ श्योणाकः काश्मर्यं पाटलिर्बला ।
पर्ण्यश्चतस्रः पिप्पल्यः श्वदंष्ट्रा बृहतीद्वयम् ॥
शृङ्गी तामलकी द्राक्षा जीवन्ती पुष्करागुरुः ।
अभया चामृता ऋद्धिर्जीवकर्षभकौ शटी ॥
मुस्तं पुंनर्नवा मेदा एला चन्दनमुत्पलम् ।
विदारीवृषमूलानि काकोली काकनासिका ॥
एषां पलोन्मितान् भागान् शतान्यामलकस्य च ।
पञ्च दद्यात् तदैकत्र जलद्रोणे विपाचयेत् ॥
ज्ञात्वा गतरसान्येतान्यौषधान्यथ तं रसम् ।
तच्चामलकमुद्धृत्य निष्कुलं तैलसर्पिषोः ।
पलद्वादशके भृष्ट्वा दत्त्वा चार्द्धतुलां भिषक् ।
मत्स्यण्डिकायाः पूतायां लेहवत् साधु साधयेत् ॥
षट्पलं मधुनश्चात्र सिद्धशीते समावपेत् ।
चतुष्पलं तुगाक्षीर्य्याः पिप्पलीद्विपलं तथा ॥
पलमेकं निदध्याच्च त्वगेलापत्रकेशरात् ।
इत्ययं च्यवनप्राशः परमुक्तो रसायनः ॥
कासश्वासहरश्चैव विशेषेणोपदिश्यते ।
क्षीणक्षतानां वृद्धानां बालानाञ्चाङ्गवर्द्धनः ॥

स्वरक्षयमुरोरोगं हृद्रोगं वातशोणितम् ।
पिपासां मूत्रशुक्रस्थान् दोषांश्चाप्यपकर्षति ॥
अस्य मात्रां प्रयुञ्जीत योपरुन्ध्यान्न भोजनम् ।
अस्य प्रयोगाच्च्यवनः सुवृद्धोऽभूत् पुनर्युवा ॥

मेधां स्मृतिं कान्तिमनामयत्वमायुःप्रकर्षं बलमिन्द्रियाणाम् ।
स्त्रीषु प्रहर्षं परमग्निवृद्धिं वर्णप्रसादं पवनानुलोम्यम् ॥
रसायनस्यास्य नरः प्रयोगाल्लभेत जीर्णोऽपि कुटीप्रवेशात् ।
जराकृतं रूपमपास्य सर्व्वं बिभर्त्ति रूपं नवयौवनस्य ॥

इति च्यवनप्राशः ।

2. Laghu Cyavana Prāśa.

लघुच्यवनप्राशोऽवलेहः ।

बिल्वादिपञ्चमूलाब्दबलापर्णीचतुष्टयम् ।
ऋद्धिवृद्धिकृष्णाशठीपथ्याजीवकर्षभकामृताः ॥
द्राक्षा पुनर्नवा मेदे जीवन्ती काकनासिका ।
उत्पलैलाजशृङ्गाश्च काकोली वृषचन्दनम् ॥
विदारीगोक्षुरव्याघ्रीपौष्करं च पलोन्मितम् ।
शतानि पञ्च धात्र्याश्च जलद्रोणे विपाचयेत् ॥
पलद्वादशके भृष्टा धात्रीस्तास्तैलसर्पिषोः ।
सिताघंतुलया युक्ताः क्वाथं लीढं पुनः पचेत् ॥
द्वे पिप्पल्याः पले वांश्याश्चत्वारः षट् च माक्षिकात् ।
चातुर्जातपलं तस्मिन् सिद्धशीते नियोजयेत् ॥
हृद्रोगश्वासहृल्लासवातरक्तक्षयार्त्तिजित् ।
सेव्योऽयं च्यवनप्राशः स्वर्यो वृष्यो रसायनः ॥

Books :—

Jīvadāna : In the Brahmavaivarta Purāṇa : Cyavana is mentioned as the author of a medical treatise called Jīvadāna (the Giver of Life). See Vol. I, 1, p. 7, foot-note. The book is not available now.

BHARADVĀJA.

A Vedic sage and composer of hymns. He was the son of Vṛhaṣpati and father of Droṇa, the preceptor of the Pāndavas. His mother was Mamatā, the wife of Utathya. "He became immortal and ascended to the heaven" (Taittirīya Brāhmaṇa). It is said that his mother, became pregnant, both by her husband Utathya and by Vṛhaspati. Dīrgha-tamas, Utathya's son, kicked his half-brother. out of her womb untimely, when Vṛhaṣpati said to his mother "Bhara-dva-jam" "Cherish this boy of two fathers," and cursed Dīrgha-tamās to be blind. See Viṣṇu Purāṇa, Sec. IV, Ch. xix. In the Mahābhārata he appears to have lived at Hardwar, but in the Rāmāyaṇa, Rama and Bharat are said to have gone to his hermitage at Allahabad. (Ayodhyākanda Ch. 54, 90-91). One of Bharadvāja's sons is Garga Ṛṣi.

In the Caraka Saṁhitā, I. i., Bharadvāja was the sage selected by the Ṛṣis, to go to Indra to learn the science of life.

दीर्घंजीवितमन्विच्छन् भरद्वाज उपागमत् ।
इन्द्रमुग्रतपा बुद्धा शरण्यममरेश्वरम् ॥

* * * *

ऋषिप्रोक्तो भरद्वाजस्तस्माच्छक्रमुपागमत् ॥

* * * *

कः सहस्राक्षभवनं गच्छेत् प्रष्टुं शचीपतिम् ।
अहमर्थे नियुज्येयमत्रेति प्रथमं वचः ।
भरद्वाजोऽब्रवीत् तस्मादृषिभिः स नियोजितः ॥

When Bharadvāja came back, the sages learned the science of medicine from him.

तेनायुरमितं लेभे भरद्वाज सुखान्वित: ।
ऋषिभ्योऽनधिकं तन्तु शशंसानवशेषयन् ॥
ऋषयश्च भरद्वाजाज्जगृहुस्तं प्रजाहितम् ।
दीर्घमायुश्चिकीर्षन्तो वेदं वर्द्धनमायुष: ॥

Ātreya Punarvasu was one of the sages and he taught his six disciples, Agniveśa and others. Some think that Punarvasu Ātreya was the same person as Bharadvāja; but this is untenable for as Cakrapāni says: "Atreya is nowhere described as Bharadvāja in the Caraka Saṁhitā."

"अत्र केचित् भरद्वाजात्रेययोरैक्यं मन्यन्ते, तन्न, भरद्वाजसंज्ञया आत्रेयस्य क्वचिदपि तन्त्रप्रदेशेऽकीर्त्तनात्" ।

Āyurveda Dīpikā, p. 15.

Cakrapāṇi also quotes from Hārīta Saṁhitā (but this is not found in the printed edition) that Bharadvāja says:

शक्रादहमधीतवान इत्यादिना मत्त: पुनरसंख्येया: विसूत्रं विप्रयोजनम् ।
अत्रात्रेयादिपर्य्यन्ता ॠद्: सप्तमहर्षय: । आत्रेयात् हारीतऋषि: इत्यन्तेन ॥

But in the Aṣṭāṅga Hṛdaya Saṁhitā, Indra is said to have taught the sons of Atri, *i.e.*, Atreya and others: and the name of Bharadvāja is not mentioned:

ब्रह्मा स्मृत्वायुषोवेदं प्रजापतिमजिग्रहत् ।
सोऽश्विनौ तौ सहस्राक्षं सोऽत्रिपुत्रादिकान् मुनीन् ॥

So there is discrepancy between the accounts given by Hārīta and Vāgbhaṭa; but this seeming anomaly is more apparent than real for in the Rasāyanapāda Samutthānīya, Indra is said to have taught the sages Bhṛgu, Aṅgirā,

Atri, Vaṣiṣṭha, Kaśyapa, Agastya, Pulastya, Vāmadeva and Asita Gautama. (See "Indra.") Here we find Atri as one of the Ṛṣis who learned the science of medicine from Indra; and the name of Bharadvāja is not mentioned. [See Caraka Saṁhitā VI, i. p. 323.] Vagbhaṭa seems to have this passage in mind when he wrote about the teachers of Āyurveda. Cakrapāṇi Datta also takes the same view: वाभटेन तु यदुक्तं "ब्रह्मा......... मुनीन्" इत्यनेनात्रेयस्य इन्द्रशिष्यत्वं, तदायुर्वेद समुत्थानीय रसायनपादे आदि शब्देन वक्ष्यमाणेन्द्र शिष्यतायोगात् समर्थनीयम्; तत्र हीन्द्रेण पुनर्म्महर्षीणामायुर्वेद उपदिष्ट इति वक्तव्यम्।

Bhāva Miśra also makes both Ātreya and Bharadvāja the disciples of Indra. On different occasions, they went separately to Indra to learn the science of medicine.

Ātreya:

चिन्तयामास भगवानात्रेयो मुनिपुङ्गवः।
क करोमि क्व गच्छामि कथं लोका निरामयाः॥
* * * *
आयुर्वेदं पठिष्यामि नैरुज्याय शरीरिणाम्।
इति निश्चित्य गतवानात्रेयस्त्रिदशालयम्॥
* * * *
आयुर्वेदोपदेशं मे कुरु कारुण्यतो नृणाम्।
तथेत्युक्त्वा सहस्राक्षोऽध्यापयामास तं मुनिम्॥

Bharadvāja:

तन्नेषां प्रशमाय कश्चन विधिश्चिन्त्यो भवद्भिर्बुधै
र्योग्यैरित्यभिधाय संसदि भरद्वाजं मुनिं तेऽब्रुवन।
त्वं योग्यो भगवन्। सहस्रनयनं याचस्व लब्धां क्रमा
दायुर्वेदमधीत्य यं गदभयान्मुक्ता भवामोवयम्।
इत्थं स मुनिभिर्योग्यैः प्रार्थितोः विनयान्वितैः।
भरद्वाजो मुनिश्रेष्ठो जगाम त्रिदशालयम्॥
तत्रेन्द्र भवनं गत्वा सुरर्षिगणमध्यगम्।
दृष्टवान् बलहन्तारं दीप्यमानमिवानलम्॥

Books : The following books are attributed to Bharadvāja :

1, He is said to have written a Tantra.

> तत्तत्वजनित ज्ञानचक्षुषा ऋषयोऽखिला: ।
> गुणाण् द्रव्याणि कर्म्मानि दृष्ट्वा तद्विधिमाश्रिता: ॥

Bhāva Prakāśa I. 1.

2. Bhāradvājīyam : Ms. : No. 13178. G.O.M.L. (Madras).

The title of the book implies that this work belongs to the medical system attributed to Bharadvāja, the teacher of Ātreya. This Ms. contains only the chapter on मेह or urinary diseases.

No. 13178. भारद्वाजीयम् ।

BHĀRADVAJĪYAM.

Beginning :

> ग्रन्थान्तरे आयुर्वेदे भारद्वाजीय प्रकरणे मेहशुक्ल आमलक्षणे
> असाध्यरोगनिर्णय: ।

> आमशुक्लं च मेहेन वायुलिप्ते न पैत्यगे ।
> दारकीलं विनाशाय निस्त्राणं च शरीरगे ॥
> वायुबन्धनदेहेन मेहज्वरविलिप्तगे ।
> अथातो वीर्यनाशं च आमशुक्लं च लक्षणे ॥
> स्वपेन मलमूत्रवेदनाच्च समस्तरोगाणि भयानि सद्य: (?) ।
> समस्तरोगा: चणमात्रनाशयेसंसेवितेद्रोगिप्रवर्तकेन (?) ॥

End

> शिर:पूरितमेहाय चलनं शिरसस्तथा ।
> परस्य विकारेणव(प)र्णमूलन्तु उदके ॥
> मेहन्तरालेन चयेन मा तिक्तज्वरे लिप्तकमेहदुर्बले ।
> स्वर्णे समानेन शरीरतोषणे शरीरमाद्यं दधुरुच्छतेन ॥

3. BHEṢAJAKALPAH.

Mss. : 13179, 13180, 13181. G.O.M.L.

This book deals with preparations of medicines for curing diseases and also treats of the various kinds of fevers.

No. 13179. भेषजकल्पः, सव्याख्यानः ।

BHEṢAJAKALPA WITH COMMENTARY.

Beginning :

अथातो भेषजकल्पं व्याख्यास्यामः इत्याह भगवान् भरद्वाजः ।

सिद्धौषधानां केषांचित् पृथक्कल्पप्रसङ्गतः ।

अथ भेषजकल्पोऽयं सामान्येन प्रकाश्यते ॥

अथ शिरोनेत्रवस्तिव्यापत्सिद्धिकल्पानन्तरम् । सिद्धौषधानाम् हरीतक्यादीनाम् । केषाञ्चित् पृथक् पार्थक्येन कल्पनाप्रसङ्गसाधारण्येनायं भेषजकल्पोऽध्यायः प्रकाश्यते । भेषजस्य कल्पः कल्पना क्रिया प्रकटीक्रियते । आदौ तस्य भेषजस्य कल्पनाप्रशंसामाह—

देशकालानुगुण्येन संगृहीतं यथाविधि ।

स्थापितं भेषजं तैस्तैः कल्पनैरमृतायते ॥

End :

नातितीक्ष्णं नातिमृदुः श्लक्ष्णपिच्छिलशीघ्रगः ।

* * *

एवमेवं दशगुणः । क्षारश्रेष्ठस्य यत्कर्म छेदनादिश्च तेजसाग्ने(ग्ने)रपि यत्कर्म पा(दा)हाश्च करोतीत्यः । लवणपाकमाह । श्लोकार्थः स्पष्टः ।

Colophon :

इति द्रव्यविशेषकभेषज्यकल्पं सम्पूर्णम् ॥

Bheṣaja Kalpa Vyākhyā : A commentary on the above treatise by Veṅkaṭeśa, son of Avadhāna Sarasvatī of Ātreya gotra.

No. 13182. भैषज्यकल्पव्याख्या।

BHAIṢAJAKALPA VYĀKHYĀ.

Beginning :

श्रीमान् दन्तिमुखो देवः श्रेयांसि विदधातु नः।
तत्प्रसादेन निर्विघ्नं सिद्ध्यन्ति कृतिनां क्रियाः॥
अवधानसरस्वत्यास्सूनरार्वेयशेखरः।
वेंकटेशो वितनुते द्रव्यकल्पस्य योजनाम्॥

अध्यायारम्भसम्बन्धमाह सिद्धौषधानामित्यादि। अथ वस्तिव्यापसिद्धिकल्पनानन्तरं सिद्धौषधानां हरीतक्यादीनां केषाञ्चित्प्रथक् पार्थक्येन कल्पनाप्रसंगसाधारण्येनायं भेषजकल्पोऽध्यायः प्रकाश्यते। भेषजकल्पनाक्रिया प्रकटीक्रियते। तथा तस्य भेषजकल्पनाप्रशंसामाह देशकालेत्यादि।

End :

सप्तवारात्परमनन्तरं प्रभाजसप्तरात्रं यवराशौ ...... नाह स(न)तीत्यादि। नतीच्ण-नातिमृदुश्लच्णापिच्छिलः चिप्रगः आशुव्यापी सितः ....तं यथा भवति तथा भ्रमयित्वा ... ... अस्मिन् पात्रे निषिच्य तुलादि

* * ° °

अच्छिद्रेऽस्मिन् चारे पादावशेषिते मति तस्मिन्.

Formulæ :—Bharadvāja is the reputed prescriber of the following formulæ :—

1. Vṛhat Phalaghṛtaṁ—Vṛnda Madhāva p. 499.
2. Phalaghṛtaṁ—Śārṅgadhara Saṁhitā p. 158.

1. VṚHAT PHALA GHṚTAM

बृहत् फलघृतम्।

कुष्ठं मुस्तं हरिद्रे द्वे पिप्पली कटुरोहिणी।
काकोली क्षीरकाकोली विशाला त्रिफलोत्पलम्.
मेदारास्नाविडङ्गानि देवदारु सहिङ्गुकम्॥१८॥

द्वे सारिवे शताह्वा च वचा यष्टी प्रियंगुका ।
अजमोदा महामेदा चन्दनं रक्तचन्दनम् ॥१९॥
जातीपुष्पं तुगाक्षीरी कट्फलं सितशर्करा ।
एतैरक्षसमैः कल्कैर्घृतप्रस्थं भिषक्तमः ॥२०॥
चतुर्गुणेन पयसा विपचेद्गोमयाग्निना ॥
शुभेऽह्नि पुष्यसंयुक्ते भाण्डे ताम्रमये दृढे ॥२१॥
कलशे हेमकल्याणे कृतकौतुकमङ्गले ।
सर्पिरेतन्नरः पीत्वा स्त्रीषु नित्यं वृषायते ॥२२॥
या च वन्ध्या भवेन्नारी या च कन्याप्रभायिना(न्या प्रसूयते) ॥
या च वाऽस्थिरगर्भा स्याद्या च सूत्वा पुनः स्थिता ॥२३॥
अल्पायुषं च जनयेद्या वा जनयते मृतम् ।
तादृशं जनयेत्पुत्रं वेदवेदाङ्गपारगम् ॥२४॥
रूपलावण्यसंपन्नं शतायुं विगतज्वरम् ।
नाम्ना फलघृतं हेद्भारद्वाजेन निर्मितम् ॥२५॥

2. PHALAGHṚTAM.

फलघृतम् ।

त्रिफला मधुकं कुष्ठं द्वे निशे कटुरोहिणी ।
विडङ्गं पिप्पली मुस्तं विशाला कट्फलं वचा ॥
द्वे मेदे द्वे च काकोल्यौ सारिवे द्वे प्रियङ्गुका ।
शतपुष्पाहिङ्गुरास्नाचन्दनं रक्तचन्दनम् ॥
जातीपुष्प तुगाक्षीरी कमलं शर्करा तथा ।
अजमोदा च दन्ती च कल्कैरेतैश्च कार्षिकैः ॥
जीवद्वत्सैकवर्णानां घृतं प्रस्थं गवां पचेत् ।
चतुर्गुणेन पयसा पचेदारण्यगोमयैः ॥
सुतिथौ पुष्यनक्षत्रे मृद्भाण्डे ताम्रजे तथा ।
ततः पिबेच्छुभदिने नारी वा पुरुषोऽथवा ॥
एतत्सर्पिर्नरः पीत्वा स्त्रीषु नित्यं वृषायते ।
पुत्रं सञ्जनयेत् धीमान् वन्ध्यापि लभते सुतम् ॥

अल्पायुसं वा जनयेत् या च मृत्वा पुनःस्थिता ।
पुत्रमाप्नोति सा नारी बुद्धिमन्तं शतायुषम् ॥
एततफलघृतं नाम भरद्वाजेन भाषितम् ।
अनुक्तं लक्षणामूलं क्षिपन्त्यत्र चिकित्सकाः ॥७९—८१॥

Bharadvāja was also known as Vitatha. He is said to have become the adopted son of the Paurava King Bhārata, and thus became a Paurava.

CHAPTER VIII.

BHṚGU.

Brahmā desiring to create living beings, produced first the ten great Ṛṣis or Maharṣis: Marīci, Atri, Aṅgirā, Pulastya, Pulaha, Kratu, Pracetas, Vasiṣṭha, Bhṛgu and Nārada (Manu Saṁhitā i, 34). They are said to have been formed from his mind, or mental sons like unto himself (Viṣṇu Purāṇa, i, pp. 4, 5, 7). The list of the mental sons differs in the different Purāṇas. In the Mahābhāratā, Ādiparva, v. 25, 17, the first six names occur, but in Sāntiparva, v. 7569, Vasiṣṭha is included, thus making a total of seven (Saptarṣi) and in v. 12685, the number becomes twenty-one. In the Śatapatha Brāhmaṇa, their names are given as Gautama, Bharadvāja, Viśvā-Mitra, Jamadagni, Vasiṣṭha, Kaśyapa, and Atri. The Vāyu Purāṇa adds Bhṛgu to the list; the Viṣṇu Purāṇa adds Bhṛgu and Dakṣa and makes them nine.

In the Rāmāyaṇa iii. 14, 7-9, seventeen Maharṣis are mentioned. Bhṛgus and Aṅgirās are the progenitors of the Brāhmaṇas. Gṛtsamada, an Âṅgirasa, son of Sunohotra, became a Bhṛgu or Bhārgava, son of Śaunaka (see Rv. Anukramaṇi). Gṛtsamada is the "Seer" of the hymns in the second maṇdala of the Ṛgveda.

Śrī, the mother of the world and wife of Viṣṇu, is said to be the daughter of Bhṛgu by Khyāti (Viṣṇu Purāṇa i, 8, 12) though she is declared to be eternal like Viṣṇu. Khyāti was the daughter of the sage Karddama; but by another account she was the daughter of Prajāpati Dakṣa. His two sons were Dhātā and Vidhātā (Bhāgavat Purāna).

It is said in the Mahābhārata, that Pulomā, wife of Bhṛgu, was carried away by the demon Puloman. She was then pregnant, and in her fright, the fœtus fell from her womb. Puloman allowed the mother to depart with her infant who developed to be the sage Cyavana (*lit.* the fallen).

In the Mahābhārata, Śāntiparva, v. 6930 ff., we find a very interesting discussion on the origin of caste between Bhṛgu and Bharadvāja. Bhṛgu was of opinion that there was no distinction of castes; the Brahmaṇa according to their work formed the four castes.

GENEALOGY OF THE BHĀRGAVAS.

Bhṛgu m. Khyāti

- Śrī m. Viṣṇu
- Dhātā m. Âyāti
  - Prāṇa
    - Vedaśira
- Vidhātā m. Niyati
  - Mṛkuṇḍa
    - Mārkaṇḍeya

Vedaśira — Mārkaṇḍeya

Bhārgāvas.

It is said that he was sent by sages to enquire as to the god of the trinity, who was highest in rank. First he went to Brahmā, but he did not salute him intentionally. He was scolded by Brahmā for his bad manners. He appeased him, and then went to Śiva, whom also he did not show proper respect. Śiva grew angry but was soon propitiated. Next he went to Viṣṇu whom he found to be asleep. In disgust, he kicked him on the breast, whereupon the latter welcomed him, apologised for his sleep and massaged his feet as the sage must have been hurt there by the kick.

Bhṛgu's acts :

1. He cursed Nahuṣa, when the king kicked Āgastya, in whose hairs he remained concealed.

2. By his favour, king Vitahavya, a Kṣatriya, entered into the state of Brāhmanhood.

3. He pierced Vala (Sāma Veda, ii, 304).

4. He invented the Science of Archery.

5. Bhṛgu is one of the sages who first kindled the sacrificial fire (see Muir's paper on Manu, the progenitor of the Aryan Indians in Vol. XXX, J. R. A. S., pp. 410-416; Ṛv., viii, 43, 13; S. V., i, 18).

6. In Ś. P. Br., xi, 6, 1, 1 ff., Bhṛgu, the son of Brahmā, is said to have visited, by his father's commands, the four directions of the world, and he saw, amongst other things, that living beings were being cut into pieces and eaten by other men as the future retribution of the slaughters performed by them.

7. Bhṛgu is one of the sages, mentioned in the Caraka Saṁhitā I. i., who assembled in the Himalayan retreat to discuss about the means of relieving human suffering and of curing men suffering from various diseases. (See C. S. I. 1).

8. In the Mānava Dharmaśāstra the sage "Bhṛgu, here called a Manava, is introduced as Manu's disciple, through whom the great teacher has his work promulgated."

NĀRADA.

Nārada is the name of a famous Ṛṣi who figures so prominently in the Purāṇas. As a physician he is not much known. He is a Devarṣi,—one of the mental sons of Brahmā. He was cursed by his father for not helping him in the act of creation. He was born again as a Gandharva, Upavarhaṇ by name, and married Mālāvatī and other Gandharva maidens. He became guilty of misdemeanour, at the sight of the celestial Rambhā while dancing before Brahmā. He was again cursed and became the son of Kalāvatī, wife of Dramila, king of the Gopas, through the grace of sage Kaśyapa, whose seed fell on the ground. Next he abandoned his body, entered into Brahmā and regained his original form. He learned a little of the science of music from his fathe; Brahmā, became proficient in it from Ulukeśvara, a Gandharva, and finally became master of the Science through Kṛṣṇa. He invented Vin, a melodious instrument of music.

Books :—Nārada is said to be the author of the following books :—

1. Dhātulakṣmaṇa : To Nārada is ascribed this treatise on humours and pulsation.

Ms. I. O. 2715.

Begins : अथ धातुज्ञानं॥

वामभागे तु नारीणां दक्षिणे पुरूषस्यतु ।
लक्षणं लक्ष्यते सर्वं शुभाशुभ फलप्रदं ॥

Ends : एवं मूल्यादिभेदेन नाड़ीज्ञेया विचक्षणै: ।
स्वर्गेऽपि दुर्लभा विद्या गोपनीया प्रयत्नत:—

Colophon : इति नारदकृत धातुलक्षणं समाप्त ।

2. Nārada Saṁhitā : on Science of Music.

3. Nārada Smṛti : on Laws. Nāradīya Dharmaśāstra is the most systematic work of all the Smṛtis and is strictly confined to Law. The text has been translated by Dr. Jolly.

4. Nāradīya Purāṇa : one of the eighteen puranas of the Hindus.

Formulæ attributed to Nārada :—

1. Mahālakṣīvilāsa Rasa	...	R. S. S., p. 331.
2. Lakṣīvilāsa Rasa	...	" p. 319. R. C. IX., p. 59. R. S. S., p. 471.

1. Mahā Lakṣmīvilāsa Rasa.

महालक्ष्मीविलासरसः।

पलं वज्राभ्रचूर्णस्य तदर्द्धं गन्धकं भवेत्।

तदर्द्धं वङ्गभस्मापि तदर्द्धं पारदस्तथा।

तत्समं हरितालञ्च तदर्द्धं ताम्रभस्मकं।

रससाम्य कर्पूरं जातीकोषफले तथा।

वृद्धदारकवीजञ्च वीजं स्वर्णफलस्य च।

प्रत्येकं कार्षिकं भागं मृतस्वर्णञ्च शाणकं।

निष्पिष्य वटिका कार्य्या द्विगुञ्जाफलमानतः।

निहन्ति सन्निपातोत्थान् गदान् घोरान् सुदारुणान्।

गलोत्थानन्त्रवृद्धिञ्च तथातिसारमेव च।

कुष्ठमेकादशविधं प्रमेहान् विंशतिन्तथा।

श्लीपदं कफवातोत्थं चिरजं कुलजन्तथा।

नाड़ीव्रणं व्रणं घोरं गुदामयभगन्दरं।

कास पीनस यक्ष्मार्शः स्थौल्य दौर्गन्ध्यरक्तनुत्।

आमवातं सर्व्वरूपं जिह्वास्तम्भं गलग्रहं।

उदरं कर्णनासाक्षिमुखवैजाड्यमेव च।

सर्व्वशूलं शिरःशूलं स्त्रीरोगञ्च विनाशयेत्।

वटिकां प्रातरेकैकां खादेन्नित्यं यथावलं।

अनुपानमिहप्रोक्तं मांसं पिष्टं पयोदधि।

वारिभक्तं सुरासीधुसेवनात कामरूपधृक्।

वृद्धोपि तरुणस्पर्द्धी न च शुक्रक्षयो भवेत्।

न च लिङ्गस्य शैथिल्यं नकेशा यान्ति पक्वतां।

नित्यं गच्छेच्छतं स्त्रीणां मत्तवारणविक्रमः।

द्विलक्षयोजनी दृष्टिर्ज्जायते पौष्टिकस्तथा।

प्रोक्तः प्रयोगराजोयं नारदेन महात्मना।

रसोलक्ष्मीविलासोऽयं वासुदेवो जगत्पतिः।

प्रसादादस्य भगवान् लक्षनारीषु वल्लभः॥

2. Lakṣmīvilāsa Rasa.

लक्ष्मीविलास रसः।

पलं कृष्णाभ्रचूर्णस्य तदर्द्धं रसगन्धके।

कर्पूरस्य तदर्द्धन्तु जातीकोषफले तथा।

वृद्धदारकवीजमुन्मत्तकस्य च

त्रैलोक्यविजयावीजं विदारीकन्दमेव च।

नारायणी तथा नागवला चातिवला तथा।

वीजं गोक्षुरकस्यापि हैज्जलं वीजमेव च।

एतेषां कार्षिकं चूर्णं गृहीत्वा वारिणा ततः।

निष्पिष्य वटिका कार्य्या त्रिगुञ्जाफलमानतः।

निहन्ति सन्निपातोत्थान् गदान् घोरान् सुदारुणान्।

वातोत्थान् पैत्तिकांश्चापि नास्त्यत्र नियमः क्वचित्।

कुष्ठमष्टादशविधं प्रमेहान् विंशतिं तथा।

नाड़ीव्रणं व्रणं घोरं गुदामयभगन्दरं।

श्लीपदं कफवातोत्थं चिरजं कुलसम्भवम्।

गलशोथमन्त्रवृद्धिमतीसारं सुदारुणम्।

काशपीनसयच्मार्शःस्थौल्यं दौर्बल्यमेव च ।
आमवातं सर्व्वरूपं जिह्वास्तम्भं गलग्रहम् ।
उदरं कर्णनासाचिमुखवैजात्यमेवच ।
सर्व्वशूलं शिरःशूलं स्त्रीणां गदनिसूदनम् ।
वटिकां प्रातरेकेकां खादेन्नित्यं यथाबलम् ।
अनुपानमिह प्रोक्तं माषं पिष्टपयोदधि ।
वारितक्रसुरासौधुसेवनात् कामरूपधृक् ।
वृद्धोऽपि तरुणस्पर्द्धी नच शुक्रस्य संचयः ।
नच लिङ्गस्य शैथिल्यं न केशा यान्ति पक्कताम् ।
नित्यं शतस्त्रियोगच्छन्मत्तवारणविक्रमः ।
द्विलचयोजनी दृष्टिर्जायते पौष्टिकः परः ।
प्रोक्तः प्रयोगराजोऽयं नारदेन महात्मना ।

रसो लक्ष्मीविलासस्तु वासुदेव जगत्पतिः ।
अभ्यासाद् यस्य भगवान् लचनारीषु वल्लभः ॥

इति लक्ष्मीविलास रसः ।

Rasendra Cintāmaṇi.

लक्ष्मीविलासोरसः ।

पलं कृष्णाभ्रचूर्णस्य तदर्द्धौ रसगन्धकौ ।
बला नागबला भीरु विदारीकन्दमेव च ।
कृष्णधूस्तूरनिचूलं गोक्षुरवृद्धदारयोः ।
वीजं शक्रागुनस्यापि जातीकोषफले तथा ।
कर्पूरञ्चैव कर्षांगु सूक्ष्मचूर्णं पृथक पृथक ।
गृहीत्वा चाष्टमांशेन स्वर्णं पर्णरसेन च ।
वटिकां स्विन्नचणकप्रमाणां कारयेद्भिषक् ।
रसोलक्ष्मीविलासोऽयं पूर्व्ववद्गुणकारकः ॥

Rasendrasāra Saṁgraha.

MARĪCI.

Marīci is described as one of the Prajāpatis (Lords of creation)—one of the seven great Ṛṣis (Saptarṣi), the mental sons of Brahmā, who are represented by the seven stars of the Great Bear in the sky. He married Kalā the daughter of Karddama Muni. He was the father of Kaśyapa.

In the Caraka Saṁhitā, I, xii, he is referred to as questioning the usefulness of a discussion on the qualities of Air in the Āyurveda :—

तच्छ्रुत्वा वार्य्योविदवचो मरीचिरुवाच। यद्यप्येवमेतत् किमर्थोऽस्यास्य वचने विज्ञाने वा सामर्थ्यमस्ति भिषग्विद्यायां भिषग्विद्यां वाधिकृत्येयं कथा प्रवृत्तेति॥

He attaches more importance to fire than air as capable of causing good and ill health in a person :—

मारीचिरुवाच। अग्निरेव शरीरे पित्तान्तर्गतः कुपिताकुपितः शुभाशुभानि करोति। तद्यथा—

पक्तिमपक्तिं दर्शनमदर्शनं मात्रामात्रत्वमूष्मणः प्रकृतिविकृतिवर्णौ शौर्य्यं भय क्रोध हृष मोहं प्रसादमित्येवमादीनि चापराणि द्वन्द्वानीति॥

C. S. I. xii.

As regards the part of the fœtus formed first, he says, that it is impossible to answer the question, as the parts cannot be seen :—

परोक्षत्वादचिन्त्यमिति मारीचिः॥

C. S. IV. vi.

KACA.

"A son of Brihaṣpati. According to the Mahābhārata, he became the disciple of Sukra or Usanas, the priest of the Asuras, with the object of obtaining from him the mystic power of restoring the dead to life, a charm which Sukra alone possessed. To prevent this the Asuras killed Kacha again and again, but on both occasions he was restored to life by the sage at the intercession of Devayāni, his daughter, who had fallen in love with Kacha. They killed him a third time, burnt his body and mixed ashes with Sukra's wine, but Devayāni again implored her father to bring back the young man. Unable to resist his daughter's importunity, Sukra once more performed the charm, and to his surprise heard the voice of Kaca come out from his own belly. To save his own life, Sukra taught his pupil the great charm. He then allowed himself to be ripped open, and Kacha, upon coming out, performed the charm and restored his master to life. This incident is said to have caused Sukra to prohibit the use of wine to Brahmans. Kacha resisted the proposal of Devayani, and refused to make her his wife. She then cursed him, that the charms he had learnt from her father should be powerless and he in return condemned her to be sought by no Brahmana and to become the wife of a Kshatriya."

Dowson's Hindu Mythology.

Formula :

Kaca is said to be the author of a formula for stoppage of urination in Cakradatta.

इत्युवाच कचः—

नलकुशकाशेक्षुशिफां क्वथितां प्रातःसुशीतलांससिताम् ।
पिबतः प्रयाति नियतं मूत्रग्रह इत्युवाच कचः ॥

मूत्राघात चिकित्सा—चक्रदत्त, p 190.

CHAPTER IX.

VIŚVĀMITRA.

Viśvāmitra is the name of an ancient physician who with other Ṛṣis, is mentioned to have learned the Science of Medicine from Bharadvāja. He flourished during the Vedic times and is said to have composed many Vedic hymns. He was contemporary to Vaśiṣṭha, with whom he often quarrelled. He was a King, a Kṣatriya rāja, but by severe penance and austerities became a Brāhmaṇa afterwards. His deeds are described in detail in the Rāmāyaṇa and the Purāṇas. He is the father of Suśruta, the disciple of Dhanvantari and the famous author of Suśruta Saṁhitā. In Susruta Saṁhi ā, V. viii, he is said to have once gone to the hermitage of Vaśiṣṭha, whom he caused to be angry. In anger the sage perspired, and drops of perspiration and other excrementitious matter fell on dried grass; and thus the different kinds of spiders are said to have been formed.

> बिश्वामित्रो नृपवरः कदाचिदृषिसत्तमं ।
> वशिष्टं कोपयामास गत्वाश्रमपदं किल ।।
> कुपितस्य मुनेस्तस्य ललाटात् स्वेदबिन्दवः ।
> अपतन्दर्शनादेव मध्यधत्ताषीच्णवर्चसः ।
> लूणे तृणे महर्षीणां धेन्वर्थं सम्भृतेऽपिच ॥
> ततो जातस्त्विमा घोरा नानारूपामहाविषाः ।
> अपकाराय वर्तन्ते नृपसाधन वाहने ।।

Viśvāmitra, the composer of ancient Vedic hymns, is said to be the same person who figures in the Rāmāyaṇa and later literature. Viśvāmitra is a *gotra* name, and any descendant of the sage is described as Viśvāmitra.

For a detailed account of the conflict between Vaśiṣṭha and Viśvāmitra see Mbh., Ramyn., R. V., Dr. Roth's "Dissertations on the Literature and History of the Veda," "Zur Litteratur und Geschichte des Weda, Stutgart," 1846 ; Muir's Original Sanskrit Texts, Vol. I, p. 317.

His parents: In the Ṛv., he is described as the son of a King named Kuśika, but in later literature he is said to be the son of Gādhi, King of Kāṇykubja, and a descendant of Puru. So he is styled as a Kauśika and also as a Paurava (Harivamṣa). In the genealogy, it would be found that Gādhi was of the Kuśika race. So he was called a Kauśika and also Gādhi-nandana. Satyavatī was the daughter of Gādhi who gave her in marriage to a Bhārgava Brāhmaṇa named Ricika. Ricika prepared two dishes of food for his wife and his mother-in-law. The dishes were exchanged and the result was that Satyavatī gave birth to Jamadagni, the warrior Brahman and the mother bore Visvāmitra, a Kṣatriya king with the qualities of a Brāhmaṇa.

Both Visvāmitra and Vasiṣṭha became the family priests of King Sudāsa. They quarrelled and cursed each other and each killed the hundred sons of his rival. Viṣvāmitra, though father of hundred sons, adopted his nephew Śunah-Śephaḥ as his heir which was objected by his fifty sons who were cursed to form the Dasyus of the frontier.

"अथैनमुवाच—वरुणं राजानं उपधाव, 'पुत्रो मे जायताम, तेन त्वा यजा, इति तथेति' स वरुणं राजानं उपससार, 'पुत्रो मे जायतां तेन त्वा यजा' इति तथेति तस्य ह पुत्रो जज्ञे 'रोहितो' नाम। तं होवाच 'अजनिवै ते पुत्रः, यजस्व मानेन' इति। स होवाच पशुः निर्दशो भवति, अथ स मेध्यो भवति, निर्दशोन्व-स्त्वथ त्वा यजा—इति तथेति—स निर्दश आस—तं हेवाच 'निर्दशोन्वभूद, यजस्व मानेन इति स होवाच 'यदा वेपशोर्दन्ता जायन्ते अथ स मेध्यो भवति, दन्तान्वस्य जीयन्तां अथत्वा यजा' इति तथेति—*

'पुत्त्रमामन्त्रयामास तथायं वैं मह्यं त्वामददात्, हन्त त्वयाहं इमं यजा' इति स ह "न" इत्युक्त्वा धनुरादायारण्यं अपतस्थौ। इति ह षष्ठं संवत्सरं अरण्ये चचार—सोऽजीगर्त्तं सौयवसिं ऋषिं अशनया परीतमरण्यमुपेयाय, तस्यह त्रयः पुत्त्रा आसुः, शुनः-पुच्छः शुनः-शेपः शुनोलाङ्गुल इति, तं हेवाच, ऋषे! अहं ते शतं ददामि, एषामेकेनात्मानं निष्क्रीणा' इति, स ज्येष्ठं पुत्त्रं निगृह्णान उवाच—'न्विमामिति' नो एवमिति कनिष्ठं माता, तौह मध्यमं सम्पादयाञ्चक्रतुः। शुनःशेपे तस्यह शतं दत्वा स तमादाय, सोऽरण्याद् ग्राममियाय, स पितरमेत्य उवाच—ततः हन्ताहमनेन आत्मानं निष्क्रीणा इति।

ऐतरेय ब्राह्मण पृ० ६७—७६,

(सोसाइटी)

"अथह शुनःशेपो विश्वामित्रस्य अङ्कमाससाद, सहोवाचाजीगर्त्तः सौयवसिं ऋषे! पुनर्मे पुत्त्रं देहीति 'नेति' होवाच विश्वामित्रो देवा वा इमं मह्यं अरासतेति स ह देवरातो वैश्वामित्र आस'

ऐतरेय ब्राह्मण—७—३—५।

In the Rāmāyaṇa, king Viśvāmitra is said to have paid a visit to the hermitage of Vasiṣṭha and was hospitably entertained by the sage. The king wanted his cow Kāmadhenu, or Nandini ; and when he attempted to take away the cow by force, his armies were defeated by the army called forth by the cow, and the sage cursed the hundred sons of Visvāmitra to be turned into ashes.

King Triśaṅku, a descendant of the race of Ikṣāku, desired to celebrate a sacrifice in order that he might ascend bodily to heaven. Vasiṣṭha declared it to be impossible but Visvāmitra by his austerities accomplished his object against the wish of the Vāsiṣṭhas and the gods.

The story of the Visvāmitra's amour with the celestial nymphs Menakā and Rambhā, and the birth of Śakuntalā is well-known to the readers of the celebrated epics.

Afterwards when Visvāmitra became a Brāhmaṇa, Vasiṣṭha welcomed him with honours.

In the Purāṇas the story of King Hariścandra, son of Triśaṅku, who was persecuted by the sage, is narrated. Vasiṣṭha cursed Viśvāmitra to become a crane, who also cursed the former to be another bird, and as birds they fought but were reconciled by Brahmā. In the Rāmāyaṇa, Visvāmitra is said to have taken Rāma and Lakṣaṇa with him to free the hermitages of Brāhmaṇas from the Rākṣasas; and it was through him that the four sons of King Daśaratha were married to the daughters of King Janaka.

Viśvāmitra ordered the river Sarasvati to deliver Vasiṣṭha to him so that he might kill him. But as Vasiṣṭha came towards Visvāmitra, the river carried away Vasiṣṭha in another direction.

The Aśvin-Rasāyaṇa as it occurs in the Navanitaka " implies (v. 781*b*) that by medical tradition the formula was ascribed to the ancient physician Viśvāmitra, apparently the respected father of Suśruta. That inscription is contradicted, however, by the initial verse (v. 773*b*) and by the name in the colophon, which attribute the formula to the Asvins," (I. A., Feb. 14, p. lx).

Visvāmitra as a medical author is qnoted in

Nivandha Saṁgraha.

1. तत्र शङ्खनाभे: प्रधानात्वादेव चार:स्यात् एवञ्च विश्वामित्रभोजोक्तभाग-
कल्पना निरस्ता ।

2. पाटल्या: पारिभद्राद्वातिलाद्वापि यवाग्रजात।
त्वगीलात्वग्युतं चूर्णं साञ्चरवारिणा पिवेत् ॥

Vyākhyā Kusumāvalī.

1. श्वेतपुष्प: कृष्णपुष्पो रक्तपुष्पस्तथैव च ।
पीतैरन्यो वरास्तेषु कालमुष्क: प्रकीर्त्तित: ॥

2. पानीयभावनायाय परिस्राव्यं चतुर्गुणम् ।
जलेऽर्धमवशिष्टं च चाराभ्ये ग्राह्यमिष्यते ॥

3. पृथ्वीकाचिचकव्योषहपुषाजाजिसैन्धवैः ।
सचव्यपिप्पलीमूलैः पिष्टैर्दीप्यकसंयुतैः ॥
मूलदाड़िमकोलानां रसे पयसि दध्नि च ।
सिद्धं घृतं जयेद्गुल्मं वातोत्थं वह्निदीपनम् ॥

4. पाटलीं परिभद्रांश्च तिलांश्चापि यवाग्रजात् ।
कणेलात्वग्युतं चूर्णं मुष्कक्षारवारिणा ।
पिबेद् गुड़ेन मिश्रं वा लिह्यान्मूत्रविघातनुत् ॥

5. विड़ङ्गफलमात्रं तु जातमात्रस्य भेषजम् ।
एतेनैव प्रमाणेन मासि मासि प्रवर्धते ॥
कोलास्थिमात्रं चीरादे दद्याभेषज्य कोविदः ।
चीरान्नादे कोलमात्रं कुमारे भेषजं हितं ॥
अन्नादे मधुसर्पिर्भ्याम् कुस्तोदुम्बर संमितं ॥

Vyākhya Madhukoṣa.

1. यदा त्वचमतिक्रम्य तद्धातुनवगाहते ।
हित्वा किलास संज्ञान्तु कुष्ठसंज्ञांलभेत्तदा ॥

Tattva Candrikā.

1. See 2, V. K. V.
2. विश्वामित्रेणापि दाड़िमरसः एवोक्तः ।
3. See 2, Ni. S.

Bhāva Prakāśa.

1. See 5, V. K. V.

VAŚIṢṬHA.

A famous Vedic Ṛṣi to whom many hymns are ascribed. He is classed among the ten Prajāpatis and the seven Maharṣis and is said to have been a mind-born son of Brahmā (Manu) or, according to another account, a son of Mitra and Varuṇa by Urvasī (R. V. vii, 33, 1). There was a special rivalry between him and the sage Viśvāmitra who wanted to take away Nandini "the cow of plenty" by force from the hermitage of Vaśiṣṭha. He appears to be the family priest of King Sudāsa (Aitareya Brāhmaṇa and R. V.) or to his son Kalmāṣpāda (Mbh.), and to Ikṣāku and his descendants (Viṣṇu Purāṇa). Muir says: "Vasistha according to all accounts must have been possessed of a vitality altogether superhuman" for the name is "used not to denote merely a person belonging to a family so called but to represent the founder of the family himself as taking part in the transactions of many successive ages." Vaśiṣṭha is a gotra name and hence arose the confusion, for all his descendants are styled as Vaśiṣṭha.

King Kalmāṣpāda, son of Sudāsa, while hunting in a forest, met Śaktri, the eldest son of the sage Vasiṣṭha, and struck him with a whip as he stood on his way. Śaktri cursed him to be a man-eating Rākhasa, and Viśvamitra ordered a man-eater to enter the body of the king. Once he offered human flesh to a Brāhmaṇa, Mitrasala by name, who also cursed him to the same effect. The king then ate Śaktri and the hundred sons of Vasiṣṭha who, however, took pity on him and restored him to his natural condition after twelve years. In the Viṣṇu Purāṇa the story is told somewhat differently. He killed a tiger, but another tiger, who disappeared, assumed the form of Vasiṣṭha, the priest, in a sacrifice performed by the King. Later, he assumed the form of a cook and served a dish of human flesh to the sage Vasiṣṭha. Thereupon the sage cursed the king, but afterwards knowing him to be innocent, limited the period of curse to twelve years. The angry king being prevented by his wife Madayanti from uttering a counter-curse upon the sage, threw the water on his feet which consequently became spotted (Kalmāṣpāda). After the term, he assumed his natural form and his wife became pregnant and gave birth to Aśmaka by an operation of Cæserian section performed by herself with a stone.

Vasiṣṭha's wife was Ūrjā, one of the daughters of Dakṣa. She gave birth to his seven sons. In the Rāmāyaṇa and Bhāgavat Purāṇa, however, Arundhatī is said to be his wife. His descendants are known as Vāsiṣṭha and Vāṣkalas.

King Nimi of the Ikṣvāku race requested him to officiate as his priest in a sacrifice. But as he already promised Indra to act as a priest, he consented to be his priest after the sacrifice of Indra was over. Nimi engaged Gautama to be his priest. Vasiṣṭha came back as he promised, became angry, and cursed the king to lose his body. Nimi uttered his curse and the energy of the sage entered into the vigour of Mitra and Varuṇa who were his fathers as their seed fell at the sight of the divine Urvasī.

Vasiṣṭha once tried to enter the house of his father Varuṇa for food by night as he tasted no food for three days. The house-dog barked as he entered and he put the dog to sleep by a hymn (Ṛv., iv. 121) which is recommended to be recited by burglars.

His name appears in the list of the sages mentioned in Caraka Saṁhitā, I.1, who wanted to learn the science of medicine.

Books : I; A Law Book is ascribed to him. In the Vaśiṣtha Dharmaśāstra we find

शोनितशुक्रसम्भव: पुरुषो मातापितृ-निमित्तक: । P. 44.

"The man is formed from blood (or ovum of woman) and semen (of man); the father and mother are accidental causes."

2. He is the reputed author of *Vasiṣṭha Saṁhitā*, a treatise on medicine.

It is quoted in Trimalla Bhatta's Yoga Taraṅgini. MSS., I. O. 2705, 2706. fol. 6a.

In the Ṛg Veda many hymns are attributed to Vasiṣṭha : we quote a few hymns below :

Ṛv. vii, 18, 4, 5, 21 to 25 : Relates the connection between Vasiṣṭha and Sudāsa.

33. 1 : Let not the Vaśiṣṭhyas be far off to help me.

2 : They have brought here Indra across the Vaisanta from the Soma offerings.

3 : Indra delivered Sudāsa through the prayer of the Vaśiṣṭhyas

4 : Vaśiṣthyas infused energy into Indra.

5 : Indra, praised by Vaśiṣṭha, helped the Tritsus.

6 : Vaśiṣṭha marched in front, and the Tritsus were deployed.

7 : Vaśiṣṭhas know the three deities.

8 : Vasiṣṭha's hymns are bright as the sun, deep as ocean, and swift as wind.

9 : Vasiṣṭhas sat down by the Apsaras.

10 : Thy birth is twofold : (1) when Mitra and Varuṇa saw thee quitting the flame of lightning. (2) When Agastya brought thee to the people.

11 : Vaśiṣṭha, the son of Mitra and Varuṇa, born from the soul of Urvasī.

12 : He was born of the Apsaras.

13 : Mitra and Varuṇa dropped their seed into the jar. Thus arose Māna (Agastya), and also Ṛṣi Vaśiṣṭha.

83. 1 to 8 : Vasiṣṭha, the priest of King Sudāsa, helped him to gain the victory in the battle of the ten kings. Both Vasiṣṭha and Sudāsa belonged to the tribe of the Tṛtsus.

86, 4 : Refers to Varuṇa's anger against Vasiṣṭha who entreats to be forgiven.

87, 4 : Vasiṣṭha received a revelation from Varuṇa.

88, 3, 1 : He embarked on the boat with Varuṇa.

2 : Varuṇa took him into the boat ; he made him a Ṛṣi, an utterer of hymn.

3 : Where is that friendship between us.

4 : If I have committed any offence, I pray Varuṇa to grant us protection.

104 : Overwhelmed with grief for the death of his hundred sons when killed by the sons of Sudasa, Vasiṣṭha contradicts the allegations that he was a Yātudhāna : 'May I die this day, if I be a Yātudhāna, or if I have destroyed any man's life ; and may Indra and Agni smite the liars who speak against me.'

The following formula is ascribed to sage Vasiṣṭha:

1. Haritakī Avaleha by Vasiṣṭha......G. N., Vol. I. p. 146.

1. Vāsiṣṭha Haritakī Avaleha.

वासिष्ठहरीतक्यवलेहः ।

यवाढकं सप्त जलाढकानि हरीतकीनां च शतं गुरूणाम् ।
दन्त्यश्वगन्धाचिरिबिल्वमूलं भल्लातकांश्चापि च पक्वबिल्वम् ॥
उभे हरिद्रे गजपिप्पली च मूलानि पत्राणि च चित्रकस्य ।
पिप्पल्यपामार्गमथात्मगुप्ता सर्वाणि कुर्यात्पलसंमितानि ॥
लौहे समादाय पचेत्कटाहे द्विपञ्चमूलं च यवप्रमाणम् ।
मृदग्निसिद्धांश्च यवान्विदित्वा शनैः प्रयत्नादवतारयेच्च ॥
निःस्राव्य तेनैव जलेन सम्यक् सार्धं पुराणस्य शतं गुडस्य ।
भूयो गुरूणामथ तत्र दद्याद्धरीतकीनां च सहस्रमन्यत् ॥
प्रस्थं पुराणस्य घृतस्य चैव नवस्य तैलस्य च तावदेव ।
शीते मधु स्नेहसमं च दद्यात्पलानि चाष्टावथ पिप्पलीनाम् ॥
पथ्ये सलेहे त्वथ भक्ष्यमाणे सर्वा रुजो नाशयती हि मासात् ।
मासद्वयेनैव च नेत्ररोगान्निहन्ति गार्ध्रं लभते च चक्षुः ॥
मासैस्त्रिभिर्नाशयती हि कुष्ठं विशीर्णतां चाङ्गुलिनासिकानाम् ।
भगन्दरश्लीपदवातगुल्मानर्शांस्यथो मासचतुष्टयेन ॥
केशान्घनाकुञ्चितदीर्घनीलांस्त पञ्चभिश्चैव करोति मासैः ।
सहस्रसङ्ख्यां च तथोपयुज्य बलं लभेदुत्तमकुञ्जरस्य ॥
स्वरं मयूरस्य जवं हयस्य शरच्छशाङ्कस्य तथैव कान्तिम् ।
सौभाग्यमेधास्मृतिसत्वतेजःशोभान्वितः पद्मसमानगन्धः ॥
जीवेत्समानां च सहस्रमन्यत्प्रयोगकालादिति सिद्धवाक्यम् ।
न चान्नपानेऽध्वनि मैथुने वा नरेण किंचित्परिहार्यमस्मिन् ॥
समीक्ष्य कल्पं तु रसायनानां चकार योगं भगवान्वसिष्ठः ॥

ATRI.

The sage Atri with his wife Anasūyā lived in a hermitage in the forest on the south of the Citra-Kuṭa mountain. It is told in the Rāmāyaṇa that when Sītā visited them, Anasūyā gave Sītā an ointment which was to keep her beautiful for ever. (See Dowson's Hindu Mythology, p. 15.) Anasūyā was the mother of the sage Dūrvāsā, the ascetic Dattātreya and Soma, the Moon.

Atri married Anasūyā, one of the daughters of Prajāpati Dakṣa.

His son is Ātreya and his sons and descendants belonging to his race are the Ātreyas.

Atri is one of the Maharṣis or great saints. He composed hymns for the magnification of Agni, Indra, Aśvins and the Viśvadevas. He is also described as one of the ten Prajapatis or lords of creation (Manu), as a mental son of Brahmā, and as one of the Saptarṣis or seven 'Seers' or Ṛṣis.

ANGIRĀ.

Aṅgirā was one of the seven Maharṣis and also one of the ten Prajāpatis. Aṅgirā is often used as a synonym of Agni, and like him, is described as the priest of the gods and as the lord of sacrifice. Aṅgira is said to have been the father of Agni in the hymns to Agni and Indra. Aṅgiras is also described as the son of Uru by Āgneyī, the daughter of Agni. A different version refers his birth from the mouth of Brahmā. He married Smṛti or 'Memory,' Swadhā, 'Oblation' and Sati 'Truth,' the daughters of Dakṣa, and Sraddhā, 'Faith,' the daughter of sage Karddama. The Ṛks or hymns were his daughters and the Manas and Haviṣmats were his sons. His other sons were Utathya, Vṛhaspati and Mārkaṇḍeya. He begot sons on the Kṣatriya Rathi-tara's wife and they were called Āngiras. He is described as the law-giver and also as a writer on astronomy. He is the regent of the planet Jupiter.

VĀMADEVA.

Vāmadeva is a Vedic sage. To him are ascribed many hymns. He is said to have come in this world with the speed of a hawk through his mother's side and not *per via naturales,* as did Buddha in his birth. In times of extreme distress he cooked entrails of a dog for his food in order to save his life.

In the Gada Nigraha, a formula for a pill is ascribed to Vāmadeva for the cure of Prameha :

प्रमेहे वामदेवेन कथिता गुटिका—

कटुत्रिकं वचा मुस्ता विड़ङ्गं चित्रकं विषम् ।

एतानि समभागानि पथ्यं च द्विगुणा विषात् ॥

पञ्चविंशद्गुड़ाद्भागा: क्राथयेन्मृदुनाग्निना ।

वदरसमाऽत्त गुटिका कार्या, एषा गुटिका प्रमेहं, आमवातं, गुल्मं, मन्दाग्नि हन्ति, विशेषतश्च लालामेहम् ॥

G. N., Vol. I, p. 237.

SANATKUMĀR.

He is said to have composed the Sanatkumār a Saṁhitā of the Pāñcarātrāgama.

MSS. G. O. M. L., Vol. XXIII No. 13102.

This is stated to form the 94th Adhyāya of the Sanatkumārasaṁhitā of the Pāñcarātrāgama and deals with treatment of eye-diseases. It is said to have been originally revealed by Sanatkumāra to Nārada. The kind of treatment explained herein is said to have met with success in the case of Bṛhadratha, son of Paribhadra, king of Kāsī (vide R. No. 1327a).

Beginning :

शुक्लाम्बरधरं विष्णुं . . विष्वक्सेनं तमाश्रये ।
सनत्कुमारं योगीन्द्रं सिद्धाश्रमनिवासिनम् ।
नारदः प्रणिपत्याथ वचनं चेदमब्रवीत् ॥
भगवन् योगिनां श्रेष्ठ सर्वतत्त्वविशारद ।
सर्वरोगहरास्त्वत्तः कल्पाश्च विविधाः श्रुताः ॥
इदानीमक्षिरोगस्य शान्तिं ब्रूहि तपोधन ।
इत्युक्तश्च मुनिश्रेष्ठस्त्रिज्ञार्थश्चर्वमन्त्रवित् ॥

सनत्कुमारः—

शृणु नारद धर्मज्ञ कल्पनारायणाख्यकम् ।
अक्षिरोगहरं पुण्यमायुष्यं पापनाशनम् ॥

नारदः—

इमं कल्पं पुरा लोके यः कृत्वा सुखमाप्नुयात् ।
तमहं श्रोतुमिच्छामि भवान्वक्तुमिहार्हसि ॥

सनत्कुमारः—

काशीपुर्यां पुरा ब्रह्मन् आसीद्राजा सुधार्मिकः ।
पारिभद्र इति ख्यातः तस्य पुत्रो बृहद्रथः ॥

* * *

भगवन् मम पुत्रस्य अचिरोगो भयावहः ।
तस्य शान्तिर्भवेत्केन तत्त्वं ब्रूहि महामुने ॥
मध्वक्तैः तिन्त्रिणीपुष्पैः चक्रगाथविया हुनेत् ।
खर्जूरं [1] नालिकेरं च द्राक्षां धात्रीं हरीतकीम् ॥

Colophon :

इति पाञ्चरात्रे महोपनिषदि सनत्कुमारसंहितायां शान्तितन्त्रे अमृतकनारायणा ... नाम चतुर्नवतितमोऽध्यायः ॥

End :

किमत्र बहुनोक्तेन सर्वसिद्धिकरो ह्यसौ ।
आचार्यादनभिप्राप्तः प्राप्तश्चादसदच्चिरः ॥
अभ्यस्तोपि सदा मन्त्रः श्रेयसे नाम कल्पते ।
इति गुह्यतमं प्रोक्तं रहस्यमतिदुर्बल(लंभ)म् ॥
एवं ज्ञात्वा भवेत्स्वस्थः किंपुनः पाठतो जनाः ।

---

[1] मातुलङ्गम् इति पाठान्तरम्

CHAPTER X

KĀMA DEVA

Kāma is the god of desire, and as such he is said in the Ṛgveda to be the cause of creation. The Atharvaveda magnified Kāma as the supreme God, and there he is identified with Agni. In the Greek mythology Eros, the god of love, is similarly described in the creation of the universe. He is the son of Dharma (Justice) and Śraddhā (Faith) (Taitt. Br.), or of Lakṣmī (Fortune) (Harivaṁśa). He is also said to have sprung from the heart of Brahmā or from water (irāja). He is also styled 'self-existent' or 'un-born.'

Rati or Revā, the daughter of Dakṣa, is his wife. She is the Venus of the Hindoos. Kāma inspired Śiva with amour for Pārvatī and was reduced to ashes by the god's angry eye on his forehead. He was born again as Pradyumna, son of Kṛṣṇa and Rukmiṇī. His son is Aniruddha and his daughter, Tṛṣā. After the death of her husband, Rati lived in the house of Śambara daitya as Māyāvatī.

He is handsome in appearance, and rides on a parrot. His bow is of sugarcane, bowstring of bees, and the arrow-tips flowery. His banner displays a Makara or a fish.

Formulæ: The following formulæ are ascribed to Kāmadeva :

1. Methī Modaka ...	Kāmadeva ...	A.R. ...	p. 53
2. Kāmadeva Ghṛta ...	„ ...	„ ...	p. 120

1. Methī Modaka.

मेथी-मोदक ।

त्रिकटु त्रिफला मुस्तजीरकद्वय धान्यकम् ।
कटफलं पौष्करं शृङ्गी यमानी सैन्धवं विड़म् ॥
तालीशकेशरं पत्रं त्वगेला च फलं तथा ।
जातीकोषं लवङ्गञ्च मराकर्पूर चन्दनम् ॥
यावन्त्येतानि चूर्णानितावदेव तु मेथिका ।
सर्वचूर्णं मोदकः कार्य्यः पुरातन गुड़ेन च ॥
घृतेन मधुना किञ्चित् खादेदग्निबलं प्रति ।
अग्निञ्च कुरुते दीप्तं स्वामि मेदं महौषधम् ॥
बलवर्णकरोह्येष संग्रह ग्रहणीहरः ।
प्रमेहान् विंशतिं हन्ति मूत्राघातं तथाश्मरीम् ॥
पाण्डुरोगं तथा कासं यक्ष्माणं हन्ति कामलाम् ।
स्तनौ च पतितौ गाढ़ौ स्यातां तालफलोपमौ ॥
दृष्टिप्रसादनश्चैष नारीनाञ्चैव पुत्रदः ।
भाषितं कामदेवेन मेथीमोदकसंज्ञकः ।

---

2. Kāmadeva Ghṛta.

कामदेवघृतः ।

अश्वगन्धापलशतं तदर्द्धं गोक्षुरस्य च ।
शतावरी विदारि च शालपर्णी बला तथा ॥
अश्वत्थास्य च शुङ्गानि पद्मबीजं पुनर्णवा ।
काश्मरीफलमेतत्तु माषबीजं तथैवच ॥
पृथग् दशपलान् भागांश्चतुर्द्रोणेऽम्भसः पचेत् ।
चतुर्भागावशेषन्तु काषायमवतारयेत् ॥
मृद्वीकापद्मकं कुष्ठं पिप्पलीरक्तचन्दनम् ।
बालकं नागपुष्पञ्च आत्मगुप्तफल तथा ॥

नीलोत्पलं शारिवे द्वे जीवनीयं विशेषतः

पृथक्कर्षसमञ्चैव शर्करायाः पलद्वयम् ॥

रसस्यपौण्ड्रकेक्षुणामाढ़कं तत्र दापयेत् ।

चतुर्गुणेन पयसा घृतप्रस्थं विपाचयेत् ॥

रक्तपित्तं क्षतक्षीणं कामलां वातशोणितम् ।

हलीमकं तथा शोथं वर्णभेदं स्वरक्षयम् ॥

अरोचकं मूत्रकृच्छ्रं पार्श्वशूलञ्च नाशयेत् ।

एतद्राज्ञां प्रयोक्तव्यं वह्वन्तःपुरचारिणाम् ॥

स्त्रीणाञ्चैवानपत्यानां दुर्व्वलाञ्च देहिनाम् ।

क्लीवानामल्पशुक्राणां जीर्णानामल्परेतसाम् ॥

श्रेष्ठं बलकरं हृद्यं वृष्यं पेयं रसायनम् ।

ओजस्तेजस्करञ्चैव आयुःप्राणं विवर्द्धनम् ॥

सम्बर्द्धयति शुक्रञ्च पुरुषं दूर्व्वलेन्द्रियम् ।

कामदेव इतिख्यातः सर्व्वरोगेषु शस्यते ॥

PULASTYA.

Pulastya is one of the mental sons of Brahmā. It is said that he was born from the ears of the creator. He is one of the Saptarṣi or seven sages. He used to practise austerities near the hermitage of the great Muni Tṛṇavindu, by the side of mount Sumeru. The Apsarās and the daughters of sages used to dance and play music there. This annoyed Pulastya. He cursed that any girl, whom he would see, would be pregnant. Havirbhu, the daughter of Ṛṣi Karddama, or of sage Tṛṇavindu by another account, thus became *prægnans*. He married her afterwards and had as his son Viśravā. Viśravā is the father of Kuvera and Rāvaṇa, and is the progenitor of the Rākṣasas. Agastya also is, according to Bhāgavat, a son of Pulastya. He received the Viṣṇu Purāṇa from Brahmā and taught it to Maitreya. Parāśara, son of Śaktri by Adṛṣyānṭi, learned it from him and made it known to the world.

Pulastya was present in the conclave of sages who desired to learn Āyurveda (C.S., I.I.). But no work of his is known to us.

JAMADAGNI.

Jamadagni, the son of Ṛcīka and Satyavatī, was a sage of the Bhṛgu race. He had five sons, Paraśurāma was the youngest. He was a warrior Brāhmin, and married Reṇukā. One day she went out to bathe and saw a loving pair, Chitraratha and his wife, sporting in water. She came home but not in her former purity of mind. The sage cursed her and asked his sons to kill her. His four sons refused and were cursed to be idiots. Paraśurāma consented and struck off his mother's head with his axe. The sage was appeased. Paraśurāma was asked to pray for a boon, and he prayed for the restoration of his mother's life and the intelligence of his brothers. The sage granted his prayer.

The Haihaya king, Kārtavīrya once came to the hermitage of the sage. He was entertained but forcibly took away Surabhi, the cow of plenty, which belonged to his host. Paraśurāma came home, followed the king and killed him in battle. The sons of Kārtavīrya killed the sage in revenge. Paraśurāma was absent then. He came back and swore to clear the earth of the Kṣatriya race. And he defeated and extirpated them twenty-one times.

Jamadagni is mentioned in Caraka Saṁhitā I. I, to have been one of the sages who learned the science of medicine. He is said to have dug up a remedy to promote the growth of his daughter's hair. It caused her hairs to grow as luxuriously as to require one's outstretched hands to measure their length (Av. vii 137).

GOTAMA.

Gotama is one of the sages mentioned in Caraka Saṁhitā I.1 who learned the science of medicine from Ātreya. In the C.S., VI.1 he appears to be one of the sages who approached Indra to learn Rasāyaṇa known as the Aindriya Rasāyaṇa. Their names are Bhṛgu, Aṅgirā, Atri, Vasiṣṭha, Kaśyapa, Agastya, Pulastya, Vāmadeva, Asita and Gotama. Indra taught them the Āyurveda and especially the Rasāyaṇa.

हिमवन्तममराधिपतिगुप्तं जग्मुः भृग्वङ्गिरोऽत्रिवशिष्ठकश्यपागस्त्यपुलस्त्यवामदेवा-सितगौतमप्रभृतयो महर्षयः ॥ * * * अथेन्द्रस्तदायुर्व्वेदामृतमृषिभ्यः संक्रम्योवाचैतः सर्व्वमनुष्ठेयञ्च ॥

C. S., Vi. I, p. 323.

The seduction of his wife Ahalyā by Indra 'has been explained mythologically as signifying the carrying away of night by the morning sun.'

Gotama or Gautama, the father of Śatānanda, is the reputed founder of the Nyāya School of Philosophy. He is also the author of a Law-book which has been edited by Stenzler.

He is quoted in the Vyākhyā Madhu Koṣa, Arśa Nidāna, p. 64.

यदाहगौतमः—

श्लेष्मा च पञ्चधावस्थः श्लेषकादिस्वकर्म्मणा ।
कफधाम्नाञ्च सर्व्वेषां यत्करोत्यवलम्बनं ॥
अतोवलम्बकः श्लेष्मा यस्त्वामाशय-संश्रितः ।
क्लेदकः सोऽनुसंघात क्लेदनाद्बोधको मतः ॥
रसनास्थः शिरसंस्थोऽक्षितर्पणात्तु तर्पकः ।
सन्धिसंश्लेषणादेव श्लेषकः सन्धिषु स्थितः ॥

Some authors write his name as Asita Gotama but Asita and Gotama are separately and jointly quoted in the Caraka Saṁhitā. I. 1.

GARGA AND GĀRGYA.

Gārgya is the name of an ancient sage, mentioned in the C.S., I.1 along with others who learned the science of medicine from Ātreya. He is the son of Garga. There were many Gargas; and we are not sure of his identity with another Garga, one of the oldest writers on astronomy. The latter was "a son of Vitatha." A grammarian Garga is mentioned by Pāṇini. The Viṣṇu Purāṇa says: "From Garga sprang Sinā (or Sīni); from them were descended the Gārgyas and Śainyas, Brahmans of Ksatriya race." The statement of the Bhāgavata is, "From Gargya sprang Sina, from them Gārgya, who from a Kṣatriya became a Brahmin." He became the preceptor of the Yādavas. His son was Gārgya, and Gārga, his daughter.

Garga as a medical author is quoted in the Prayoga-ratnākara by Kavikaṇṭhahāra.

Garga describes the anomalies of normal pregnancy thus:

गर्ग उवाच।

अकालप्रसवा नार्य्यः कालातीत प्रजास्तथा।
विकृतप्रसवाश्चैव युग्मप्रसवनास्तथा॥
अमानुषा अवन्ताश्च न जात व्यञ्जनास्तथा।
हीनाङ्गा अधिकाङ्गाश्च जायन्ते यदिवा स्त्रियः॥
पशवः पक्षिणश्चैव तथैव च सरीसृपाः।
विनाशं तस्य देशस्य कुलस्य च विनिर्दिशेत्॥

Matsya Purāṇa, Ch. 209.

Books :—

1. Garga Saṁhitā : The book is not available now. But there is a book called *Jvaraśānti* on the cure of Fever according to Garga Saṁhitā.

MSS. L. 4086, 4115.

2. Vṛddha Gārgīya Jyotiḥśāstra. This work on Astronomy by the ancient sage Garga is referred to in Bhāndārkar's Report of a Second Tour (1904-6) in search of Sanskrit Manuscripts in Rajputana and Central India, p. 46.

VYĀSA.

Vyāsa is the son of sage Parāsára and Satyavatī, an unmarried Śūdra girl. So he is known as Pārāśara, Sātyavata and Kānīna. As he was born in an island in the Jamunā, he is styled Dvaipāyaṇa, and from his black complexion, Kṛṣṇa. Satyavatī married king Sāntanu afterwards and became the mother of two sons, Citrāṅgada and Vicitra-vīrya. The former died in battle, and the latter married Ambikā and Ambālikā, the daughters of Kāśirāja, and died untimely without any child. Vyāsa performed severe austerities. According to law and at the special request of his mother, Vyāsa had two sons by the widows,—by Ambikā, Dhṛtarāṣṭra, and by Ambālikā, Pāṇḍu, whose sons are known as the Kauravas and the Pāṇḍavas respectively. He had another son, Vidura, by the maid-servant of Ambālikā. He married Arunī and had a son, the famous Śukadeva.

According to the Purāṇas, Vyāsa (*lit.*, an arranger) incarnated himself to arrange the Vedas in different ages. He is thus known as Veda Vyāsa or arranger of the four Vedas. He is also said to be the compiler of the great epic, the Mahābhārata, and the arranger of the eighteen Purāṇas: *viz.*, Brahma, Viṣṇu, Śiva, Bhāgavat, Nārada, Markaṇḍeya, Agni, Bhaviṣya, Brahma-vaivarta, Liṅga, Varāha, Skanda, Vāmana, Kūrmma, Matsya, Garuḍa and Brahmāṇda. He is a Vedāntakṛt, the founder of a school of the Vedānta. Veda-vyāsa was the same person as Vādarāyaṇa, the celebrated author of the Brahma-sūtra. Vyāsa is also the author of Mimāmsā.

As Ganeśa consented to be the writer of the ślokas of the Mahābhārata on condition that his pen must continue to write without any interruption, Vyāsa is said to have composed intentionally many obscure couplets as it was settled beforehand that the writer must understand the import of each śloka before writing it. Afterwards he prayed to God to be forgiven for sins committed by him; (1) for assigning shape to the formless God, (2) for describing qualities of the indescribable and (3) for locating the omnipresent in sacred places.

रूपं रूपविवर्ज्जितस्य भवतो ध्यानेन यत्कल्पितम् ।
स्तुत्यानिर्व्वचनीयताऽखिलगुरो दूरीकृता यन्मया ।
व्यापित्वञ्च निराकृतं भगवतो यत्तीर्थयात्रादिना ।
क्षन्तव्यं जगदीश ! तद्विकलतादोषत्रयं मत्कृतम् ॥

महाभारतम् ।

There were many Vyāsas in ancient times. No less than eighteen sages became Vyāsas during the Dvāpara Yuga: (1) Svayambhuba, (2) Prajāpati, (3) Uśanā, (4) Vṛhaspati, (5) Savitā, (6) Mṛtyu, (7) Indra, (8) Vasiṣṭha, (9) Sārasvata, (10) Tridhāma, (11) Trivṛṣo, (12) Bharadvāja, (13) Antarikṣa, (14) Dharmmī, (15) Trayyāruṇa, (16) Dhanañjaya, (17) Kṛtañjaya, (18) Ṛṇajyo. There were other sages who received the surname 'Vyāsa,' and even in modern times we find some learned Brāhmins styled as Vyāsa. This fact would explain how the authorship of all the books was ascribed to Vedavyāsa; probably these works were composed by different sages in different times.

Vyāsa as a medical author is quoted in Sarvāṅga Sundarī:

तथा च भगवतो व्यासस्य :—

यश्च निःस्वं परशुना यश्चैनं मधुसर्पिषा ।
यश्चैनं गन्धमाल्येण सर्व्वस्य कटुरेव सः ॥

Sarvāṅga Sundarī, I. xiv.

Formulæ attributed to Vyāsa:

1. Gaṇḍīrāsava—G. N., Vol. I, p. 194.

1. Gaṇḍīrāsava.

गण्डीरासवः ।

जातसारं तु गण्डीरं सपुष्पं परिशोषयेत् ॥

खण्डशः चोदितं कृत्वा तस्य पञ्चाढकं पचेत् ।

त्रींश्चैव त्रिफलाप्रस्थान् दशमूलीतुलां तथा ॥

दद्यात्कुटजवल्कस्य पलानां पञ्चविंशतिम् ।

भल्लातकानीन्द्रयवं विड़ङ्गं घनमेव च ॥

अर्धप्रस्थसमान् भागानेकैकस्य समावपेत् ।

पाठा मधुरसा दन्ती षड्ग्रन्था चित्रकस्तथा ॥

एषां दशपलान् भागान्म्हद्वीकायास्तथाढकम् ।

तोयद्रोणेषु दशसु पचेद्द्विद्रोणशेषितम् ॥

तस्मिन्कषाये पूते तु गुड़स्यैकां तुलां क्षिपेत् ।

तथा तु शोधितस्यापि, शुभे भाण्डे निधापयेत् ॥

द्वौ प्रस्थौ मधुनश्चैव द्वावयोरजसस्तथा ।

अर्धप्रस्थो विड़ङ्गानां कुड़वो मरिचस्य च ॥

एतयोः सूक्ष्मचूर्णानि प्रतिवापार्थमाहरेत् ।

चूर्णं मरीचकानां च मधुना सह योजयेत् ॥

भाण्डप्रलेपः कर्तव्यः समासिच्य निधापयेत् ।

एष मासस्थितः पेयो यथाव्याधिबलाबलम् ॥

गण्डीरारिष्ट इत्येष व्यासतः परिकीर्तितः ।

एष शोषान् प्रमेहांश्च गुल्मांश्च उठराणि च ॥

क्रिमिकुष्ठानि वर्माणि प्लीहार्शांसि भगन्दरन् ।

श्वयथून् पाण्डुरोगांश्च ग्रहणीदोषमेव च ॥

ग्रन्थींश्च गलगण्डं श्च गण्डमालां तथैव च ।

विषमज्वरकासांश्च विद्रीधीन वातशोनितम् ।

अरिष्टः शमयत्याशु युधि शक्र इवासुरान् ॥

There is a difference of opinion as regards the identity of Vādarāyaṇa and Vedavyāsa, but there exist proofs, both external and internal, that the names refer to the same person and that Brahma-Sūtra of Vādarāyaṇa must have been composed before the age of Pāṇini who, according to Goldstucker, flourished about six centuries B.C., if not earlier. Windischman doubted this identity as Śaṅkarācārya in his commentary mentions Vādarāyaṇa but never the name of Vyāsa as the author of the Sūtra. The glossators of Śaṅkara Bhāsya,—Govindānanda, Vācaṣpati Miśra and Ānanda Giri—have ascribed the authorship to Vyāsa. Rāmānuja, Madhava, Vallabha, Śrinibāsa and Valadeba have similarly expressed their opinion. The Skanda Purāṇa and the Bhāgavat also identify the two authors. Hemcandra, the lexicographer, in his Abhidhāna Cintāmaṇi gives Māṭhara, Dvaipāyaṇa, Pārāśarya, Kānīna Vādarāyaṇa as synonyms.

His date : In the Mahābhārata, which in its old recension Bhārata dates back to 3000 B.C., it is said that he had five disciples, *viz.*, Vaiśampāyana, Paila, Sumantu, Jaimini and Śūkadeva. The first four names occur in the Gṛhya Sūtras (Sāṅkhyāyana and Aśvalāyana), the first two names in Pāṇini (ii, 4, 5, 9 ; iv, 3, 104) and the first name in Taitt. Āranyaka. Vyāsa and Jaimini quote each other in their works—the two Mimāṁsās, as teacher and disciple, as noticed by the commentator Śavara Svāmin (I, i, 5), and also by Govindānanda and Ānanda Giri, the tikākārs of Śaṅkara Bhāsya. He used to live with his disciples at his Himalayan retreat, the Vadarī or Nara-Nārāyaṇa Sthāna of the Mahābhārata, and possibly he derived his name Vādarāyaṇa from Vadarī the locality of his residence. According to Skanda Purāṇa, he was a resident of Vadarikāraṇya (Brahma Khaṇḍa, Ch. 31, Śloka 93). The term Vādarāyaṇa does not occur in Pāṇini but it finds a place in its Ganapāṭha. Pāṇini, however, refers to Bhikṣu-Sūtra of Pārāśarya. Vādarāyaṇa is mentioned in the Bhāgavata, Sāṇḍīlya Sūtra and in the Caraka Saṁhitā (Sūtra Sthāna) as the source of divine knowledge. Caraka refers to the doctrines of the Advaita school of the Vedānta. There were other teachers of Vedānta and Caraka refers to three of them, *viz.*, Ātreya, Āśvārthya and Vādarāyaṇa. The Buddhistic work Brahma-jāla-sutta presupposes the Brahma-Sūtra. Thus we find that Vyāsa flourished long before Buddha.

PĀRĪKṢI.

He is the son of the sage Parīkṣi and was called Maudgalya; and so he is referred to as Pārīkṣi Maudgalya. In a discussion as to the origin of disease, a question raised by the royal sage Vāmaka (C. S., I. xxv), he says "Both the body and the disease owe their origin to the soul."

पारीक्षिस्तत् परीक्ष्याग्रे मौद्गल्यो वाक्यमब्रवीत् ।

आत्मजः पुरुषो रोगाश्चात्मजाः कारणं हि सः ॥
न चिनोत्युपभुङ्क्ते च कर्म्म कर्म्मफलानि च ।
न ह्यते चेतना धातोः प्रवृत्तिः सुखदुःखयोः ॥

He is again referred to in the Caraka Saṁhitā, I. xxvi as holding with the other sages a discourse on Taste and Food. There he is styled as पूर्णाक्ष मौद्गल्य or the Full-eyed Maudgalya.

He says: त्रयो रसा इति पूर्णाक्षो मौद्गल्यश्छेदनीया उपशमनीयः साधारणश्चेति। "There are three kinds of Tastes: Chedanīya (corrective, *i.e.*, corrects the faults of the body), upaśamanīya (calmative, *i.e.*, pacifies the faults without correcting them) and sādhāraṇa or the ordinary taste.

CHAPTER XI

DHANVANTARI

Dhanvantari is the name of the physician of the gods in heaven. He appeared in this world as Divodāsa, king of Kāsī, surnamed Dhanvantari. In Suśruta Saṁhitā he is referred to as the teacher of Śalya Tantra or Major Surgery and he imparted this knowledge to Suśruta, the representative of an assembly of Ṛṣis or sages. He said : "It was I who cured the diseases of the gods and prevented their deaths and decrepitude. I have now come to this world to teach Śalya Tantra and the other divisions of the Āyurveda in detail."

अयं हि धन्वन्तरिरादिदेवो जरारुजामृत्युहरोऽमराणाम् ।
शल्याङ्गमङ्गैपरैरुपेतं प्राप्तोऽस्मि गां भूय इहोपदेष्टुम ॥

He taught the science of Śalya or Major Surgery to Aupadhenava, Vaitaraṇa, Aurabhra, Pauṣkalavata, Karbīrya, Gopura-Rakṣita, Suśruta and others in his Himalayan retreat. In S. S., I. 1 the origin of medical science is thus described :—

Once upon a time Aupadhenava, Vaitaraṇa, Aurabhra Pauṣkalavata, Gopura-Rakṣita, Suśruta and other sages approached Lord Divodāsa, the king of Benares, surnamed Dhanvantari, as he sat amidst the sages in his retreat, and said "O Lord! Diverse sorts of pain arise from bodily, mental, sudden and natural calamities. We are very sorry to see men, though full of resources, act when afflicted by these diseases, as if quite helpless; they remain apathetic and shout words of despair. We wish to learn Āyurveda from you to cure diseases of these pleasure-seeking men, to protect our own bodies, and for the general good of the animated creation. Please do thou teach us this science. Upon it depends our welfare in this and the next world. Therefore we approach you as disciples." Dhanvantari replied: "It is pleasure to meet you here, O my dear students! you are well-versed in many sciences and so are fit subjects to impart the knowledge of Āyurveda. I shall teach you the Āyurveda divided into eight branches. Now what shall I lecture on? And to whom?" The sages replied: "O Lord, please teach us the Śalya Tantra or the Science and Art of Surgery with notes." He said: "Be it so." They further said: "O Lord, we are of the same opinion, and so representing us, Śusruta will suggest our doubts and difficulties. We shall hear your words attentively." He said: "Be it so."

"My dear Suśruta, Āyurveda is necessary in this world to cure diseases of the sick and to protect the healthy. By this science we can prolong or know Āyu or Life. I will teach you the Science of Surgery in conformity to facts, knowledge, theories and analogy. Be attentive. According to its rules, ulcers heal up and wounds unite. In the days of yore, the separated head of Dakṣa was united to his body by its aid. Of all branches of medicine, the Science of Surgery is the most useful, for by its help we can gain our objects soon, and it treats of the practical uses of surgical instruments, caustic and cautery. By its practice we may acquire fame and piety here, and secure heaven after death. First of all Bramhā narrated this Veda; Dakṣa learned it from him. The Aśvin twins were taught by Dakṣa. They in their turn taught Indra, from whom I learned it. Now I will for the good of all men lecture on this science for those who want to learn it

In the Suśruta Saṁhitā, Dhanvantari, Divodāsa and Kāśirāja are the different names of the same individual. But in the Viṣṇu Purāṇa and Harivaṁśa we find that the names belonged to two different kings :—

VIṢṆU PURĀṆA (IV. viii).

Purūravā
|
Āyu + Bāhu's daughter
|
Nahuṣa | Kṣatravṛdha | Rambha (childless) | Raji (500 sons) | Anena.

Kṣatravṛdha
|
Kāśa | Lāśa | Gṛtsamad (Originator of caste)

Kāśa
|
Kasīrāja
|
Dīrghatamā
|
Dhanvantari
|
Ketumāna
|
Divodāsa
|
Pratardana (Śatrujit, Kuvalayāśva or Vatsya).
|
Alarka
|
Sannati
|
Sunītha
|
Suketu
|
Dharmaketu
|
Satyaketu

HARIVAMŚA (CH. XXIX).

Anena
|
Pratikṣatra
|
Sañjaya
|
Bijaya
|
Kṛti
|
Haryaśvan
|
Sahadeva
|
Nadīn
|
Jayat sena
|
Saṁkṛti
|
Kṣatradharmā
|
Sunohotra

- Kāś
- Sal
  - Arṣṇi Sena
    - Kāśya
      - Kāśyap t
      - Dīrghatapā
        - Dhanva
          - *Dhanvantari* (disciple of Bharadvāja)
            - Ketūmāna
              - Bhīmrath
                - *Divodāsa*
                  - Pratardana
- Gṛtsamada
  - Śunaka
    - Śaunaka (Brahmin, Kṣatrya, Vaiśya and Śudra sons)

Here we find that Divodāsa was either the grandson or great-grandson of Dhanvantari. Again Kāśirāja appears to be the grandfather of Dhanvantari. It is difficult to say whether Kāśirāja means king of Kāśi or is the name of a king. "The work called Navanitaka (in the Bower MS.) professes to be by Susruta, to whom it was declared by the Muni Kāsiraja. The latter is clearly a proper name, not a title 'a king of Kāsi'." (Hoernle.)

Again it is dificult to say whether Dhanvantari the progenitor of the present race of Vaidyas was identically the same Dhanvantari who propounded the science of life in this world. In the Skanda, Gaḍura and Mārkaṇdeya Purāṇas, it is stated that Dhanvantari flourished in the Tretā Yuga. His birth is thus narrated :—

Once upon a time the sage Gālava became greatly fatigued in search of Kuśa grass, etc., in a forest. He was very thirsty, but finding no water, he came out of the forest. He met a young maiden going home with a pail full of water on her waist. He said: "O maiden! I am very thirsty; kindly save my life by giving me water to drink." She presented the pail to the sage. He bathed and quenched his thirst to his satisfaction. He was highly pleased and uttered this benediction: "May you be the mother of a worthy son." She blushed and informed him that she was still unmarried, and that she was Vaiśya by caste and Vīrbhadrā by name. The sage then ordered her to follow him to the society of the Munis (hermits) who said "Be it so, and let Dhanvantari be born of this girl." So they prepared an effigy of kuśa, threw it on her lap, animated it with life by chanting Vedic mantras; and the boy in beauty and splendour proved an ornament to sweet Vīrbhadrā. The boy was called Vaidya because he was born by the Veda mantras and became the famous Ambaṣṭha, from the circumstance of his lying in his mother's lap.

युधिष्ठिर उवाच।

धन्वन्तरिमहाभाग अमरेशः कथं पुरा।
अभवच्छूल्वतो विप्रस्तन्मेवद महामुने ॥

मैत्रेय उवाच।

भो राजेन्द्र यथा जातो धन्वन्तरिरिहैवतु।
महर्षिर्गालवो नाम काष्ठदर्भाहरोवनम् ॥
जगाम तत्रभ्रमणादतिश्रान्तोबभूव सः।
ततोनिरीक्षयामास तृषातुर कलेवरः ॥
वनस्यच वहिर्भागे कन्यामेकां ददर्श सः।
जलपूर्णं घटं नीत्वा गच्छन्तीं पितृमन्दिरं ॥
तां दृष्ट्वा हृष्टचित्तोऽसौ वभासे मुनिपुङ्गवः।
हे कन्ये त्वं जलं देहि प्राणरक्षां कुरुष्व मे ॥
ततः सा कलसं भूमौ निधायातिष्ठदुत्तमा।
गालवश्चाद्रैतोयेन स्नात्वा तोयं पपौच तत्।
प्रोवाच चापि हे कन्ये त्वं सत्पुत्त्रवती भव ॥
ततः प्रोक्तवती कन्या न मे पाणिग्रहोऽभवत्।
ततोमुनिवरश्चाह का त्वं किं नाम ते वद ॥
उवाच पुनरन्येषा वैश्यकन्याह्यहं विभो।
वीरभद्राभिधानाच जानीहि मुनिपुङ्गवः ॥
ततो विचिन्त्य स मुनिस्तामादाय जगामह।
ऋषीणामग्रतो नीत्वा वृत्तान्तमवदत्तदा ॥
उत्कर्णस्ते महाराज उच्चुर्हर्षित मानसः।
भद्रं कृतं मने नूनमानीतेयं यतस्त्वया ॥
वैश्यायां वीरभद्रायां धन्वन्तरिर्भविष्यति।
इत्युक्तातेऽपि मुनयः कुशपुत्तलिकां ततः ॥
कृत्वा क्रोड़े ददुस्तस्या वेदमुच्चार्य्य तत्क्षणे।
प्राणप्रतिष्ठामप्यस्याचक्रुः पुरुषकाकृतिम् ॥

ततोऽभवत् काञ्चनराशि गौरं
वालोति सौम्याकृतिरेव तस्याः ।
क्रोड़े विलोक्यैव सुतं मुणीन्द्राः
प्रापुर्मुदं वेदृतः एष जातः ।।
वैद्य स्ततोऽयं जननी कुलेच
स्थितस्ततोऽम्बष्ठ इति प्रसिद्धः ।
एवमुक्ता ततः सर्व्वे मुनयो देवरूपिणः
अमृताचार्य्यमस्याख्यां चक्रुर्वैश्याभिधानकम् ॥

अम्बष्टाचारचन्द्रिकोद्धृत पुराणवचनानि ।

In the Skanda Purāṇa, a similar story is narrated. Here the father of the girl Vīrbhadrā is said to have ffered the maid to the sage Gālava for marriage. Gālava declined the offer but fulfilled his benediction by giving her a son, Dhanvantari, the celebrated physician.

Thus we find that the origin of Dhanvantari is a mystery,—and this story got currency by the description of supernatural incidents about his birth, so that he might be respected as a god. औषधः जाह्नवीतोयं वैद्यनारायणः स्वयम् । "The medicines are like sacred water of Ganges and the doctor is like God himself." The truth appears to be that the girl was married to Gālava with the consent of the sages and she gave birth to Dhanvantari in due time. The boy was taught Āyurveda by Bharadvāja and others. That the progenitor of Vaidyas was born of a Vaiśya mother and Brāhman father can be proved by the following passages from the Law books and the Purāṇas :

शूद्राविशोस्तु करणोऽम्बोष्ठो वैश्याद्विजन्मनोः ।

Brahma Vaivarta Purāṇa, Brahma Khaṇḍa, Ch. X.

वैश्यायां ब्राह्मणाज्जातोऽम्बष्ठो गन्धको बणिक् ।

Vṛhat Dharma Purāṇa, Uttara Khanda, Ch. XIII.

The renowned Dhanvantari is said to have married the three daughters of Aśvini Kumāra : Sidhavidyā, Sādhyavidyā and Kaṣtasādhyavidyā. He became the father of fourteen sons, Sena, Dāsa, Gupta, Datta, etc. He learned the Āyurveda well but became indifferent to worldly prosperity. So he was made king of Benares by Bharadvāja, Gālava and other sages at the request of Brahmā. He taught Suśruta and other disciples, *viz.*, Aupadhenava, Aurabhra and others.

Now we have here two stories of the birth of Dhanvantari. According to the Purāṇas, he was a Kṣatriya king of Benares. He taught Āyurveda to Suśruta. In the second version, he was the son of a Brāhmana father and Vaiśya mother; and he was afterwards made a king of Benares. In Susṛuta Saṁhitā there is internal evidence in support of the latter view. He has been styled निमित्तान्तरऽ भूभिप: (S.S., II. ix.), and this remark could not apply to a Kṣatriya king, the son of a reigning family. It has also been objected that Suśruta the son of the royal sage Viśvāmitra by a vaiśya mother could not possibly offer a salutation to a Kṣatriya king but could do so to Dhanvantari the son of Gālava, a Brahmana.

Another version of the birth of Dhanvantari is that he rose from the ocean when it was churned by Devas and Asuras for Amṛta or nectar.

[See Visnu Purana, William's translation quoted in Dowson's Mythology, p. 13.]

"Then, seated on a lotus,
Beauty's bight goddess, peerless Srī, arose
Out of the waves ; and with her, robed in white,
Came forth Dhanwantari, the gods' physician.
High in his hand he bore the cup of nectar—
Life-giving draught—longed for by gods and demons.

Then had the demons forcibly borne off
The cup, and drained the precious beverage,
Had not the mighty Vishnu interposed.
Bewildering them, he gave it to the gods;
Whereat, incensed, the demon troops assailed
The host of heaven, but they with strength, renewed,
Quaffing the draught, struck down their foes, who fell
Headlong through space to lowest depths of hell!"

नारायणांशो भगवान् स्वयं धन्वन्तरिर्म्महान्।
पुरा समुद्रमथने समुत्तस्थौ महोदधेः॥
सर्व्ववेदेषु निष्णातो मन्त्र-तन्त्र-विशारदः।
शिष्योहि वैनतेयस्य शङ्करस्योपशिष्यकः॥

Bramha Vaivarta Purāṇa, III. li.

Again it has been argued that perhaps there were two men called Dhanvantari,—one is the Kṣatriya king of Benares, and the second is the progenitor of the Vaidya caste; and that both of them were medical men who propagated the science to the public. Bhāvamiśra held the view that the teacher of Suśruta was Dhanvantari, the Kṣatriya prince born in the family of Vāhu.

अधीत्य चायुषो वेदमिन्द्राद्धन्वन्तरिः पुरा।
आगत्य पृथिवीं काश्यां जातो वाहुजवेश्मनि।
नाम्ना तु सोऽभवत् ख्यातो दिवोदास इति क्षितौ।
वालएव विरक्तोऽभूच्चचार सुमहत्तपं।
यत्नेन महता ब्रह्मा तं काश्यामकरोन्नृपम्॥

Bhāva Prakāśa, I. i.

विश्वामित्रो मुनिस्तेषु पुत्रं सुश्रुतमुक्तवान्।

*   *   *

तत्र नाम्ना दिवोदासः काशीराजोऽस्ति वाहुजः।
स हि धन्वन्तरिः साक्षादायुर्व्वेदविदां वर॥

Ibid.

The theory of two Dhanvantaris no doubt reconciles both the versions but there is no evidence for believing that there were two such men. Both in Suśruta Saṁhitā and Purāṇas, mention is made of a single Dhanvantari, the heavenly physician ; as for example we find in Suśruta Saṁhitā :

धन्वन्तरिं धर्म्मभृतां वरिष्टं अमृतोद्भवं ।
चरणावुपसंगृह्य सुश्रुतः परिपृच्छति ॥

S. S., II. i.

चिकित्सितात् पुण्यतमं न किञ्चिदपि सुश्रुतः ।
ऋषेरिन्द्र प्रभावस्यामृतयोनिर्भिषकगुरोः ॥

S. S., V. viii.

येनामृतपां मध्यादुष्कृतं पूर्व्वजन्मनि ।
यतोऽमरत्वं संप्राप्तस्त्रिदशास्त्रिदिवेश्वरात् ॥

S. S.,VI. xxxix.

Disciples of Dhanvantari.—He is said to have initiated and taught one hundred disciples in the science of medicine. In Suśruta Saṁhitā, I. i, we find the names of Aupadhenava, Aurabhra, Pauṣkalāvata, Karabīrya, Gopura Rakṣita (some commentators think Gopura and Rakṣita to be two persons), Vaitaraṇa, Suśruta and others. By "others" are meant such persons as Bhoja, Nimi, Kāṅkāyaṇa, Gārgya and Gālava. So we get names of twelve students.

औपधेनवादयः सुश्रुतान्ताः सप्तशिष्या उचुः उक्तवन्तः। प्रभृति शब्देन भोजादयः। अन्ये तु गोपूररक्षितौ इति नामद्वयं मन्यन्ते। इत्यौपधेनवादयोऽष्टौ। प्रभृति ग्रहणात् निमि-काङ्कायन-गार्ग्य-गालवा इति। एवमेते द्वादश शिष्याः प्राहुः स्म।

Dallvanācārya I. i.

In the Bower MS., Muni Kāśirāja appears as the teacher of Suśruta. Dhanvantari is again referred to there as teaching Keśava (or Visṇu) the doctrine of Plumbago plant (Bower MS., Ch. XIII, p. 169).

Formulas attributed to Dhanvantari :—

	Name.	Author.	Book.	Page.
1.	Dhānvantara Ghṛta or Clarified Butter.	Dhanvantari	V. M., Śataślokī Bower MS.	101
2.	Pāśupatarasa	„	R. S. S.	227-8
3.	Mṛtuñjaya Lauha	„	„	396-7
4.	Vāriśoṣaṇarasa	„	„	404-6
5.	Rasa Rājendra	„	„	138-9
6.	Vṛhat Purṇa Candra Rasa	Kāsinatha	„	476-8
7.	Pittāntaka rasa	Kāśirāja	„	335
8.	Rasābhra Guggula	Dhanvantari	A. R.	261
9.	Aśvagandhādya Taila	„	G. N., I.	47-8
10.	Saptaviṁśati Guggula Vatikā	„	„	129-30
11.	Dvātriṁśaka	„ „	„	130-1

1. Dhānantara Ghṛta.

धान्वन्तरम् घृतम् ।

दन्तीचित्रकमूलानामष्टौ कुर्व्वीत सन्नखाम् ।
अभयाविंशतिं गुर्व्यः षटपलम् देवदारु च ॥
निम्बकदम्बं वरणम् राजवृक्षम् पुनर्न्नवाम् ।
चिरिविल्वत्वचाश्चैव पृथक् षट्पलिकाः स्मृताः ॥
द्वे पञ्चमूले संहृत्य पृथगाढ़कसम्मिते ।
विपाचयेदपान् द्रोणे सारसे मृदुनाग्निना ॥
चतुर्भागावशेषम् तत्कषायमवतारयेत् ।
घृताढ़के पचेत तस्मिं न पेश्यं श्रेमान प्रदापयेत् ॥
पिप्पली पिप्पलीमूलम् चव्यञ्च मरिचानि च ।
लवणानञ्च पञ्चानामवपेदेक कर्षिकान् ॥

एतद्धान्वन्तरम् सर्प्पिः सर्व्वरोगनिवारणम् ।
पञ्चगुल्मानभिव्यक्तानष्टौ चोदरवृद्धयः ॥
श्वयथुं शोषमर्शांसि प्रमेहम स्चैकविंशति ।
दीपयेत् ग्रहणीम् मन्दां कुष्ठान् वहुविधान् जयेत् ॥
अहीनाम् मूषिकानाम् च यच्च स्यात् कृत्रिमां विषम् ।
सर्व्वाहारेष्वनियमो वृंहनो देहमात्मानः ।
एतद्द धान्वन्तरम् सर्पिः श्रेष्ठं ब्रह्माभिपूजितम् ।
यथावत् समप्रयुञ्जानः प्राप्नुयात् सिद्धिमुत्तमम् ॥

THE DHĀNVANTARA CLAṚIFIED BUTTER.[1]

(232-240) Take eight handfuls of Dantī (*Baliospermum Montanum*) and plumbago-root, twenty choice chebulic myrobalans, six pala of deodar, (233) also six pala each of the larger and smaller kinds of Kadamba (*Anthocephalus Cadamba*), Varaṇa (*Cratæava religiosa*), Rājavṛiksha (*Euphorbia nerifolia*), Punarnavā (*Boerhaavia diffusa*) and rind of Chirivila (*Pongamia glabra*), (234) and add one āḍhaka each of the two Pancha-mūla (or 'sets of five drugs'). Then boil *the whole* in one droṇa of tank-water over a gentle fire, (235) till it is reduced to one-fourth *of the original quantity*. Now, boil this decoction once more in one āḍhaka of clarified butter, throwing in also pastes of one Karsha each of the following drugs : (236) long pepper, root of long pepper, Chavya (*Piper Chaba*), black pepper and the five salts. (237) This *preparation of* clarified butter called the Dhānvantara (or 'Composed by Dhanvantari') is a remedy for all diseases. It cures the five *kinds of* abdominal tumours, the eight *kinds of* enlargements of the abdomen, (238) swellings, consumption, piles, and the twenty-one *kinds of* morbid secretion of urine. It also relieves chronic diarrhœa and dyspepsia,

[1] **Bower Manuscript, Hoernle's Edition, pp. 101-2.**

and cures the many kinds of skin-diseases. (239) It counteracts the venom of snakes and mice, also every sort of artificial poison. Taken with any meal it is an unfailing agent for increasing the bulk of one's body. (240) This clarified butter, composed by Dhanvantari, is most excellent and highly esteemed by Brahman. Whoever makes suitable use of it will attain the highest prosperity.

2. Pāśupata Rasa.

पाशुपतरसः ।

शुद्धसूतं द्विधागन्धं त्रिभागं तीक्ष्णभस्मकं ।
त्रिभिः समं विषं देयं चित्रकक्वाथभावितं ।
धूर्त्तवीजस्य भस्मापि द्वात्रिंशद्भागसंयुतं ।
कटुत्रयं त्रिभागं स्यात् लवङ्गैला च तत्समं
जातीफलं तथा कोषमर्द्धभागं नियोजयेत् ।
तथार्द्धं लवणं पञ्च चूर्ण्यर्कैरम्लतिन्तिड़ी ।
अपामार्गाश्वत्थजञ्च क्षारं दद्याद्विचक्षणः ।
हरीतकी यवक्षारः स्वर्ज्जिका हिङ्गु जीरकं ।
टङ्कणञ्च सूततुल्यं चाम्लयोगेन मर्द्दयेत् ।
भोजनान्ते प्रयोक्तव्यो गुञ्जाफलप्रमाणतः ॥
रसः पाशुपतो नाम सद्यः प्रत्ययकारकः ।
दीपनः पाचनो हृद्यः सद्यो हन्ति विसूचिकां ।
तालमूलीरसेनैव उदरामयनाशनः ।
मोचरसेनातीसारं ग्रहणीं तक्रसैन्धवैः ।
सौवर्च्चल-कणा-शुण्ठीयुतः शूलं विनाशयेत् ।
अर्शों हन्ति च तक्रेण पिप्पल्या राजयक्ष्मकं ।
वातरोगं निहन्त्याशु शुण्ठी-सौवर्च्चलान्वितः ।
शर्कराधान्ययोगेन पित्तरोगं निहन्त्ययं ।
पिप्पलीक्षौद्रयोगेन श्लेष्मरोगञ्च तत्क्षणात् ।
अतः परतरो नास्ति धन्वन्तरिमतो रसः ॥

3. Mṛtyuñjaya Lauha.

मृत्युञ्जयलौहं ।

शुद्धसूतं समं गन्धं जारिताभ्रं समं समं
गन्धकाद्द्विगुणं लौहं मृतताम्रञ्चतुर्गुणं ।
द्विक्षारं टङ्कणं विड़ं वराटमथ शङ्खकं ।
चित्रकं कुनटी तालकटुकी रामठन्तथा ।
रोहितकन्त्रिवृच्चिञ्चा विशालाधवमङ्कोठं ।
अपामार्गं ताललग्डमल्लिका च निशायुगं ।
कानकन्तुत्थकञ्चैव यक्षकर्द्दमं रसाञ्जनं ।
एतानि समभागानि चूर्णयित्वा विभावयेत् ।
आर्द्रकस्वरसेनैव गुड़ूच्याः स्वरसेन च ।
मधनः कुड्ढैर्भाव्यं वटिका माषमात्रतः ।
अनुपानं प्रदातव्यं बुद्ध्वा दोषानुसारतः ।
भक्षयेत् प्रातरुत्थाय सर्व्वरोगकुलान्तकं ।
प्लीहानं ज्वरमुग्रञ्च कासञ्च विषमज्वरं ।
चिरजं कुलजञ्चैव श्लीपदं हन्ति दारुणं ।
रोगानीकविनाशाय धन्वन्तरिकृतं पुरा ।
मृत्युञ्जयमिदं लौहं सिद्धिदं शुभदं नृणां ॥

4. Vāriśoṣana Rasa.

वारिशोषणरसः ।

चतुर्विंशतिभागाः स्युर्गन्धाद्वङ्गं तदर्द्धकं ।
वङ्गभागाद्द्विवेदर्द्धः पारदः कृष्णमभ्रकं ।
चतुर्द्दशविभागं स्यान्मृतं तद्दीयते पुनः ।
मृतलौहमष्टभागं मृतताम्रं नवात तत् ।
मृतहेमद्वयं तेषां मृतरूप्यञ्च सप्तकं ।

अतिशुद्धमतिस्थूलं मृतं हीरं त्रयोदश।
भागा ग्राह्या माक्षिकस्य विशुद्धस्यात्र षोड़श।
अष्टादशमितं ग्राह्यं नवकाशीशकं पुनः।
तुल्यकञ्च षड़ेवात्र नवीनं ग्राह्यमेवच।
तालकञ्च चतुर्भागं शिला योज्यास्त्रयो बुधैः।
शैलेयं पञ्च दातव्यं सर्व्वमेकत्र नूतनं।
मृतमौक्तिकभागैकं सौभाग्यं द्वयमेवच।
कुट्टयित्वा विचूर्ण्याथ जम्बीरस्य रसेन वै।
भावयेत् सप्तधा गाढ़ं गुड़िकान्तस्य कारयेत्।
पानकद्वितये कृत्वा मुद्रयेत् पानकद्वयं।
घटमध्ये निवेश्याथ दत्त्वा पूर्व्वञ्च बालुकां।
ऊर्द्धञ्च तां पुनर्दत्त्वा वालुकां मुद्रयेन्मुखं।
अहोरात्रं दहेदग्नौ स्वाङ्गशीतं समुद्धरेत्।
वकुलस्य च वीजेन कण्टकारीद्वयेन च।
गुड़ूची त्रिफलावारा भावयेत् सप्तसप्ततः।
वृद्धदाररसेनापि तथा देयास्तु भावनाः।
गिरिकर्ण्णारसेनापि रोहितमत्स्यपित्ततः।
एवं सिद्धो भवेत् सम्यक् रससौवारिशोषणः।

देवान् गुरून् समभ्यर्च्च्य यतिनो गुरवस्तथा।
रक्तिकाद्वितयं देयं सन्निपाते समुत्क्रये।
मरिचेन समं देयं तेन जागर्त्ति मानवः।
श्लैष्मिके च गदे देयं ग्रहण्यामग्निमान्द्यके।
प्लीह्नि पाण्डौ प्रयोक्तव्यं त्रिकटुत्रिफलाम्भसा।
शूलरोगे प्रयोक्तव्यमुदावर्त्ते विशेषतः।
कुष्ठे सुदुष्टे देयोयं काकडुम्बरिकाम्भसा।
अतिवह्निकरः श्रीदो वलवर्णाग्निवर्द्धनः।
धन्वन्तरिकृतः सद्यो रसः परमदुर्लभः।

सर्व्वरोगे प्रयोक्तव्यो निःसन्देहं भिषग्वरैः॥

5. Rasa Rājendra.

रसराजेन्द्रः ।

पलं शुद्धस्य सूतस्य पलं ताम्रमयस्तथा ।
अभ्रं नागं पलं वङ्गं पलं गन्धकतालकं ।
पलं शुद्धविषं चूर्णं सर्व्वमेकत्र कारयेत् ।
मर्द्दयेत् काकमाच्याश्च आर्द्रकस्य रसेन च ।
मात्स्यवाराहमायूरछागमाहिषपित्तकैः ।
मर्द्दयेच्छिन्नभिन्नाश्च विकटीरम्भोभिस्तथा ।
सिद्धोऽयं रसराजेन्द्रो धन्वन्तरिसुसंस्कृतः ।

गुञ्जामात्रं रसं दद्यात् सुरसारससंयुतं ।
मेघवारिप्रवाहेण धारितं वारि मस्तके ।
अनिवारो यदा दाहस्तदा देया च शर्करा ।
भोजनं दधिसंयुक्तं वारमेकन्तु दापयेत् ।
ईश्वरेण यथाकामः केशवेन च दानवः ।
पावकेन यथा शीतमनेन च तथा ज्वरः ॥

6. Vṛhat Purna Candra Rasa.

बृहत्पूर्णचन्द्र रसः ।

द्विकर्षं शुद्धसूतस्य गन्धकञ्च द्विकार्षिकं ।
लौहभस्मपलञ्चाभ्रं जारितञ्च पलांशिकं ।
द्वितोलं रजतञ्चैव वङ्गभस्म द्विकार्षिकं ।
सुवर्णं तोलकञ्चैव ताम्रं कांस्यञ्च तत्समं ।
जातीफलञ्चन्द्रपुष्पमेलाभ्रङ्गञ्च जीरकं ।
कर्पूरं वनितामुस्तं कर्षं कर्षं पृथक् पृथक् ।
सर्व्वं खल्लतले क्षिप्त्वा कन्यारसविमर्द्दितं ।
भावयित्वा वरातोयैः केवुकानं रसेन च ।
एरण्डपत्रैरावेष्ट्य धान्ये रात्रिदिनोषितं ।

उद्धृत्य मर्द्दयित्वा तु वटिकां चणसम्मितां ।
खादेच्च पर्णखण्डेन संयुक्तां व्याधिनाशिनीं ।
सर्व्वव्याधिविनाशाय काशीनाथेन भाषितः ।
पूर्णचन्द्ररसोनाम सर्व्वरोगेषु योजयेत् ।
बल्यो रसायनो वृष्यो वाजीकरण उत्तमः ।
अयमष्ठीलिकां हन्ति कासश्वासमरोचकं ।
आमशूलं कटीशूलं हृच्छूलं पित्तशूलकं ।
अग्निमान्द्यमजीर्णञ्च ग्रहणीं चिरजामपि ।
आमवातमम्लपित्तं भगन्दरमपि द्रुतं ।
कामलां पाण्डुरोगञ्च प्रमेहं वातशोणितं ।
नातः परतरः श्रेष्ठो विद्यते वाजिकर्म्मणि ।
रसस्यास्य प्रसादेन नरो भवति निर्गदः ।
मेधाञ्च लभते वाग्मी सर्व्वशास्त्रसमन्वितः ।
मदनस्य समां कान्तिं मदनस्य समं बलं ।
मीयते मदनेनैवं मदनस्य समं वपुः ।
स्त्रीणान्तथानपत्यानां दुर्व्वलानाञ्च देहिनां ।
क्षीणानामल्पशुक्राणां वृद्धानां वातरेतसां ।
ओजस्तेजस्करश्चायं स्त्रीषु कामविवर्द्धनः ।
अभ्यासेन निहन्ति मृत्युपलितं सर्व्वामयध्वंसिनो ।
वृद्धानां मदनोदयोदयकरः प्रौढ़ाङ्गनासङ्गमे ।
नित्यानन्दकरः सुखातिसुखदो भुपैः सदा सेव्यते ।
दृष्टः सिद्धफलो रसायनवरः श्रीपूर्णचन्द्रोरसः ॥

7. Pittāntaka Rasa.

पित्तान्तकोरसः ।

जातीकोषफली मांसी कुष्ठं तालीशपत्रकं ।
माक्षिकं मृतलौहञ्च अभ्रं दिव्यं समांशिकं ।
सर्व्वतुल्यं मृतं तारं समं निष्पिष्य वारिणा ।
द्विगुञ्जाभा वटी कार्य्या पित्तरोगविनाशिनी ।

कोष्ठाश्रितञ्च यत् पित्तं शाखाश्रितमथापिवा।
शूलञ्चैवाम्लपित्तञ्च पाण्डुरोगं हलीमकं।
दुर्नाभं भ्रान्तिवान्तिञ्च चिप्रमेव विनाशयेत्।
रसः पित्तान्तकोह्येष काशीराजेन भाषितः॥

8. Rasābhra Guggulu.

रसाभ्रगुग्गुलुः।

कर्षद्वयं पारदस्य लौहं गन्धञ्च तत्समम्।
लौहगन्धसमं चाभ्रं गुग्गुलुं कुभरद्वयम्॥
अमृताया रसप्रस्थे रसप्रस्थे फलत्रिके।
सान्द्रीभूतेरसे तस्मिन् गभंदत्त्वाबिचचणः॥
त्रिकटु त्रिफलादन्तो गुडूचि चेन्द्रवारुणी।
विडङ्गं नागपुष्पञ्च त्रिवृता च सुचूर्णितम्॥
प्रत्येकं कर्ष मादय सर्व्वमेकत्र कारयेत।
भचयेत्कोलमात्रन्तु छिन्नाक्काथानुपानतः॥
वातरक्तं महाघोरं रुकुटीतं गलितं जयेत।
अष्टादशविधं कुष्ठं क्रिमिरोगाश्मरीं तथा॥
भगन्दर गुदभ्रंशं श्वेतकुष्टं सकामलम्।
अपचीं गण्डमालाञ्च पामाकण्डूविचर्चिका:॥
चर्म्मकिलं महादद्रु नाशयेन्नात्र संशयः॥
वातरक्तविनाशाय धन्वन्तरिकृतः पुरा॥

रसाभ्रगुग्गुलुः ख्यातो वातरक्तेऽमृतोपमः॥

9. Aśvagandhādya Taila.

अश्वगन्धाद्यं तैलम्।

मूलानि चाश्वगन्धायाः शतं स्यात्खण्डशः कृतम्
द्विद्रोणेऽपां पचेत्क्वाथमष्टभागावशेषितम्।
तैलाढकं समावाप्य चीरं दद्याच्चतुर्गुणम्।
एतत्समालोड्य पचेत्कल्कांश्चेमान् समावपेत्॥

तगरं शतपुष्पां च मुस्तं व्याघ्रनखं त्वचम् ।
मधुकं शृङ्गवेरं च पृश्निपर्णीं ; बलां स्थिराम् ॥
रास्नां पुष्करमूलं च भूतीकं सपुनर्नवम् ।
मञ्जिष्ठां नलदं पत्रं द्रवन्तीं सुरसां वचाम ॥
श्वदंष्ट्रां च मृणालं च वयस्थां वहुपुत्रिकाम् ।
श्लक्ष्णपिष्टार्धपलिकान् दत्त्वा गर्भं विपाचयेत् ॥
तत्सिद्धमविदग्धं च ततः समवतारयेत् ।
वस्तौ पाने तथाऽभ्यङ्गे नस्यकर्मणि भोजने ॥
यत्र यत्र विधातव्यं तन्मे निगदतः शृणु ।
खञ्जमूकजडत्वे च तिमिरे च तथाऽर्बुदे ॥
पक्षाघाते तथाऽऽयामे च्युतभग्नास्थिसन्धिषु ।
विधेयं पृष्ठभग्नेषु हनुमन्याग्रहे तथा ॥
स्तम्भकम्पेषु शोफेषु रुजासु विविधासु च ।
ज्वरे च विषमे गुल्मे तथा मारुतशोणिते ॥
प्लीह्नि प्लीहोदरे चैव विद्रधिग्रन्थिशोषु च ।
क्षीणेन्द्रिया नष्टशुक्रा ये चान्ये षण्टका नराः ॥
भूतोपहतचित्ताश्च शस्यते तेषु नित्यशः ।
व्यापन्नयोनौ वन्ध्यासु पाययेत तदा भिषक् ॥
पुत्रदं परमं प्रोक्तं धन्वन्तरिवचो यथा ।

---

10. Dhanvantari's Guggulu Pills containing 27 ingredients for Leprosy.

धन्वन्तरीया सप्तविंशतिका गुग्गुलुगुटिका ।

त्रिकटुत्रिफलामुस्तं विडङ्गं चव्यचित्रकौ ।
सूक्ष्मैला पिप्पलीमूलं माक्षिकं सुरदारु च ॥
तुम्बरु पौष्करं कुष्ठं विषा च रजनीद्वयम् ।
सौवर्चलं विडं चैव सैन्धवं हस्तिपिप्पली ॥
यावन्त्येतानि द्रव्याणि तावन्तं गुग्गुलुं पचेत् ।
प्रक्षिप्य सर्पिषा सार्धं गुटिकां कारयेद्बुधः ॥

अजमोदा विड़ङ्गं च दाड़िमं साम्लवेतसम् ।
वाष्पिका पौष्करं दारु त्वगेलापत्रकेसरम् ॥
एषामर्धपलं भागैः पलानि दश गुग्गुलोः ।
संमिश्र्य सर्पिषा सार्धं गुटिकां कारयेद्बुधः ॥
भक्षयित्वा ससर्पिष्कां जीर्णे च प्रमिताशनम् ।
वातश्लेष्मविकारेषु नाड़ीदुष्टव्रणेषु च ॥
श्लेष्मकासे च शोफे च योगमेनं प्रयोजयेत् ।
जठरं योनिशूलं च ह्यान्तभूतं च विद्रधिम् ॥
पार्श्वशूलं क्रमीन् गुल्मान्प्रमेहांश्चार्द्य रोचकौ ।
केवलानिलजान्रोगान् शीतजान् श्लेष्मिकानपि ॥
सेविता नाशयत्याशु रसायनमनुत्तमम् ।

11. Guggula Pills containing 32 ingredients for Amavāta.

धन्वन्तरीया द्वात्रिंशका गुग्गुलुगुटिका ।

त्रिकटुत्रिफलामुस्तं विडङ्गं चित्रकं वचा ।
चव्येलापिप्पलीमूलं हपुषा सुरदारु च ॥
तुम्बुरु पौष्करं कुष्ठं विशाला रजनीद्वयम् ।
वाष्पिका जीरकं शुण्ठी सपत्ना च दुरालभा ॥
सैन्धवं च विडं चारौ विषा च हस्तिपिप्पली ।
भागानेषां समान्कृत्वा तुल्यं कृत्वा तु गुग्गुलुम् ॥
ततो बदरमात्रां तु गुटिकां कारयेद्बुधः ।
तां भक्षयित्वा तु मेधावी मधुना सह योजिताम् ॥
आमं हन्यात्सुदुर्वारमन्त्रवृद्धिं गुदक्रमीन् ।
आनाहं च तथोन्मादं कुष्ठानि गुदजानि च ॥
गृध्रसीं च हनुस्तम्भपक्षाघातापतानकाम् ।
शोफं प्लीहामयं मेहं कामलामपचीं तथा ॥
नाम्ना द्वात्रिंशकोह्येष गुग्गुलुः कथितो महान् ।

धन्वन्तरिकृतो योगः सर्व्वरोग निसूदनः ॥

His works :—

In the Bramhavaivarta Purāṇa, three medical treatises are ascribed to three authors : Dhanvantari, Divodāsa and Kāśirāja. This is in agreement with the genealogy given in the Viṣṇu Purāṇa. These books are, however, not extant.

1. Cikitsā-Tattva-Vijñāna—by Dhanvantari.
2. Cikitsā-Darśana— by Divodāsa.
3. Cikitsā-Kaumūdī— by Kāśirāja.

See *Ward's Hindus, 1. 497.*

To Kāśirāja is ascribed another work :

4. Ajīrnāmṛtamañjarī, *i.e.*, Nectar of Indigestion by Kāśirāja.

5. Roga Nidāna : Pathology of Diseases—by Dhanvantari.

6. Vaidya Cintāmaṇi : by Dhanvantari. It treats of nervous affections and derangements of the urinary system.

7. Vidyā Prakāśa Cikitsā : by Dhanvantari, but it is undoubtedly a modern work.

MS. : L. 1446. A treatise on the treatment of diseases :

Beginning :

यस्योदयास्तसमये पुरमुकुटनिष्ठचरण कमलोऽपि ।
कुरुतेऽञ्जलिं त्रिनेत्र: स जयतु धाम्नां निधि: सूर्य्य: ॥

End :

अमृतं त्रिफलाक्काथ: पिप्पलीचूर्णसंयुत: ।
* सौभ शीतलो नित्यं सद्योनेत्रव्यथां जयेत् । इति नेत्ररोग: ॥

Colophon :

इति श्रीधन्वन्तरि विरचिता विद्याप्रकाशचिकित्सा समाप्ता ।

8. Dhanvantari Nighantu: A Dictionary of Materia Medica and Therapeutics,—by Dhanvantari. Dr. Mitra says: "It is a modern compilation" in nine chapters (Vargas). This work has been printed in the Ānandāśrama Sanskrit Series.

Beginning:

अनेकदेशान्तरभाषितेषु सर्वेष्वपि प्राकृतसंस्कृतेषु।

गूढेष्वगूढेषु च नास्तिसंख्या द्रव्याभिधानेषु तदौषधीनाम् ।

... ...

इत्येवामतक्रमशो (?) नववर्गाः प्रकीर्त्तिताः ॥

End:

इति धन्वन्तरि निघण्टु रसवीर्य्यसहितः समाप्तः ॥

Mss.: Bik.: 1392.
I.O.: 2736, 2737.
Ox. Cat.: 451.
GOML.: 13283—13294.

9. Vaidyakabhāṣkarodaya: a treatise on medicine attributed to Dhanvantari.

Reference: Bhandarkar's second Report of Rajputana Mss.. P. 59.

10. Cikitsāsāra Saṁgraha: A Treatise on Pathology. The eight different ways of diagnosing diseases are explained in the beginning. In the colophon the author is stated to be Dhanvantari.

Mss.: GOML., 13137-13145.

Beginning:—

यस्य द्विरदवक्त्राद्याः ... ...

... ... विष्वक्सेनं तमाश्रये ॥

आदौ समस्तरोगेषु अष्टस्थानं परीक्षयेत्।

नाडीमूत्रमलं जिह्वा शब्दस्पर्श (च) रूपदृक् ॥

नाड़ीपरीक्षा—

मूलमाश्रित्य अङ्गुलवयपीड़नम् ।
आदौ वायुः कफो मध्ये अन्ते पैत्यश्च वर्तते ॥
यवस्य बीजमात्रं च नाड़ी सर्वाङ्गसङ्गतिः ।
नारीणां वामभागे च पुंसां दक्षिणशोधयेत् ॥

End :—

फलसर्पिश्च कल्याणघृतमत्र प्रदापयेत् ।
ऊर्ध्वमग्निमथो गर्भं मध्ये तु जलसंग्रहम् ॥
वायुना किं न नीतोऽसौ कथं गर्भं न जीर्यते ।
नाभिप्रदेशे कमलमष्टकोणं तथा भवेत् ॥
तन्मध्ये वीर्यपतनं तत्पुष्पं मुकुलं भवेत् ।
तन्नालमध्ये क्रिमिजं तच्छुक्लं भक्षितं भवेत् ॥

Colophon :—

इति श्रीचिकित्सासारसंग्रहे धन्वन्तरिकृतौ सर्वरोगनिदानं नाम प्रथमविलासः ।

In the GOML. Mss., we find the following names cited as authorities: Dhanvantari, Judhiṣṭhira and his four brothers, Rāma, Aśvins, and in the Ms. No. 13145: Rasārṇava, Bāhaṭa, Pārijāta, Kaumūdī, Nāgarjuṇa, Kāpāla, Dāmodara, Rasa Prasidhasāra, Pillaṭa, Kalyāṇabheṣaja, Saṃgraha, Kāpālamindunātha, Guṇacintāmaṇi, Vīrbhadrīya, Vedadīpaka, Somnātha, Nandanātha, Cikitsitam, Vaidyamuktāvalī, Keruṭa Cakravarti, Somarājīya, Candrajñāna, Caraka, and Nighantu. So the work is modern.

In the Brahma Vaivarta Purāṇa, III, li, the following story is narrated about the dispute between Manasā, the goddess of the snakes, and the king Dhanvantari, the celebrated physician. Once upon a time, Dhanvantari, while going to Kailāsa, accompanied by his thousand students, saw on his way the hideous snake Takṣaka coming towards them in an angry mood. One of his disciples, proud of his attainment in medical science, caught hold of the snake, took the jewel from the snake's head and threw it on the ground. Vāsuki, the king of the snakes, was informed, and he sent a large number of poisonous snakes under the command of five generals, *viz.*, Droṇa, Kālīya, Karkkoṭa, Puṇḍarīka and Dhanañjaya. he disciples of Dhanvantari became panic-stricken, and being unable to withstand the poisonous gases evolved by their respiration, became unconscious. Dhanvantari stimulated them to life again by the nectar that he had in his possession, and caused the snakes to be senseless. Vāsuki soon became aware of the danger in which his army of snakes had fallen and sent the goddess Manasā, the disciple of Śiva. Both she and Gaḍura were Śiva's pupils and Dhanvantari was a follower of Gaḍura. She went where the physician was and caused his students to fall in a trance from which the physician failed to resuscitate them. Manasā tried her best to injure Dhanvantari with the help of her charms and arms, but without success. A' last she took the jāvelin which Śiva gave her. The instrument was invulnerable, and as she attempted to throw it on the physician, Brahmā and Śiva appeared in the battle-field and appeased both the parties. Dhanvantari worshipped Manasā who also blessed him in her turn. The snakes returned home, Manasā and Dhanvantari went to their retreat, and the Devas to their heavenly abode.

In the Mahābhārata I. xlii and xliii, we find another story about Takṣaka, a snake, and Kāśyapa, a physician well-versed in the science of Ophiology. Śingī Muni, son of the sage Śamīka cursed Rājā Parīkṣita to die of snake-bite within seven days, as a retaliation against an insult to his innocent father in the shape of twining a dead snake round his neck by the king. To fulfil the Brāhmaṇa's curse, Takṣaka, as he was going to kill the king, met Kāśyapa on the way. Kāśyapa was going to the king to save him from the effects of snake-bite, and thus gain honour and riches. He domonstrated his skill by imparting life to a tree, after it was destroyed by the bite of Takṣaka. The snake won over the Brāhmaṇa by giving him riches and presents. Kāśyapa then went home. The Nāgas assumed the shape of Brāhmaṇas, and Takṣaka contracted himself into a minute filiform worm and remained concealed in a fruit which was offered to the king. The king accepted the gift of the Brāhmaṇas, and as he attempted to eat the fruit, the snake appeared in its own shape and killed the king.

In both these stories, we find that the enemies of the kings were the Nāgas who are described as snakes. It is difficult to tell whether these stories have any sub-stratum of truth, but the legends may possibly be relics of stories of battles fought between the two kings and some foreign race, called Nāgas, who may represent the snakes of the Purāṇas. But there is no doubt that the science of treatment of snake-bite was successfully cultivated by the Ancient Indians, as we learn from the records of historians who came to India with Alexandar the Great. The marvellous cure of snake-bite by the Hindus was also well-known to foreign travellers. Even now, stories are told of men who possess this power of curing patients from the effects of bite by poisonous snakes. The science, is known as Sarpa-vidyā, Ophiology, or Viṣa-vidyā, Toxicology, and is described in the Vedas and in the Āyurvedic works. Snake-charmers are now commonly found in all parts of India, and they are said to be provided with medicines which cure them when bitten by snakes.

—o—

NIMI

Nimi, a native of Videha, is the name of an ancient physician, who is quoted as an authority on Sālākya Tantra. Videha is the modern Trihut and he is styled as निमिश्च राजर्षि वैदेहो । C. S., I. xxvi, 'Nimi, the Royal sage of Videha' In Aṣṭāṅga Hṛdaya Saṁhitā he is also mentioned as an eye doctor and called there a muni or 'Sage' (VI. xiii) मुनिना निमिनोपदिष्टमेतत् परमं रचणमीचणव्य पुंसाम् । But a little earlier he is quoted as विदेहपति or King of Videha, शस्त्रं सर्व्वाचिरोगेषु विदेहपतिनिर्म्मितम् । And in Caraka Saṁhitā (I. xxvi) he is described as Rājā Videha or King Videha, or Nimi Vaideha. *i.e.*, Nimi of Videha षड्रसा इति निमि वैदेहो (C. S., I. xxvi). But we are not certain as to whether Videhādhipa, *i.e.*, King of Videha, may not refer to King Janaka of Mithilā. In Suśruta Saṁhitā VI. i, Videhādhipa is quoted as an authority on eye diseases : शालाक्य शास्त्रभिहिता विदेहाधिपकीर्त्तिता: । Dallaṇa understands by Videhādhipa a reference to Nimi : विदेहाधिपकीर्त्तिता इत्यादि । निमिप्रणीता: षट्सप्ततिनेत्ररोगा: । But he mentions a rival reading in Śusruta Saṁhitā and its commentary by Dallaṇa who refers Janaka to be the King of Videha and the authority in Śālākya Tantra : अस्याग्रे केचित् । विदेहाधिपति: श्रीमान जनको नाम विश्रुत इत्यादि पाठं पठन्ति व्याखानयन्ति च । But this reading is not accepted by Pañjikākāra and so Dallaṇa rejects it : तच्च बृहत्पञ्जिकाकारो न पठति तस्मान्मयापि न पठितो न व्याख्यातश्च । The King of Videha is again mentioned in Aṣṭāṅga Hṛdaya Saṁhitā (VI. xxii) विशेषतो रोहिणिकास्यशोषगन्धान् विदेहाधिपप्रणीता: । and also in Vaṅgasena, L. viii.

In Caraka Saṁhitā (I. xxvi) he is mentioned as one of the conclave of nine physicians who disputed about the questions on the number and nature of the "rasa" or taste. He maintained the existence of seven tastes, *viz.*, the six tastes usually recognised, with the addition of kṣāra or caustic (as distinguished from lavana or saline): सप्तरसा इति निमिर्वैदेहो मधुराम्ललवणकटुतिक्त कषायक्षारा:—sweet, acid, saline, pungent, bitter, astringent and caustic.

In Aruṇadatta's Commentary 'Sarvāṅga Sundarī' Janaka is mentioned as the authority for Sālākya: ऊर्ध्वाङ्ग-चिकित्सा च जनकप्रणीतात्तन्त्रादयथावगम्यते।न तथा सुश्रुतप्रणीतात्।

In Caraka Saṁhitā IV. vi, the opinion of Janaka of Videha is mentioned as regards the part of the fœtus formed first. He is said to have held the view that the organs of sense being the seat of intelligence, are the parts formed first: इन्द्रियाणीति जनकोवैदेहस्तान्यस्य बुद्ध्यधिष्ठानानीति कृत्वा।

Now who was Nimi? He is generally identified with Nimi, the twelfth son of Ikṣāku the founder of the dynasty of Mithilā, about whom the myth is told that he died in consequence of a curse of Vaśiṣṭha, and was then placed by the Gods, in spirit form, in the eyes of living creatures (see Dowson's Classical Dictionary of Hindu Mythology, p. 222). For the legends of Nimi see Muir's Sanskrit Texts, Vol. I, p. 316; Wilson's Viṣṇu Purāṇa, 4to ed., p. 388; Bhāgavat Purāṇa, IX, 13, 1-13. The myth had its origin in the fact of his being an oculist. But do the names Nimi, Janaka and Videha refer to the same person? We should remember that Janaka was a family name used by many kings of Videha. In the Videha line we find Mithi-Janaka and Śīradhvaja Janaka. The latter is the famous Janaka of Mithilā—the father of Sītā and a contemporary of Daśaratha and

Lomapāda. There is no reference in the Rāmāyaṇa that Śīradhvaja was proficient in eye diseases. Whereas if we take Janaka to be the family name, Nimi, Janaka and Videha may refer to a single person.

That Mithi Janaka, Videha and Nimi might have referred to the same king, we have the testimony of Rāmāyaṇa (vii. lxvii) where we find that, owing to the curse of Vasiṣṭha "विदेहो भव" "Be thou without your body", Nimi ceased to have any corporeal body. The sages then performed ceremonies in the forest, and a son was born to him who was styled Mithi, Janaka and Videha.

मुनिः क्रोधात्तं शशाप त्वं विदेहो भव ।
दृष्ट्वा विदेहं राजानमृषयः सर्व्व एव ते ।
तञ्च ते याजयामासुर्यज्ञदीक्षां मनीषिणः ।
नरेन्द्रस्यापि तं देहमरक्षन्नृषिपुङ्गवाः ।
वस्त्रैर्माल्यैश्च गन्धैश्च पूज्यमानं मुहुर्मुहुः ॥
ऋषयोऽपि महात्मानो निमिदेहं समान्यिरे ।
अरणिन्तस्य देहात्तु मन्थानञ्चापि चक्रिरे ॥
मन्त्रहोमैर्महात्मानः पुत्रहेतोर्निमेस्तथा ।
अरण्यां मथ्यमानायां प्रादुर्भूतो यतश्च सः ॥
यतो मिथिरिति ख्यातो जननाज्जनकोऽभवत् ।
विदेहस्त्वाभवद्यस्मान्महात्मा स महातपाः ॥
तस्माद्विदेहाः प्रोच्यन्ते सर्व्वे तद्वंशजा नृपाः ।
एवं विदेहराजस्तु पूर्व्वकोजनकोऽभवत् ॥
मिथिर्नाम महावीर्य्यो येन सा मैथिलीऽभवत् ।

But elsewhere in the same book (Rāmāyaṇa I, lxxi) Nimi is said to be the father of Mithi and grand-father of Janaka.

There is another name quoted in the commentaries, Mahā-videha or Videha the Great; and as such he is twice quoted in Vyākhyā Kusumā Valī. In the later commentaries, however, Nimi, Janaka, Videha and Mahāvideha are often quoted separately by name without supplying us any clue as to their identity. Sometimes they are quoted one after another, as in Vyākhyā Madhu Koṣa : चयादिक्रमेण जनकमपि दोषदर्शयन्नाह, and a few lines after यदाह विदेहः। (Nāsāroga Nidāna). In Śiraroga Nidāna Nimi is quoted तथाचाह निमिः, and immediately afterwards विदेहे, etc. Again the same subject is differently written by Nimi and Videha; compare couplets No. 6 Nimi in Vyākhyā Madhu Koṣa and No. 19 Videha in Nivandha Saṁgraha. So it is highly probable that there were different persons निमि वैदेह, विदेह, and महाविदेह। King Janaka was also a very learned man and he became a Brāhmaṇa. (See Śatapatha Brāhmaṇa; Muller's Anc. Sansk. Lit., pp. 421 ff. Rāmāyaṇa, MBH., Muir's Original Sanskrit Texts, Vol. I, p. 426.)

In the Mahā Bhārata, Nimi is said to have introduced the Śrādh ceremony (offering oblations to fathers) in honour of the dead relations. He belonged to the family of Atri, who taught him the efficiency and desirability of performing Srādh. (Anuśāsana Parva, Ch. 92.)

Genealogy of Nimi (Rāmāyaṇa I, ch. 71)

Nimi
|
Mithi
|
Janaka
|
Udāvasu
|
Nandivardhana
|
Suketu
|
Devarāta
|
Vṛhadratha
|
Mahavīra
|
Sudhṛti
|
Dhṛṣṭaketu
|
Haryyaśva
|
Maru
|
Pratīndhaka
|
Kīrtiratha
|
Devamīḍha
|
Vivudha
Mahīdhraka
Kīrtirāta
|
Mahāroman
|
Svarṇaroman
|
Hrasvaroman

Sīradhvaja		Kuśadhvaja	
Sītā m. Bāma	Urmmīte m. Lakṣaṇa	Māṇḍavī m. Bharata	Śruta kīrti m. Śatrughṇa

The following books are ascribed to King Janaka :—

1. Vaidyaka-Sandeha Bhañjanī or "Solution of Doctor's Difficulties" by Rajā Janaka of Mithilā.

Reference.—Bramhavaivarta Purāṇa.

2. Janaka Tantra.—A quotation from this book occurs in the glosses on the margin of MS. of Aṣṭāṅga Hṛdaya Saṁhitā. See I. O. 2653, fol. 38a.

No work of Nimi is available now. We have collected the quotations from Nimi, Videha, Mahā Videha and Janaka as given in the following books :—

Nimi in Vyākhyā Kusumā Valī —

1. आयसी रौप्यी ताम्री लौह्ये हैमी प्रसादने ।
शैषा अपि यथादोषं प्रयोज्या रसकोविदैः ॥ p. 452

2. अस्विन्नं स्वेदयेद्धीरं पुनरास्विन्नलक्षणादिति । p. 540

3. अर्धहीनं त्रिभागं वा भोजयित्वाऽनुवासयेदिति । p. 564

4. धूमो हि वक्त्रकुष्ठाभ्यां विललयति शक्तितः ।
मस्तिष्कं तद्धि विध्यन्नं नाशाय प्रतिपद्यते ॥ p. 586

5. स्नेहधूमप्रयोगे तु सुखेन वमनीयं न कथमपि नासया । p. 589

6. धूमपाने तु विज्ञेय उच्छ्वासास्त्रिगुणः कलाः ।
तिस्रः कलाश्चात्र मात्राप्रमाणं स्यात्त्रिमात्रिकम् ॥
पिबेत् स्वस्थविधौ मात्रां दुर्बलस्तु कलां पिबेत् ।
अभिष्यन्ने प्रमाणं स्यात् प्रमाणं च पिबेद्रुजि ॥ p. 590

Videha in Vyākhyā Kusumā Valī :—

1. तीर्थायतनदेवाग्नि गुरुवृद्धोपसर्पणैः ।
ज्वरश्च पूजनैश्चापि महसैवोपशाम्यति ॥ p. 57

2. खर्जिंकाविश्वञ्जिष्ठालाक्षामूर्वानिशामयैः ।
तैलं षड्गुणतक्रेण सिद्धं ज्वरहरं परम् ॥ p. 62

3, चर्णितान्प्रपिबेच्छीतैर्वारिभिर्गुडमिश्रितैरिति । p. 85

4. अजाविमूत्रे पक्वा तु आर्द्रवंशावलेखने ।
व्यत्यासात्सर्पिषा कार्य्यं कर्णशूले तु पूरणम् ॥ p. 437

5 कर्पासीतुल्फिकेरीणां स्वरसो मधुसंयुतः ।
युक्तः सर्जकषायेण कर्णस्रावस्य भेषजम् ॥ p. 440

6. प्रागेवात्यामये भक्तं विरात्रमगुरु स्मृतम् ।
उपवासस्त्र्यहं वा स्यात्तिक्तं वाऽप्यशनं हितम् ॥ p. 448

7. अभिष्यन्देऽधिमन्थे च नेत्रयोः कफसंभवे ।
उत्पत्तावेव कर्त्तव्यं नेत्रयोः कफनाशनम् ॥
तीक्ष्णशाच्योः परीषेकस्तीक्ष्णं चाऽऽश्चोतनादिकम् ॥ p. 449

8. कण्टकारी शिफैरण्डमूलत्वक्पक्व साधितं ।
चीरमाजं हितं सेके रुक्षु स्यन्दाधिमन्थयोः ॥ p. 450

9. प्राणवात्यामये कार्य्यं विरावं लुप्तभोजनम् ।
उपवासस्त्र्यहं वा स्यान्नक्तं वाऽप्यशनं लघु ॥
ततश्चतुर्थे दिवसे व्याधिं संजातलक्षणम् ।
समीक्ष्याऽऽश्चोतनैः सेकैर्यथास्वमुपपादयेत् ॥ p. 454

10. वल्मीक शिखराकारं भङ्गे नीलोत्पलद्युति ।
स्रोतोञ्जनं प्रशंसन्ति चक्षुर्वेदार्थचिन्तकाः ।
अञ्जनं मधुरं स्निग्धं कषायं लेखनं हिमम् ।
पित्तरक्तविषच्छर्दिहिक्कां हन्ति सुदृष्टिदम् ॥
तत्र स्रोतोञ्जनं श्रेष्ठं तस्मात्सौवीरकाञ्जनम् ॥ p. 476

11. अतितीक्ष्णैर्निरूढस्य हृतदोषस्य सर्वतः ।
कंचिद्देवानभिप्रेतं मार्गं स्नेहोऽनुगच्छति ॥ p. 569

12. प्रयोगपाने पूर्वं वा नस्ततो (नासया) धूमामाचरेत् । p. 589

13. प्रदेशिन्या निमग्रे द्वे पर्वणी च मतोऽखिलः ।
नस्य कर्मणि तैलादि विज्ञेयो बिन्दुसंज्ञितः ॥ p. 594

14. चतुरश्चतुरो बिन्दुन्नैकैकस्मिन्समाचरेत् ।
एषा लघ्वी मता मात्रा तथा शीर्षं विरेचयेत् ॥
अध्यर्धां द्विगुणां वाऽपि त्रिगुणाम् वा चतुर्गुणाम् ।
यथाव्याधि विदित्वा तु मात्रां समवचारयेद् ॥ p. 595

15. निष्ठीवेन्न पिबेन्नस्यं व्यापदः पिबतस्त्विमाः ।
भवन्ति कासश्छर्दिश्च क्लमाऽन्ने वमथुस्तथा ॥ p. 595

16. क्षीणं मांसं बलं यस्य वातार्तिश्चोर्ध्वजत्रुजा ।
सुदीप्ताग्निः स्नेहसात्म्यः स नस्यं नस्ततः (नासया) पिबेत् ॥
धातूंश्च तर्पयेद्द्वे हि पीतं नस्यंतु नस्ततः (नासया) ॥ p. 595

17. सूर्य्यस्य उदयात्पूर्वमायामत्प्रथमान्निशः ।
कालोऽस्य दाने सर्वः स्यात्तायं प्रातर्विशेषतः ॥ p. 597

18. इत्येवं स्नेहनस्याख्यः प्रतिमर्शः प्रकीर्तित. ,
स्नेहेनासंस्कृतेनैष कर्त्तव्यः संस्कृतेन वा ॥
नस्यं तु संस्कृतेनैव दातव्यं भिषजां वरैः ॥ p. 598

19. नाड़ी षड़ङ्गुलायामा द्विमुखी च तया धमेत् ।
चिशूर्णं सुचुटीमात्रमेष प्रधमने विधिः ॥
शक्तिमात्रं तु जिघ्रेद्वा बद्धं सूक्ष्मेण वाससा ॥ p. 599

20. गण्डुषः शर्करा चौद्रघृतोत्पलपयस्तिलैः ।
व्यस्तैः समस्तैर्योज्यस्तु मुखे चारादितापितः ॥ p. 601

Mahāvideha in Vyākhyā Kusumā Vali :—

1. चत्वारिंशत्तथाऽष्टौ च प्रमाणेनाङ्गुलानि हि ।
नेवं प्रायोगिकं कार्य्यं द्वाविंशत्स्नैहिकं भवेत् ॥
चतुर्विंशत्यङ्गुलकं वैरेचनिकमिष्यते ॥
कासघ्ने कर्दमीये च कर्त्तव्यं षोड़शाङ्गुलम् ॥ p. 588

2. भीतः क्रुद्धः शोकवांश्च दृष्टिहानिं भ्रमं क्लमम् ।
वक्त्रार्ककर्मक्लान्तस्तु तथा दौर्बल्यमाप्नुयुः ॥

तृष्णास्यशोषमोहांस्तु क्षीणधातुः पुनः क्षयम् ।
रुजः पित्तानिलकृतान्व्याधीन्दौर्बल्यमेव च ॥
रक्तोल्वणः पैत्तिकस्य विरुद्धौ रक्तपित्तयोः ।
पिपासार्तस्तालुशोषी मूर्च्छार्तश्चलचेतनः ॥
तेषां हृद्विर्निशिरेण वाग्घातं मौनमेव च ।
ज्वरी मद्यात्ययी मद्यं पीत्वा च लभते नरः ॥
मोहं तृष्णां वक्त्रशोषं दृष्टिहानिं शिरोरुजम् ।
प्रजागरी शिरोरोगं तिमिरी दृष्टिवैकृतम् ॥
विरिक्तो हृतदोषस्य शोषं तृष्णां शिरोरुजम् ।
दत्तबस्तिर्हृष्टिहानिं क्षतो भूयः क्षतामयान् ॥
धूमो गर्भस्य गर्भिण्याः शोषतापेन्द्रियव्यथाः ।
क्षौद्रसेवी प्राणरोधं तन्दोषं वा समाप्नुयात् ॥
दधिक्षीरं पयोमस्त्वाम्भुक्त्वा वा धूममाचरेत् ।
हृन्दोषमूर्च्छाहृल्लासच्छर्दीः प्राप्नोति मानवः । p. 590

Videha in Nivandha Samgraha :—

1. युग्मेषु तु दिनेष्वासां भवत्यल्पतरं रजः ।
संयोगं तत्र या गच्छेत् सा पुमांसं प्रसूयते ॥
अयुग्मेषु दिनेष्वासां भवेद्बहुतरं रजः ।
संयोगं तत्र यो गच्छेत् सा तु कन्यां प्रसूयते ॥ p. 702

2. See 15 Videha in V. K. V. p. 1199

3. See. 16 „ „ p. 1199

4. अश्रुस्रावः शिरा गत्वा नेत्रसन्धिषु तिष्ठति ।
ततः कनीनकं गत्वा चाश्रु कृत्वा कनीनके ॥
ततः स्रवत्यथास्रावं यथादोषमवेदनम् ।
अश्रुस्रावशब्देनात्र तत्सहितो दोषाऽभिधीयते । p. 1308

5. वर्त्मोत्सङ्गेऽप्यधावन्तो सन्निपातात्प्रजायते ।
अभ्यन्तरमुखाः स्थूला बाह्यान्तश्चापि दृश्यते ॥

पिण्डकापिड़काभिश्च चितान्याभिः समन्ततः।
उत्सङ्गपिड़का नाम कठिना मन्दवेदना ॥
सा प्रभिन्ना स्रवेत् स्रावं कुक्कुटाण्डरसोपमम्। p. 1310

6. श्लेष्मदुष्टेन रक्तेन क्लिष्टमांसमिवोभयं।
वन्धुजीवनिभं वर्त्म क्लिष्टवर्त्म तदुच्यते ॥ p. 1312

7. प्रक्षालितेऽथवा स्पृष्टे आनह्यते पुनः पुनः।
अपरिक्लिन्न वर्त्मानं पिञ्जाख्यमिति निर्द्दिशेत् ॥ p. 1312

8. समन्ताद्विस्तृतः श्यावो रक्तो वा मांससञ्चयः।
सान्निपातेन दोषाणां प्रस्तार्य्यर्म्मतदुच्यते ॥ p. 1315

9. रक्तराजीनिभं कृष्णे विद्रुमाभं प्रलक्ष्यते।
सूच्यग्रेणेव तत् शुक्लमुष्णांशुस्रावि सव्रणम् ॥ p. 1318

10. चोषकृत् स्रावदाही च कृष्णे पिड़िकोद्गमः।
व्यक्तामुद्गफलाकारं शुक्लं द्वित्वाश्रितं भवेत् ॥ p. 1319

11. अन्तर्गतशिराणान्तु यदा तिष्ठति मारुतः।
स तदा नयनं प्राप्य शीघ्रं दृष्टिं निरस्यति ।।
तस्यां निरस्यमानायां निर्म्मन्थन्निव मारुतः।
नयनं निर्व्वर्मत्याशु शूलतो दाहि मन्थनैः ॥
अथवा शोषयेदक्षिणी तेजो वलावलम् ॥
तत्तमसीव संशुष्कमवसीदति लोचनम्।
हताधिमन्थं तं विद्यादसाध्यवातकोपत ॥ p. 1324

12. नक्तमन्ध्यास्तु चत्वारो ये पूरस्तात् प्रकीर्त्तिताः।
तेषामसाध्योनुकुलो कृस्वजाद्यस्तथैव च। p. 1333

13. प्रागेवात्त्यामये भक्तं चिराचगुरुस्मृतं।
उपवासस्त्र्यहं वा स्यात् नक्तं व्यापाशनं हितं।
ततश्चतुथ दिवसे व्याधौ सञ्जात लक्षणे।
यथोक्तास्तु क्रियाः कार्य्याः नस्यसेकाञ्जनादिकाः।

शिरोमोचणे तव शिरा उपनासिका ललाटया वा।
अपां चोष्णं आश्चोतने च शीतमेव।
सैन्धवादौ नस्य षष्ट्याह्न पिप्पलीभिः।
घृतं पयः हितमर्द्धोदकं सेके आश्चोतने एव च। p. 1338

14. निरन्तरं दिनान्तरं द्व्यन्तरं त्र्यन्तरं वा।
योज्यं तर्पणं सन्निपातोच्छेद्यन्तरं वान्तरं कफे॥ p. 1388

15. प्रागेवात्यामये कार्य्यं विरात्रं लघुभोजनम्।
उपवासस्त्र्यहं वा स्यात् नक्तं वाप्यशनं त्र्यहम्॥
ततश्चतुर्थे दिवसे व्याधिं सञ्जातलक्षणम्।
समीक्ष्याश्चोतनैः सेकै यथास्वमुपपादयेत्॥ p. 1393

16. तीक्ष्णाञ्जनैरतिक्लिष्टेषु नेत्रेषु वातातपधूमरजःकीटमक्षिकामशकस्पर्शादिभिरभिहतेषु सलिलक्रीड़ाजागरणलङ्घनाद्यभिभूतेषु वा परिश्रमक्लान्तेषु भयाद्दितेषु दिवाकराग्निचन्द्रग्रहनक्षत्रक्रमणकर्म्मविविधरूपप्रेक्षणाद्यभिहतेषु दुर्व्वलेषु नेत्रेषु रागदाहतोदशोफपाकघर्षादिवेदनास्विति। p. 1405

17. गव्येन दध्ना पिष्टाभ्यां शङ्खसैन्धवाभ्यां स्रोतोऽञ्जनं रसाञ्जनं अर्द्धपक्षं सार्द्धसप्तरात्रमसकृत् लेपयेत् ततोऽनन्तरं तत् स्रोतोऽञ्जनरसाञ्जने पिष्टा वर्त्तिः कोर्पासाञ्चलेन शिशोः शुक्रं नुदति स्फोटयतीर्थः। p. 1408

18. मारुतकफवाताभ्यां संसृष्टशोणितेन च।
कर्णे क्ष्वेड़ं सञ्जनयेत् क्ष्वेड़नं वेणुघोषवत्॥ p. 1411

19. तत्र वातानुगं पित्तं चितं शिरसि तिष्ठति।
मध्याह्ने तेजसार्कस्य तद्विदग्धं शिरोरुजम्॥
करोति पैत्तिकीं घोरां संशाम्यति दिनक्षये।
अस्तं गते प्रभाहीने सूर्य्ये वायुर्व्विवर्द्धते।
पित्तं शान्तिमवाप्नोति ततः शाम्यति वेदना।
एष पित्तानिलकृतः सूर्य्यावर्त्तविपर्य्ययः। p. 1435

Videha in Vākhyā Madhu Koṣa :—

1. ज्वरस्तु पूजनैर्व्वापि सहसैवोपशाम्यति। p 16

2. क्रोधशोकौ स्मृतौ वातरक्तपित्तप्रकोपणाविति । p. 27

3. मृद्भक्षणाद्भवेत् पाण्डुस्तन्द्रालस्यनिपीड़ितः ।
सश्वासकासशोषार्शः सदारुचिसमन्वितः ।
शूनपादाननकरः कृशाङ्गः क्षमपावक ॥ p. 79

4. पित्तेन तिक्तास्य विदाहकृत् स्यात्
स्वाद्वास्यहृल्लासकरः कफेन ॥ p. 109

5. निःस्वप्नं सत्यसंस्कृतभाषिणमिति । p. 136

6. क्रोधनं स्वस्त सर्व्वाङ्गो लालाफेणाविलाननः ।
निद्रालुः कम्पनो मूको गणमातृभिरर्द्दितः ॥ p. 136

7. देवविप्रगुरुद्वेषी वेदवेदाङ्गवित् शुचिः ।
आत्मपीड़ाकारी हासी ब्रह्मराक्षस सेवित । p. 138

8. मेढ्प्रवृत्तः क्षतजः सास्राक्षः स्रुतनासिकः ।
रुग्नजिह्वः पतिगर्भो हतवागतिदुर्व्वलः ॥ p. 138

9. एक एव वायुः स्थानकर्म्मभेदात् पञ्चधेवोच्यते । p. 146

10. अत्यन्त सुकुमाराङ्गी रजो दुष्टं स्रवन्ती च ।
अव्यायामवती यस्मात्तस्मान्न स्खलितः स्त्रियाः ॥ p. 297

11. यदव पटलाभासं सरुजस्कं शिरस्त्वचि ।
परुषं जायते जन्तोस्तस्यरूपं विशेषतः ॥
तोदैः समन्वितं वातात् सकण्डूगौरवं कफात् ।
सपिपासं सदाहार्त्तिं रागं पित्तासजं तथा ॥ p. 297

12. मूर्च्छा दाहो ज्वरः श्वासः क्लमोऽथ वमथुस्तथा ।
उपद्रवाः कर्णशूले भवन्त्येते मरिष्यत ॥ p. 322

13. शिरोगतो यदा वायुः श्रोत्रयोः प्रतिपद्यते ।
तदा तु विविधान् शब्दान् समीरयति कर्णयोः ॥
झङ्कार क्रौञ्चनादं वा मण्डूकारण्डयो स्तथा ।
तन्त्रीमृदङ्गशब्दं वा सामसूर्य्यस्वनन्तथा ॥

पीताध्ययनवंशानां निर्घोषं चूडनन्तथा।
अपामिव पतन्तीनां शकटस्येव गच्छत: ॥
श्वसतामिव सर्पाणां सदृश: श्रुयते स्वन ॥ p. 322

14. See 18 in Ni. S p. 323.

15. कफाद्वा मारुताद्वापि सन्निपातेन वा पुन: ॥ p. 323

16. कफपित्तमसृङ्मिश्रं सञ्चितं मूर्ध्नि देहिनां।
विदह्यमुषमणोद्गाढं व्रणां कृताचिरशङ्कजां।
तत: प्रस्यन्दते घ्राणात् सरक्तं पूतिपीतकं।
पूनितस्यन्तु तं विद्यादघ्राणकण्डू ज्वरप्रदं ॥ p. 328

17. पूर्व्वरूपाणि दृश्यन्ते प्रतिश्याये भविष्यति।
घ्राणधुमायनं मन्थ: क्षवथु स्तालुदाहनं।
कण्ठोध्वंसी मुखस्राव: शिरस: पूरणन्तथा ॥ p. 332

18. नृणां दुष्टप्रतिश्यायस्त्वसाध्य: सर्व्वज: स्मृत:। p. 333

19. मन्यानामन्तरे वायुरुन्नत: पृष्ठतोऽपि वा।
करोति भेदं निस्तोदं शङ्खं ग चाक्ष्णोर्भ्रुवोस्तदा।
तमाहुरन्यतीवातं रोगं दृष्टिविदो जना: ॥ p. 340

20. एकत्वग गतमेवं स्याद्वित्वग्गतमिदं भवेत्।
चोषंपाकासदाहस्तु तृष्णा च पिड़कोद्गम। p. 343

21. व्यक्तमुक्ताफलाकारं अर्म्म द्वित्वग्गतं भवेत्। p. 343

22. कृष्णेऽक्ष्णोर्यद्भवेच्छुक्लं छागलीविट् समप्रभ:।
नान्त: पिच्छिलरक्ताश्रु स्त्रिलग्गतमजकाजातं ॥ p. 344

23. यथास्वं रज्यते दृष्टिर्दोषैस्त्रिपटलस्थितै:।
चतुर्थपटल प्राप्तैर्मण्डलं रज्यते तु तै: ॥ p. 346

24. "पित्तं रक्तप्रसादेन मूर्च्छयित्वा तु मारुत" इत्यारभ्य "एष
याप्य: स्मृत: काचो ग्लायि नाम्ना शरीरिणां" इति ॥ p. 349

25. See 12 Videha in Ni. S.

विशेषेण भवेयातां तौ चतुःपटलाश्रितौ ।

च सम्प्राप्तरागत्वादसाध्यौ परिकीर्त्तितौ ॥ p. 353

26. मारुतोत्पीड़ितः श्लेष्मा शुक्लभागे व्यवस्थितः ।

जलविन्दुरिवोच्छूनो ह्यमृदुःकफसम्भवः ।

बलासग्रथितं नाम तं शाथं वृत्तमादिशेत् ॥ p, 357

27. शोथ क्लेदसमाविष्टं तोदभेदसमाकूलं ।

पूरालसन्तु तं विद्यात् सन्धौ कालीनिकं नृणां ॥ p. 358

28. वायुः श्लेष्माणामादाय दृष्टिसन्धौ व्यवस्थितः ।

अरुणं कठिनं ग्रन्थिं जनयेदल्पवेदनं ।

श्लेष्मोपनाहं तं विद्यात् स्रावान् वत्यामतःपरं ॥ p. 358

29. चत्वार एवोक्ताः सन्निपातात् कफाद्रक्तात् पित्तात् स्रावोऽचिसन्धिषु ।

p. 359

30. वर्त्मशुक्लस्य सन्धौ तु ग्रन्थिः पित्तकफात्मकः ।

उष्मणा पच्यते गाढ़ं तत्र मूर्च्छन्ति जन्तवः ।

सुसुक्ष्मा जालचारणा वर्त्मपक्ष्मसमाश्रयाः ।

ततस्ते पूयसंसृष्टाः पतन्ति क्रिमयस्तथा ।

लक्षणैर्विविधैर्युक्ताः सन्निपातसमुत्थिता ।

क्रिमिग्रन्थिन्तु तं विद्याद्देहिनां नेत्रदूषण ॥ p. 360

31. शुक्लकृष्णान्तसन्धौ तु चीयन्तेऽसृक कफानिलाः ।

पर्व्वणिपिड़का तैस्तु जायते त्वङ्कुरोपमा ।

ताम्रास्रदाहचोषोष्णपीतकाश्रुसमाकूलाः ।

कफपित्ते तु संमूर्च्छ सह रक्तेन मारुतः ।

शुक्लकृष्णान्त सन्धौ तु जनयेद्गोस्तनाकृतिं ।

पिड़कामलजीं तान्तु विद्धि तोदाश्रु संकुलात् ॥ p. 360

32. See 5 Videha in Ni. S. p. 361

33. सुसूक्ष्मा पिड़काकीर्णा या स्थूला पिड़का खरा।
जायते सन्निपातात्तु वर्त्म शर्करिकेति सा॥ p. 362

34. नीरुजा कठिना वर्त्म पश्चान्तवाह्यतोऽपि वा।
पिड़का सन्निपातेन तदर्शोवर्त्म निर्दिशेत्॥ p. 362

35. वर्त्मोऽभ्यन्तर्गतं त्वर्शः शुष्कं स्थूलञ्च दारुणं।
जायते सन्निपातेन तच्छुष्कार्शः प्रकीर्त्तितं॥ p. 362

36. See 6 Videha in Ni. S. p. 363

37. दुष्टश्लेष्मा मरुत् पित्तं वर्त्म नोन्नीयते यदा।
अग्निदग्धानिभं श्यावं श्याववर्त्मेति तद्विदुः॥ p. 364

38. प्रक्षालितेऽथवा स्पृष्टे आनह्यते पुनः पुनः।
अपरिक्लिन्नवर्त्मानं तत्पिन्नमिति निर्दिशेत्॥ p. 364

39. वायुः शोणितमादाय शिराणां प्रमुखे स्थितः।
जनयत्यङ्कुरं ताम्रं वर्त्मनि छिन्नरोहणं।
तच्छोणितार्शोऽसाध्यं स्याद्रक्तस्राव्यथ नीरुजं॥ p. 366

40. यस्य वातसम्बन्धे न दोषाः प्रकुपितास्त्वयत्यादि। p. 367

41. शून्यं भ्रमति तुद्येत शिरोविभ्रान्तनेत्रता।
मूर्च्छागात्रावसादश्च शिरोरोगे चयात्मके॥ p. 370

42. सूर्य्यावर्त्तविपर्य्ययो मध्याह्नात् प्रभृति वर्द्धते दिनक्षये च प्रशाम्यतीति।
p. 371

43, शिरसोऽन्यतरे पार्श्वे कुपितो मारुतो यदा।
श्लेष्मणा रुध्यते जन्तो स्तोदस्फुटनदालनैः।
शूलावदावरणैर्गाढ़मर्द्धान्तदवरुध्यते।
नयनञ्चावदीर्य्यते सोऽर्द्धभेदः कफानिलात्।
तथा त्र्यहात् स पक्षाहात् पक्षान्मासाच्च देहिनां॥ p 373

44. चीयते तु तदा पित्तं शङ्खयोरनिलाचितं।
निरुणद्धि ततो मर्म्मपरिपूपित मूलकं।

ततः शङ्खौ प्रयुज्येते दह्येते इव वह्निना ।
सूचीभिरिव तुद्येते निकृत्येते इवासिना ।
शङ्खको नाम शिरसि व्याधिरेष सुदारुणः ।
तृष्णामूर्च्छाज्वरकरस्त्रिरात्रात् परमन्तकृत् ।
कुशलेन तूपक्रान्तस्त्रिराचादेव जीवति ॥ p. 373

Nimi in Vyākhyā Madhu Koṣa :—

1. श्लेष्म पित्तजलोन्मिश्रे कोथः शोणितमांसजे ।
जायन्ते जन्तवस्तच कृष्णास्ताम्राः सितारुणाः ।
भक्षयन्ति तु ते कर्णं कुर्व्वते विविधा रुजः ।
क्रिमिकर्णन्तु तं विद्यात् सन्निपात प्रकोपजम् ॥ p. 324

2. पञ्चभूतात्मिका दृष्टिर्मसूरार्द्धदलोन्मितिः । p. 344

3. नेत्रायामत्रिभागश्च कृष्णमण्डलमुच्यते ।
कृष्णात् सप्तममिच्छन्ति दृष्टिं दृष्टिविदो जनाः ॥ p. 344

4. काच इत्येष विज्ञेयो याप्य स्त्रिपटलेस्थितः ।
चतुर्थपटलप्राप्तो लिङ्गनाशः स उच्यते ।
प्रत्याख्येयश्च कफजो व्याधिः साध्यस्तु तद्विदा ॥ p. 347

5. प्रस्तारिणोऽर्म्मणः स्रावं निरुणद्धि शदानिलः ।
भिन्नस्रावं हि शुष्कं तं स्नायुर्म्मेति प्रकीर्त्तितं ॥ p. 356

6. हिमशीतात्मको नित्यमहेतुकफमारुतौ ।
कुर्व्वाते वेदनां तीव्रां दिनात् पूर्व्वाह्न एव तु ।
आदित्य तेजसायुक्ते निवृत्तेऽपि च भास्करे ।
स्रोतसां विवृतत्वाच्च ततः श्लेष्माधिगच्छति ।
उद्रिक्तौ मातरिश्वा च स्वमार्गं प्रतिपद्यते ।
तस्मान्मध्यदिनादूर्द्ध्वं वेदनाच प्रशाम्यति ॥ p. 371

Videha in Tatta Candrikā :—

1. दशभिर्द्दशभिः शश्वत् पिप्पलीभिस्तु वर्द्धयेत् ।
पञ्चभिः पञ्चभिर्वापि शतादवतरेत् पुनः ॥ p. 210

2. बंशावलेखकल्केन मूत्र श्राजे तथाविके।
   पचेत् तैलं रुजः शान्त्यै कर्णयोः पूरणं भिषक्॥ p. 290
3. उपवासस्त्र्यहं वा स्यात्। p. 296
4. See 8 Videha in V. K. V. p. 297
5. सिद्ध वातहरक्काथे कल्के मधूरके घृतम्।
   पाने नस्ये विधातव्यं शिरोरोगे चयोद्भवे॥ p. 317

Videha in Bhāva Prakāśa :—

1. See 20 Videha in V. M. K.
2. एकैकमनुपद्यन्ते पर्य्यायात् पटलान्तरम्। p. 976
3. See 19 Videha in V. M. K., p. 1002.

Nimi in Navanītaka (Bower MS.) :—

1. See formula 1 : Remedies against Cataract. p. 161

Janaka in Vyākhyā Madhukoṣa :—

1. जनकमपि दोषं दर्शयन्नाह चयं गता इत्यादि। चयं गता इत्याभिधानं स्वे स्वे स्थाने स्वस्थाने वृद्धिर्द्दोषाणाम् "चय इत्यभिधीयत" इति वचनात्। p. 331

The following formulæ are ascribed to Nimi, Janaka or Videha :

	Formula.	Author.	Book.	Page.
1.	Remedies against Cataract	Nimi	Bower Ms.	161
2.	Mahātraiphala Ghṛta.			
	महात्रैफलघृतम्	,,	G. N., I	13
3.	Triphalādya Ghṛta			
	त्रिफलाद्यघृतम्	,,	,,	21
4.	Prasaraṇī Oil			
	तृतीय प्रसारणी तैलम्	Janaka	,,	36
5.	Triphalā Yoga			
	तिमिरे त्रिफलायोगः	Nimi	,, II.	450

	Formula.	Author.	Book.	Page.
6.	Cūrnañjaṇa			
	चूर्णाञ्जणम्	Nimi	G. N., II	459
7.	Kunkumādya Oil			
	कुङ्कुमाद्य तैलम्	Videha	V. M.	412

1. Remedy against Cataract.

(883 and 884.) Take one part each of white antimony and cuttlefish bone, also one part each of white pepper and long pepper, (884) and add one part of salt, equal to an aksha. This, in the form of a fine powder, makes a capital remedy against cataract, highly esteemed by Nimi, and fit for people of respectability.'

स्रोतोऽञ्जनस्य भागो भागश्च भवेत् समुद्रफेनस्य ।
श्वेतमरिचस्य भागो भागोऽप्यथ पिप्पलीनाम् च ।
लवणाच्चभागयुक्तम् निमिना परमार्च्चितम् हितमुदारम् ।
तिमिरापहम् सुसूक्ष्मम् चूर्णम् स्यादार्य जन योग्यम् ॥

2. Mahātraiphala Ghṛta.

वैदेहाक्ष्निरोगे महात्रैफलं घृतम् ।
त्रिफलाया रसप्रस्थं प्रस्थं भृङ्गरसस्य च ।
पीडयित्वा वृषं वालं रसप्रस्थं च दापयेत् ॥
अजाक्षीरस्य च प्रस्थं, प्रस्थं तैः सर्पिषः पचेत् ।
त्रिफला चन्दनं द्राक्षा पिप्पली मधुकं वला ॥
काकोलीक्षीरकाकोलीमेदामरिचसैन्धवैः ।
शर्करा पुण्डरीकं च हरिद्रोत्पलनागरैः ॥
कल्कैः सिद्धं भिषग्दद्यान्नेत्ररोगविनाशनम् ।
काचं शुक्रं नीलिकां च वर्त्मरोगांश्च नाशयेत् ॥
नक्तान्ध्यं नकुलान्ध्यं च कण्डुं पिल्लमथापि च ।
अजकां तिमिरांश्चैव नेत्रस्रावांश्च दारुणान् ॥

त्रिफलासर्पिरेतद्धि पाननावनतर्पणैः।
विदेहराज्ञा निर्दिष्टं दृष्टिनैर्मल्यकारकम् ॥ १२९ ॥

---

3. Triphalādya Ghṛta.

विदेहात्सर्वतैत्ररोगे त्रिफलाद्यं घृतम्।

त्रिफलाया रसप्रस्थं प्रस्थं भृङ्गरसस्य च।
पीडयित्वा वृषं बालं रसप्रस्थं प्रदापयेत् ॥
अजाक्षीरस्य च प्रस्थं कार्षिकैः सुक्ष्मपेषितैः।
पिप्पली शर्करा द्राक्षा त्रिफला नीलमुत्पलम् ॥
मधुकं क्षीरकाकोली मधुपर्णी निदिग्धिका।
मञ्जिष्ठापद्मकोशीरसारिवादारुचन्दनैः ॥
घृतं प्रस्थं पचेत् प्राज्ञः कल्कैरेभिः समन्वितम्।
ऊर्ध्वं पानमधः पानं मध्ये पानं विशिष्यते ॥
अति प्रदुष्टे रक्ते च रक्ते वातिस्रुते तथा।
नक्तान्ध्ये तिमिरे काचे सर्वनेत्ररुजासु च ॥
बकविद्योतितं भ्रान्तं सूर्यतेजोद्विषं तथा।
गृध्रदृष्टिकरं धन्यं बलवर्णाग्निवर्धनम् ॥
त्रिफलाया घृतं सिद्धं सर्वनेत्ररुजान्तकृत ॥

4. Prasāraṇī Taila.

वातरोगे तृतीयं प्रसारणीतैलम्।

समूलपत्रामुत्पाद्य जातसारां प्रसारणीम्।
कुट्टयित्वा पलशतं कटाहे समधिश्रयेत् ॥
दशमूली बला रास्ना तथा सहचरास्तते।
शतावरी श्वदंष्ट्रा च एरण्डः कपिकच्छुका ॥
पृथग्दशपलान् भागांस्तथैव समधिश्रयेत्।
वारिद्रोणे समायुक्तं चतुर्भागावशेषितम् ॥
कषायसमभागं तु तैलमत्र प्रदापयेत्।
प्रशस्ते च दिने कार्यं नक्षत्रे चापि शोभने ॥

देवदारु वचा मुस्तं शताह्वा मधुयष्टिका।
पिप्पली मधुकं रास्ना ह्यष्टवर्गेण संयुता ॥
चित्रकं पद्मकोशीरे कुष्ठं व्याघ्रनखं शठी।
शुण्ठीसैन्धवमञ्जिष्ठाः कल्कपेष्याणि कारयेत् ॥
दधिमस्त्वम्लशुक्तानां तथा मांसरसस्य च।
आढकाढकमादाय शनैर्मृद्वग्निना पचेत् ॥
एतदभ्यञ्जनं पानं नस्यकर्मानुवासनम्।
पृष्ठपार्श्वग्रहे शूले सक्थिवङ्क्षणयोस्तथा ॥
एकाङ्गके पक्षवधे हनुमन्याशिरोग्रहे।
बाधिर्ये कर्णशूले च कर्णनादे च दापयेत् ॥
अभ्यङ्गात्त्वग्गतं हन्ति पानान्मांसगतं तथा।
पक्वाशयगते बस्तिर्निरूहः सार्वकामिकः ॥
अशीतिर्वातजान् रोगांश्चत्वारिंशच्च पैत्तिकान्।
विंशतिः श्लेष्मजांश्चैव सर्वानेवापकर्षति ॥
गृध्रसीं वातभग्नं च ऋतुदोषं तथैव च।
ये नरा नष्टशुक्राश्च ऋतुहीनाश्च याः स्त्रियः ॥
वन्ध्या च लभते गर्भमृतुस्नाता न संशयः।
(यस्मात्प्रसारयत्येषा मेधाग्निजनता शुभा ॥
आयुर्वृद्धिकरा चैव तथा जनकपूजिता। ?)

---

5. Triphalā Yogā.

तिमिरे त्रिफलायोगाः।

तिमिरं रागतां याति रागाः काचत्वमेव च।
काचात्संजायते नीली तदाऽन्धो जायते नरः ॥
लिह्यात्सदा च त्रिफलां सुचूर्णितां
घृतप्रगाढां तिमिरे च पित्तजे।
समीरजे तैलयुतां कफात्मके
मधुप्रगाढां विदधीत युक्तितः ॥

कल्कः क्वाथोऽथवा चूर्णं त्रिफलाया निषेवितम् ।
मधुना हविषा वाऽपि समस्ततिमिरान्तकृत् ॥
त्रैफलेनाथ हविषा लिहानस्त्रिफलां निशि ।
यष्टीमधुकसंयुक्तां मधुना च परिप्लुताम् ॥
मासमेकं हिताहारः पिबन्नामलकोदकम् ।
सौपर्णं लभते चक्षुरित्याह भगवान्निमिः ॥

त्रिफलाक्वाथकल्केन सपयस्कं घृतं शृतम् ।
तिमिराण्यचिराद्धन्यात्पीतं निशामुखे ॥
शतावरीपायस एव केवलस्तथा कृतो वाऽऽमलकेषु पायसः ।
प्रभूतसर्पिस्त्रिफलोदकोत्तरो यवौदनं वा तिमिरं व्यपोहति ॥
त्रिफलाऽयोरजोयष्टीसर्पिःक्षौद्रसमन्विता ।
दिनान्ते शीलिता हन्त्या सर्वनेत्रगदाञ्जयेत् ॥
घृतं पुराणं त्रिफलां शतावरीं पटोलमुद्गामलकं यवानपि
निषेवमाणस्य नरस्य यत्नतो भयं सुघोरात्तिमिरान्न विद्यते ॥
यस्त्रैफलं चूर्णमपथ्यवर्जी
सायं समश्नाति हविर्मधुभ्याम् ।
स मुच्यते नेत्रगतैर्विकारै-
र्भृत्यैर्यथा क्षीणधनो नरेन्द्रः ॥
जाता रोगा विनश्यन्ति न भवन्ति कदाचन ।
त्रिफलायाः कषायेण प्रातर्नयनधारणात् ॥
जलगण्डूषैः प्रातर्बहुशोऽम्भोभिः प्रपूर्य मुखम् ।
निर्दयमुच्चनुच्चि क्षपयति तिमिराणि ना सद्यः ।
भुक्त्वा पाणितलं घृष्य चक्षुषोर्यदि दीयते ।
अचिरेणैव तद्वारि तिमिराणि व्यपोहति ॥

6. Cūrṇāñjana.

चूर्णाञ्जनम् ।

द्राक्षा मृणालीक्षुरसे क्षीर मद्यव साम्बु च ।
पृथग्दिव्याम्बु स्रोतोजं सप्तकृत्वो निषेचयेत् ॥

तच्चूर्णं संस्थितं शङ्खे दृक्प्रसादनमञ्जनम् ।
शस्तं सर्वाक्षिरोगेषु विदेहपति निर्मितम् ॥

7. Kuṅkumādya Taila.

कुङ्कुमाद्य तैलम् ।

कुङ्कुमं चन्दनं लाक्षा मञ्जिष्ठा मधुयष्टिका ॥
कालीय कमुशीरं च पद्मकं नीलमुत्पलम् ॥
न्यग्रोधपादाः प्लक्षस्य शुङ्गाः पद्मस्य केसरम् ॥
द्विपञ्चमूलसहितैः कषायैः पालिकैः पृथक् ॥
जलाढ़कं विपक्तव्यं पादशेषमथोद्धरेत् ॥
मञ्जिष्ठा मधुकं लाक्षा पत्त (ना) ङ्गं मधुयष्टिका ॥
कर्षप्रमाणैरेतैस्तु तैलस्य कुड़वं पचेत् ॥
अजाक्षीरं तद्विगुणं शनैर्मृदग्निना पचेत् ॥
सम्यक्पक्वं परं ह्येतन्मुखवर्णप्रसादनम् ॥
नीलिकपिटिकाव्यङ्गानभ्यङ्गादेव नाशयेत् ॥
सप्तरात्रेण वदनं भवेत्कमलसन्निभम् ॥
कुङ्कुमाद्यमिदं तैलं श्रेष्ठं वैदेहनिर्मितम् ॥

ŚĀLIHOTRA.

Āyurveda according to Caraka (I. xxx), is the science of life. It gives us an insight into the phenomena and different manifestations of life; its origin, development, and decay; its existence in man and other animals, and plants, in health and diseases with prophylaxis and treatment; its duration and the means of prolonging it; its relations with the body and mind and the inter-relation between them; its misery and how to avoid it, and its happiness and the means of its augmentation. This definition is sufficiently comprehensive and includes for its consideration the various divisions of medical science as a whole (Pūrnāṅga) and its various branches, the octopartite (Aṣṭāṅga) and the three-shouldered (Triskandha). The Āyurveda in its narrow sense treats man as its object, and we have well-known treatises dealing with it, *viz.*, Caraka Saṁhitā, Suśruta Saṁhitā, and other works, too numerous to mention here. For a detailed list of such works I would refer my readers to my contributions to "History of Indian Medicine," which is in course of publication by the University of Calcutta. The treatment of plants or Sthāvara Jīva or 'Fixed Beings' is a subdivision of Indian medical science, and notices of it (Vṛkṣa Āyurveda) are to be found in works on Botany, which are only available to us in a fragmentary condition in the writings of Varāha Mihira (Chapter LIV), in the Agni and other purāṇas, in the Upavana Vinoda by Sāraṅgadhara, and in the contributions of Caraka, Suśruta, Rāghava Bhatta, and others, in the Amarakoṣa, and in the Nighantus of medicine, *e.g.*, Śabda Pradīpa, a dictionary of medical Botany by Sureśvara, Court Physician to King

Bhīmapāla of Bengal, and '*Nigtantu-Śeṣa*,' a botanical glossary by Hemcandra.

In my work on the *Surgical Instruments of the Hindus*, Vol. I, pp. 130-1, I remarked: "In the Siddhisthāna, Chapter XI of the Caraka Saṁhitā, there is a passage showing that veterinary medicine was well-known to the ancient Hindus at a very early period. This portion was edited by Dṛḍhvala and it is impossible to decide whether the passage refers to Agniveśatantra or not. It runs as follows: Then the disciples asked: 'how are clysters to be made in cases of animals such as elephants, camels, cows, horses, lambs, and goats'? To this the sage Ātreya explained the clysters for animals, etc." In the *Hārīta saṁhita* (III. ii. P. 113), Ātreya is said to have delivered his lectures on the science of treatment for men, horses, elephants, deer, buffaloes, camels, snakes, mice, trees and plants

तस्माद्वत्त्यामि चादौ ज्वरतुलगदं वाजीनां कुञ्जराणां
मर्त्त्यानां वा पशूनां मृगमहिषखरोष्ट्रादिकानां तरूणां ।
वल्लीनामोषधीनां चितिधरफणिनां पक्षिणां मूषिकाणां
एष प्राणापहारी ज्वर इति गदितो दुर्निवारो हि लोके ॥

Hārīta Saṁhitā, III. ii.

Animal anatomy was thoroughly understood in the Vedic India as each part of the body of animals had its own distinctive name. Thus we find that in Ancient India, veterinary science was a subject in the curriculum of studies to be learned by the young aspirant to medical fame. Treatisès on the treatment of horses, elephants and cows exist even to the present time. Of all the sages whose names are mentioned in connection with the teaching of the veterinary science, Śālihotra stands pre-eminent. He is said to have learned the science from

Brahmā, the fountain-head of all medical lore, and to have expounded and taught the science to his disciples. He lectured on the subject of 'Horse and its treatment,' the '*Hayāurveda*,' '*Aśvāyurveda*,' or '*Turaṅgama Śāstra*.' Some chapters of his book are quoted in the *Agni Purāṇa* (ch. 281). *Hayāurveda* is also described in *Matsya* (ch,. 189 and 191) and *Gadura* (chs. 197 and 207) *Purāṇas*. Garga was another ancient writer on horse. His work is not available to us now, but he is quoted by Gaṇa in his work on *Aśvāyurveda*. Śukrācārya in his *Nītisāra* treated the subject in detail, and he is largely quoted in the commentary on the *Aśva-Vaidyaka*. King Nala had a surname 'Aśvavit,' *i. e.*, versed in the science of horse. Nakula and Sahadeva, the twin-sons of Mādrī, were taught by Droṇa in the art of training, managing and curing horses and cattle respectively. In the *Mahābhārata*, *Virāt Parva, Chapter III*, when the Pāṇḍavas entered into the services of King Virāta, Nakula declared himself well-versed in the science of management and treatment of horses, and Sahadeva referred to his scientific knowledge about the cows. To Nakula is ascribed the work called '*Aśvacikitsā*' or 'Treatment of Diseases of the Horse' which is still extant. This book is also called *Śālihotra*. It has been edited by Pandit Umeschandra Gupta Kaviratna and printed in the *Bibliotheca Indica*, as a supplement to the *Aśva Vaidyaka* by Jayadatta Suri in 1887. Reference is also made in the *Aśvalakṣaṇa śastra* to a big treatise on the subject by Siṁhadatta (अश्वशास्त्रसमुद्रं तं सिंहदत्तेन भाषितम्) G.O.M.L., Vol. xviii, Ms. No. 13318. Vātsya was another sage, versed in the veterinary science. Jayadeva also wrote on the treatment of horses and he is quoted by Jayadatta. Mallinātha Sūrī has quoted verses from *Haya Lilāvatī*. Bhoja was a writer on the same subject (*Vāji Cikitsā*), but no such work of his is known to scholars. In *Juktikalpataru*, draught and other animals are described by King Bhoja. This book has been printed in the *Calcutta Oriental Series.* There is another work *Aśvavaidya śāstra* by Dīpaṅkara. In *Kavi Kalpalatā* we find some descriptions of horses, and in *Basantarāja* (13th Varga), prognostications are indicated from the characteristics of horses (*Haya Śakūna*). Sāraṅgadhara is the author of *Turaṅga Parīkṣā* and *Vājī-Cikitsā.* Even as late as 1812, King Indusena wrote his *Sārasaṁgraha*, a short treatise on veterinary medicine, based on Śailhotra's work. *Manapriyamataṁ* is a book on the characteristics of good and bad horses with hints for ascertaining their age, etc.,

Pālakāpya expounded the science of treatment of elephants. He lectured on this science—*Gajāyurveda* or *Hasti-Āyurveda*—to King Romapāda, the contemporary of King Daśaratha of Ayodhyā. This work has been edited and published in the *Ānandāśramą Sanskrit Series*, Poona. Another book on the 'Treatment of Elephants' is quoted by Alberuni (see Sachau's *Preface to Indica*, p. xi). '*Gaja-Nirūpana*,' '*Mātaṅga Lilā*' (published in the *Trivaudrum Sanskrit Series*) and '*Gaja Cikitṣā*' are other works on the subject. The topic also finds a place in the various Purāṇas, *e.g.*, *Agni Purāṇa* (chs. 289-91), and in Kauṭilya's '*Artha Śāstra*' and Kāmandakī's *Nītisāra*. *Gajapaddhati* and *Aśvapaddhati* are chapters in the *Subhāṣitasudhānidhi*, an anthology compiled by Sāyaṇa.

The fifth chapter of the *Śyainika Sāstra*, a book on hawking by the royal poet Rudradeva of Kumaon (*Bib. Ind.*) is devoted to the considerations of the kind and quality of the hawk's food, their tending in different seasons, and the treatment of their diseases. In the *Tanjore Cat.*, Lix, (12, 305) D, ff. 8, is noted '*Aśvalaksana*' said to be from the *Akāśabhairava Tantra* and '*Gajaśants* (12, 297) D. ff. 4 from *Akāśabhairavāgama*.

In the literature of the Jains we find descriptions of vegetable kingdom and a comparison of the life-history of plants with that of man. It is said that the cultured women of the time were versed in the different kinds of sciences (72 in number), in the list of which, mention is made of the science of horsemanship, management of elephants, medicine, chemistry, and tarucikitsā or 'Treatment of Trees.' The women were also proficient in the 64 *kalās* or arts which are enumerated, and in the list we find *Āranaropana* (Gardening), *Gajaparīkṣā* (Examination of elephants), *Aśvaparīkṣā* (Examination of horses) and Vaidyakriyā (Practice of Medicine).

In Magadha, horses and elephants were used for war. Rhys Davids remarks: "The testimony of Indian records ascribe the pre-eminence in the training of horses to the extreme north and west which then belonged to Magadha, and the pre-eminence in the training of elephants to the east, which is precisely Magadha. This use of elephants in war may have been an important factor in the gradual rise of Magadha to the supreme power."

That the Indians were proficient in horsemanship, we have the testimony of foreign writers on the subject, *e.g.*, Megasthenes and Arrian. "The greatest proficients use their skill by driving a chariot round and round in a ring; and in truth it would be no trifling feat to control with ease a team of four high mettled steed when whirling round in a circle."

The *Atharva Veda* is the repository of the medical science in its infancy, and we may trace the origin of veterinary medicine in its pages. In II. 32, we find a charm against worms in cattle (cows): it really describes some parasitic diseases of cows and their treatment. I have described the scientific explanation of the hymn in my contribution, '*The Hnman Parasites in the Atharva Veda*' which is in course of publication. The treatment of cows had always been a fascinating and useful subject for study in India, and *Go-Vaidyas* or cattle-doctors still practise their profession. But to such a disgrace has the practice fallen in recent times, that the word *Go-Vaidya* is rather a term of reproach to physicians who are not sufficiently proficient in their art. Voelcker truly observes: "Comparatively little is known in India on the subject of cattle disease, and yet it is one of great agricultural importance, for, when an epidemic breaks out, the cattle perish in thousands, and do not seem to have a power of resisting it equal to that possessed by English cattle. The Natives believe the cattle epidemics are visitations of the goddess Mata, and they can only get rid of the epidemic by propitiating the goddess. The variety of names by which diseases are known to the Natives in different parts makes it hard to ascertain how far they really recognise the particular ones and the respective symptoms. To a certain extent it appears that the people are aware of the advantages of isolation, and make some use of it. The herding together of a lot of miserable half-starved cattle on the 'village waste' is, as I have previously remarked, one of the most potent means of spreading disease." *Report on the Improvement of Indian Agriculture, Second Edition*, Calcutta, 1897, p. 212) But such was not the condition of its practice in ancient times. In the Law Books we have unmistakeable testimony of the practice of the science according to scientific method. In the *Manu Saṁhitā* public lands for pasture are described (VIII, pp. 237-8). Todd (*Rajasthana*, Vol. II. *Marwar*, ch. xvi, p. 145) describes the Gaswali to be a graduated tax on cattle, or as the term imports, the right of pasture. A sheep or goat is estimated at one anna, a buffalo eight annas, and each camel three rupees.

In the *Parāśara Saṁhitā* it is ordained : "If a cow is kept confined for treatment of her diseases, or for the rectification of any abnormal presentation during delivery, and, notwithstanding all possible precautions taken for its prevention, the cow dies, then no expiation would be necessary. But if a number of diseased cows are kept under control, and if one of them dies, after being treated by a cattle-doctor who is not proficient in his art, expiatory ceremony must be performed." Apastamva and Sambarta also give us similar directions. Viṣṇu lays down that "those who have hurt a man or a domestic animal shall pay the expense of his cure" (vs. 75 and 76). "A physician who adopts a wrong method of cure in the case of a patient of high rank, shall pay the highest, in the case of another patient, the second, and in the case of an animal the lowest amercement" (Vs. 175-177). Parāśara again remarks : "If a cow is killed by any man, the blood of the dead cow must be examined, for it becomes necessary to know whether the cow was diseased or weak before her death. For the ceremony of expiation would vary according to the state of health and disease of the cow." Such an examination of the dead cow to determine her health and disease during life foreshadows our post-mortem reports in a court of law. But it seems strange that though such an examination is recommended by the law-givers in cases of accidental death of cows, no such procedure is mentioned in the law books as far as I am aware of in cases of accidental death of human beings. It may be due to the fact that cows were held in high veneration by the ancient Hindus as the modern Hindus do at the present time. But human life was always held sacred by the Hindus, and possibly similar post-mortem examinations were the practice in cases of accidental and homicidal death of man, but notices of such practice are not forthcoming.

But though we do not find any reference to post-mortem examinations in the law-books and medical literature of the Hindus, we find it mentioned in the *Arthaśāstra* of Kauṭilya as *Āśumṛtakaparīkṣā* "Examination of bodies of men who have recently died." Report of such an examination was necessary in higher courts of law "Kaṇṭakaśodhana Courts" during the reign of Candra Gupta. Bodies of men who committed suicide by hanging, drowning, poisoning, etc., were kept in an "Examination Room" which was set apart for the purpose. Such examination rooms, corresponding to our morgues, were established in the different provinces of the empire. Here all accidental cases, homicidal or suicidal, were kept for examination and reported as to the cause of death to higher authorities who dealt with the cases accordingly. To prevent decomposition, dead bodies were kept immersed in oil or oleagenous preparations (*Āśumṛtaka-parīkṣā* in the *Arthaśāstra*, pp. 215-217). At least we know of two instances of the use of oil as a preservative to dead bodies: when Daśaratha died, as Rāma was away in the forest and Bharata was away in the house of his maternal uncle, the dead body of his father was kept by the ministers immersed in oil in an iron pan. Similarly the dead body of Nimi was preserved in oil.

"तैलद्रोण्यां तदामात्याः संवेश्य जगतीपतिम् ।
राज्ञः सर्व्वाण्यथादिष्टाश्चक्रुः कर्म्माण्यनन्तरम् ॥"

Rāmāyaṇa, Ayodhyākāṇḍa, Ch. 66.

आशुमृतक परीक्षा।

"तैलाभ्यक्तमाशुमृतकं परीक्षेत—

निष्कीर्णमूत्रपुरीषं वातपूर्णकोष्ठत्वक्कं शूनपादपाणिमुन्मीलिताक्षं

सव्यञ्जनकण्ठं पीड़ननिरुद्धोच्छ्वासहतं विद्यात् ॥

तमेव सङ्कुचितबाहुसक्थिमुद्बन्धनहतं विद्यात् ॥

शूनपाणि पादोदरमपगताक्षमुद्वृत्तनाभिमवरोपितं विद्यात् ॥

निस्तब्धगुदाक्षं सन्दष्टजिह्वामध्मातोदरमुदकहतं विद्यात् ॥

शोणितानुसिक्तं भग्नभिन्नगात्रं काष्ठै रश्मिभिर्वा हतं विद्यात् ॥

सम्भग्नस्फुटितंगात्रं विक्षिप्तं विद्यात् ॥

श्यावपाणिपाददन्तनखं शिथिलमांसरोमचर्माणं फेनोपदिग्धमुखं

विषहतं विद्यात् ॥

तमेव सशोणितदंशं सर्पकीटहतं विद्यात् ॥

विक्षिप्तवस्त्रगात्रमतिवांतविरिक्तं मदनयोगहतं विद्यात् ॥

अतोऽन्यतमेन कारणेन हतं हत्वा वा दण्डभयादुद्बन्धनिकृत्तकण्ठं विद्यात् ॥

विषहतस्य भोजनशेषं पयोभिः परीक्षेत।

हृदयादुद्धृत्याग्नौ प्रक्षिप्तं चिटचिटायदिन्द्रधनुर्वर्णं वा विषयुक्तं विद्यात् ॥

दग्धस्य हृदयमदग्धं दृष्ट्वा वा तस्य परिचारकजनं वा दण्डपारुष्यादतिमार्गेत।

दुःखोपहतमन्यप्रसक्तं वा स्त्रीजनं दायनिवृत्तिस्त्रीजनाभिमन्तारं वा बन्धुम्।

तदेव हतोद्बन्धस्य परीक्षेत ॥

स्वयमुद्बन्धस्य वा विप्रकारयुक्तं मार्गेत ..

सर्वेषां वा स्त्रीदायाद्यदोषः, कर्मस्पर्धा प्रतिपक्षद्वेषः

पण्यसंस्थासमवायो वा विवाद पदानामन्यतमद्वा रोषस्थानं ;

रोषनिमित्तो घातः ॥

Examination of Sudden Death.

"In cases of sudden death, the corpse shall be smeared over with oil and examined.

"Any person whose corpse is tainted with mucus and urine, with organs inflated with wind, with hands and legs swollen, with eyes open, and with neck marked with ligatures may be regarded as having been killed by suffocation and suppression of breathing.

"Any person with contracted arms and thighs may be regarded as having been killed by hanging.

"Any dead person with swollen hands, legs, and belly, with sunken eyes and inflated navel may be regarded as having been killed by hanging.

"Any dead person with stiffened rectum and eyes, with tongue bitten between the teeth, and with belly swollen, may be considered as having been killed by drowning.

"Any dead person, wetted with blood and with limbs wounded and broken may be regarded as having been killed with sticks or ropes.

"Any dead person with fractures and broken limbs, may be regarded as having been thrown down.

"Any dead person with dark-coloured hands, legs, teeth and nails, with loose skin, hairs fallen, flesh reduced, and with face bedaubed with foam and saliva, may be regarded as having been poisoned.

"Any dead person of similar description with marks of a bleeding bite, may be considered as having been bitten by serpents and other poisonous creatures.

"Any dead person, with body spread and dress thrown out after excessive vomiting and purging, may be considered as having been killed by the administration of the juice of the *madana* plant.

"Death due to any of the above causes is, sometimes under the fear of punishment, made to appear as having been brought about by voluntary hanging, by causing marks of ligature round the neck.

"In death due to poison, undigested portion of meal may be examined in milk. Or the same extracted from the belly and thrown on fire may, if it makes 'chitchita' sound and assumes the rainbow colour, be declared as poisoned.

"Or when the belly (Hṛdayaṃ) remains unburnt, although the rest of the body is reduced to ashes, the dead man's servants may be examined as to any violent and cruel treatment they may have received at the hands of the dead. Similarly such of the dead man's relatives as a person of miserable life, a woman with affections placed elsewhere or a relative defending some woman that has been deprived of her inheritance by the dead man may also be examined.

"The same kind of examination shall be conducted concerning the hanging of the body of an already dead man.

"Causes such as past evils or harm done to others by a dead man, shall be inquired into regarding any death due to voluntary hanging.

"All kinds of sudden death, centre round one or the other of the following causes :—

"Offence to women or kinsmen, claiming inheritance, professional competition, hatred against rivals, commerce, guilds and any one of the legal disputes, is the cause of anger ; anger is the cause of death."

Kautilya's Arthaśāstra—Translation by R. Shamasastry, B.A., M.R.A.S., Librarian, Government Oriental Library, Mysore.

Śālihotra's works :

Now let us consider about Sālihotra, the veterinary surgeon who is described as the father of the veterinary science in India. The complete work of Sālihotra is not available to us.

1. Śālihotra.: Mss. : I. O. : 2762.

Dietz : A. M. : 2041, p. 155.

Begins :

श्रीवत्सवक्षसः कांतां प्रणम्य तुरगारणिं (!)।
श्रियं देवीं प्रवक्ष्यामि तुरंगाणां चिकित्सितं ॥१॥
कृताग्निहोत्रमासीनं शालिहोत्रं महामुनिं।
सुश्रुतः श्रुतसंपन्नः पप्रच्छ पितरं सुतं ॥२॥
भगवन् सर्वधर्मज्ञ हयायुर्वेदकोविद।
कथमेतत्समुत्पन्नं तुरंगाणां चिकित्सितं ॥३॥
तमुवाच महातेजाः शालिहोत्रोऽर्थतत्त्ववित्।
आसन् विहगमाः पूर्वं तुरगाः कामचारिणः ॥४॥
कामाहारविहाराणां तेषां सच्छंदचारिणां।
शरीरमात्यात्सर्वेषामासीद्रोगसमुद्भवः ॥५॥
यतः प्रभृति ते नीता वाहनत्वं मया सुत।
ततः प्रभृति वैरुद्धात्पीड्यंते व्याधिभिर्भृशं ॥६॥
ततस्तेषां दयापन्नः कृत्वाहं सुमहत्तपः।
आराध्य देवं ब्रह्माणं प्राप्तवांस्तच्चिकित्सितं ॥७॥
यतः प्रभृति वाहानां पक्षच्छेदी मया कृतः।
पक्षिसंक्षिप्तवेगाच्च मह्यां पद्भ्यां चरंति ते ॥८॥
ततः प्रभृति ते रुद्धा वाहने बंधनेषु च।
क्षुत्पिपासासहास्तेऽश्वाः शीतवातनिपीड़िताः ॥९॥
परवश्यागतास्तेऽश्वा पीड्यंते व्याधिभिस्तु ते।
ततस्तेषां दयापन्ना ब्रह्मपार्श्वं गता वयं ॥१०॥

ब्रह्मोवाच—

शालिहोत्र किमायातो हयघोषसुतः शुचिः।
सर्व्वधर्म्मविदां श्रेष्ठो हयरक्षासु तत्परः ॥११॥
ब्रह्मप्रोक्तमिदं वाक्यं मयोक्तं ब्रह्मणा सह।
वेदं किमात्मकः प्रोक्तः केनासौ परिकल्पितः ॥१२॥
त्वदुद्भवः कथं स्वामिन् मां प्रति ब्रूहि सुव्रत।
एवं प्रोक्त मया पुत्र ब्रह्मप्रोक्तं शृणुष्व तत ॥१३॥

ब्रह्मोवाच—

वेद स्वयंभूरित्युक्तो न केनापि प्रकल्पितः ।
मया हि पठितो यस्मात्स्वयंभूस्तदहं मुने ॥१४॥
धाता स्रष्टा जगत्कर्त्ता वैदिकः स चराचरे ।
मया हि पठितो यस्मात् कर्त्ता तेनाप्यहं मुने ॥१५॥
नैकाननेन शक्तोऽहं वेदसंचारधारणे ।
तस्माद्विभाज्य सहसा निक्षिप्तश्चातुराननै ॥१६॥
पूर्वं ऋग्वेदसंभुतिर्यजुर्व्वेदस्य दक्षिणे ।
पश्चिमे सामवेदस्य अथर्वसौत्तरे(!) तथा ॥१७॥
इतिहास ऋचो वेदात् धनुर्व्वेदो यजोर्षतः (!) ।
गंधर्व्ववेदः सामस्य (!) आयुर्वेदस्त्वथर्वणः ॥१८॥
अथर्ववेदस्योपांगमायुर्वेदं प्रचक्षते ।
श्लोकाः शतसहस्राणि पंचविंशतिकानि च ॥१९॥
सपादलक्षं तेनैतद ब्रह्मणा परिभाषितं ।
अष्टादशसहस्राणि आरदाचसुदाहृतं (!) ॥२०॥
उत्तरायां तु संभूतं तेन वै कूलमुत्तरं ।
मागधे मागधे (!) देशे सहस्राणि चतुर्दश ॥२१॥
पूर्वाशायां तु संभूतं पूर्व्वंकूलं तु तेन बि (! वै)।
गांधारं दक्षिणे देशे ब्रह्मणा परिकल्पितं ॥२२॥
द्वादशैव सहस्राणि कुलं तेन तु दक्षिणं ।
श्रीपाटं पत्तने (!) देशं शालिहोत्रस्य भाषितं ॥२३॥
दशचैव सहस्राणि कुलं चैव तु पश्चिमं ।
आराध्य देवं ब्रह्माणं उपांगं प्राप्तमष्टधा ॥२४॥
अंगान्यष्टौ ततः पुत्त्र सांगोपांगं चिकित्सितम् ।
शल्यं कायचिकित्सा च तथा शालक्यमेव च ॥२५॥
किशोरवालचिकित्सा विषतंत्रं तथैव च ।
रसायन भूतविद्या वाजीकरणमष्टमं ॥२६॥
ह्यायुर्व्वेद इत्येष अष्टांगः परिकीर्त्तितः ।
अङ्गान्यष्टौ विजानीयाः शृणु शुश्रुत विस्तरं ॥२७॥

शलं तृणं च काष्टं च पांशु पाषाणलोष्टकं ।

रोमवालनखाः केशाः शास्त्राणि विविधानि च ॥२८॥

अंत्राणि चास्थिनिचयं गर्भमुक्तं च शल्यकं ।

यंत्रचाराग्निशस्त्राणां व्रणान् यदुपशामयते ॥२९॥

औषधादचियोगेषु शल्यतंत्रं तदुच्यते ।

कायजांश्च विकारांश्च सर्वांगांश्च श्रुतांस्तथा ॥३०॥

ज्वरातिसाररोगाश्च उन्माद शोष एव च ।

कुष्ठान्यर्शों रक्तं पित्तं मूत्ररोगांश्च दारुणान् ।

एवं कायचिकित्सा च हयतंत्रे प्रतिष्ठित ॥३१॥

शालक्यं नाम यच्चांगः ऊर्द्धमनुगता (ऊर्द्धजानु) रुजः ।

श्रवणे नयने घ्राणे वदने मस्तके तथा ।

येन ते प्रशमं यांति शालाक्यं तदुदाहृतं ॥३२॥

किशोरकचिकित्सा च किशोरी येन वर्धते ।

आरोग्यं जायते येन स्तन्यं येन विशुध्यति ॥३३॥

गुर्विण्यो येन पुष्यंति वृषा येन तथैव न ।

योगाद्यौ

(There is evidently a lacuna here, the definition of the other 4 headings being omitted).

अष्टाङ्गस्यास्य कात्स्न्येंण शृणु स्थानानि पुत्रक ॥२४॥

उन्नयं प्रथमं स्थानं द्वितीयं स्यात्तयोत्तरं ।

शारीरकं तृतीयं तु चतुर्थं तु चिकित्सितम् ॥२५॥

पञ्चमं शिशुभैषज्यं षष्ठं स्यादुत्तरोत्तरं ।

नाम्ना च तत् क्रियापन्नं सिद्धिस्थानं तु सप्तमं ॥

रहस्यमष्टमं स्थानमित्यायुर्वेदसंग्रहः ॥२६॥

Analysis.

This MS. contains only the first sthāna, of which the chapters are :—

अध्यायानां क्रमं सम्यक् स्थाने स्थाने निबोध मे ।

आयुर्वेदसमुत्पत्ति विद्याध्यायनमेव च ॥१७॥

1. उत्नये संभवः पूर्वं ततः स्याद्गर्भसंभवः ।
प्रकृतिवर्णविज्ञानं चातुर्वर्ण्यं तथैव च ॥३८॥
सर्वाङ्गसंपरीक्षा च प्रदेशो व्यंजनानि च ।
आवर्ता वयसो ज्ञानं शरीरोतकर्षणं गतिः ॥३९॥
गन्धाः पुष्पाणि पुंद्राणि सज्ञानुकाणि सारदा ।
मानसूत्रं कुलाध्यायो विकृताविकृतं तथा ॥ ४०॥
दशांगाभिजनं मिश्रं वर्णलक्षणमेव च ।
मात्रज्ञानं विधायोगः शोभा शूकल धावितं ॥
क्रयो राजोपवाह्यश्च सौगंधी वेधनं तथा ॥४१॥

2. उत्तरे तु महाप्रश्नः अण्डजसंभवस्तथा ।
त्रिविधं रागविज्ञानं दुर्भनो ज्ञानमेव च ।
वर्तातिसारो वर्तांश्च प्रस्कन्नो लिङ्गितानि च ।
चतर्दोषास्त्वभिष्यन्दननुष्यन्दषड़्तुकं ।
पादरोगाभितापश्च हिक्काश्वासस्तथा ज्वरः ॥
हारिद्रकं तथा ज्ञानं कृमिशूलं तथैव च ।
सिंघानकश्च कासश्च तथातीसारं एव च ॥
क्षीरसंब्रहणं चैव तथा कट्कपिच्छिका ।
वालादकोशूदभ्रंशं तथा शोणित पैत्तिकं ॥
अधिदन्तचिकित्सा च पादोल्कचिकित्सितं ।
विज्ञानं सर्पजातीनां दष्टव्यंजनभेषजम् ॥
तथा विगर्हणीयं च वेगविज्ञानमेव च ।
व्यंजनं विषपीतस्य दिग्धं विद्धस्य चोभयोः ॥
ग्रहणीवंधविधश्च (!) विषोपशममेव च ।
एतावदुत्तरं प्रोक्तं द्वितीयं स्थानकं तथा ॥

3. शारीरकं तृतीयं तु वक्ष्यतेऽत परं तव ।
गर्भोत्पत्तिश्च महती शरीरनिचयस्तथा ॥

कायोत्पत्तिः शिरोव्यूहस्तथा दंशप्रमाणिका ।
हीनानि रिक्तमध्यात्मा कार्य्याकार्य्य निपानिकं ॥
अधिकार चिकित्सा च जड़ांधवधिराणि च ।
रसस्कंधश्च चत्वारो यवसानां रसास्तथा ॥
श्वयथुर्द्विव्रणीयश्च मूत्रकावरणानि (?) च ।
लंघणं वृंहणं चैव मूढ़गर्भचिकित्सितं ॥
प्रनष्टशल्योद्धरणं शल्योद्धरणमेव च ।
नाड़िभग्नचिकित्सा च तथार्वुदचिकित्सितम् ॥
वातार्दितात् योनिदोषा वृषशुक्रा च चिकित्सितम् ।
लक्षणं प्रसूतानां च शारीरं तु प्रकीर्त्तितं ॥

4. व्यानकः प्रथमो व्याधिस्तथाश्वान्योनिराणकः (!) ।
अवालुकिरवातंकौ (! अलाबुक) जिह्वास्तम्भो तृषितस्तथा ।
शालुकी शिरसन्तापो ॥ slokas ending.
आध्मानश्चाप्यतीसारः स्थानमेतच्चिकित्सितम् ॥

5. किशोरकचिकित्साया मिश्रकं प्रथमं भवेत् ।
ग्रहभूपस्ततः प्रोक्तो जराध्यायस्ततः परः ॥
पामाध्यायः कृमि कोष्ठे 4 slokas ending.
तथा भग्नचिकित्सा च किशोरकचिकित्सितं ॥

6. हयमारी वास्तुविद्यारेवं (!) तस्य च पूजनं ।
ग्रहाणां शांतिकं चैव श्रियः संपूजनं तथा ॥
तथा च स्वातिसंपातो रम्या नीराजनक्रिया ।
लोहाभिहरणं, चैतमश्वाणां च विचेष्टितं ।
एतत्ते षष्ठमुद्दिष्टं स्थानं वै उत्तरोत्तरं ॥

7. स्नेहक्षीरसुराधान्यलवणादिसमुत्थिताः ।
विज्ञेया व्यापदश्चैता नाड़ीव्यापत्तथैव च ।
सिद्धस्थानमिदं प्रोक्तं रहस्यं शृणु चाप्यथ ॥

8. रेखानिर्य्याणकार्य्यं व आयुर्ज्ञानं ततः परं ।
रिष्टिकाध्यायस्तथोक्तं कल्पारिष्टकमेव च ॥
उपसर्गारिष्टकं च नक्षत्राहतरिष्टकम् ।
हरीतकीनां कल्पस्तु रसोनस्य च गुग्गुलोः ॥
सार्षपाणां तथा कल्पो लाक्षायाः कल्प एव च ।
त्रिफलायास्तथा कल्पः स्वर्जिकाकल्प एव च ॥
रसायनानि दिव्यानि वाजीकरणमेव च ।
शिक्षा चैव तथाश्वानां बालानां दमनक्रिया ॥
भारादानं तथा प्रोक्तं विविधा रणकल्पना ।
रथवंधश्च विज्ञेयस्तथा वाससर क्रिया ॥
मन्त्रयोगः क्रियायोगो रहस्योपनिषत्तथा ।
इत्येतदष्टमं स्थानं रहस्यं परिकीर्त्तितम् ॥
अष्टाङ्गमेतद्विदयं (? विदधौ) स्थानैः सर्वैस्तमाष्टभिः ।
हयायुर्वेदमखिलं ब्रह्मा शुभं चतुर्मुखः ॥
इति श्रीश्री शालिहोत्रे आयुर्वेदोत्पत्ति प्रथमः ॥
अथोवाच पुनः पुत्रं शालिहोत्रस्तु सुश्रुतं ।
शिष्योपनयनं नाम सुश्रुताय श्रृणुष्व मे ॥

The MS. is called *Śālihotra*, a work on veterinary medicine. Śālihotra is described to be the son of Hayaghoṣa, and the father of Suśruta, in answer to whose questions he expounded the *Haya-Āyurveda* revealed to him by Brahmā himself. It is a work on the treatment of horses. It is a practical farriery, a complete guide to all that relates to the horse; its history, varieties, and uses; breaking, training, feeding, stabling, grooming; how to buy, keep and treat a horse in health and disease, etc., forming a complete system of veterinary art as practised in ancient India, and there it was accepted as the standard work on the subject. Śālihotra gives his name to the art, and to this day horse and cattle doctors are known in the North-West Provinces under the name of Saluter.

The work is divided into eight divisions, as we find the Āyurvedic system of medicine to be composed of eight aṅgas or parts (Aṣṭāṅga or octopartite), namely, Śalya or Major Surgery, Śālākya or Surgery of parts above clavicles. Kāya-cikitsā or Inner Medicine, Bhūtavidyā or Demonology, Kaumārabhṛtya or the Science of Pāediatrics (described as Kiśora-vāla-cikitsā), Viṣatantra or Toxicology, Rasāyana or Treatment to prolong life, and Vajīkaraṇa or Treatment to stimulate sexual power. There are eight sthānas or main sections which treat of these eight aṅgas. Each section is virtually a book in itself; it is sub-divided into many chapters dealing exhaustively with every phase of its subject.

In the Introductory chapter, Suśruta is represented to have requested his father Śālihotra to teach him the origin and treatment of horses. Śālihotra addressed Suśruta as his son and said that "horses were birds originally. (आसन् विहगमाः पूर्व्वं तुरगाः कामचारिणः ॥). But as they came to be submitted by men as beasts of burden, diseases began to attack them in their captivity. Then out of kindness to the equine race, I performed austerities and learned the science of their treatment from Brahmā himself. I severed their wings, and now they roam over the earth on their legs, retaining their former speed. The Vedas were uttered by the Sayambhu and I learned it from the Self-existent. He described its four-fold divisions by his four mouths to the four directions of this world. Āyurveda was developed from the Atharva Veda:

इतिहास ऋचो वेदात धनुर्वेदो यजोर्षतः (?) ।
गान्धर्व्ववेदः सामस्य (?) आयुर्वेदस्त्वथर्वणः ॥

Brahmā originally described the science in one *lac* and twenty-five slokas but I abridged it and described in 18,000 ślokas."

The eight sthānas mentioned above are:—1. Unnaya, 2. Uttara, 3. Śārīrika, 4. Cikitsita, 5. Śiśu-Bhaiṣajjya, 6. Uttara-uttara, 7. Siddhisthāna, and 8. Rahasya. Only the first of these eight sthānas, and even this not quite complete, is contained in the I.O. Ms. 2762. It appeared necessary to transcribe the whole of Sanskrit passages from the *I. O. Cat.*, that the reader may form a just estimate of Śālihotra's work. I have also attempted an analysis of its contents in English with my identification of diseases described therein. The other sections are not available. In the Monthly General Meeting of the Asiatic Society of Bengal held on the 4th March, 1925, MM. H. P. Śāstrī showed us a valuable find of manuscript in the shape of the eighth sthāna of Śālihotra's work, the *Rahasya sthāna,* from Udaipur in Rajputana. The MS. is in very good preservation and well-written. The manuscript is no doubt unique, but his opinion that this was the only part of Śālihotra's work known to exist, required modification, and when I pointed out the *I. O. MS.* and *Tanjore Cat. MS.*, the MSS. were afterwards verified by him. The MS. consists of 5,000 slokas and is in the possession of MM. Śāstrī. Afterwards I learned from him that with the instinct of a scholar he made a gift of the MS. to the Library of the Society and it is now available to scholars. The entire MS, of Śālihotra exists in Baroda and will be published soon. In the *Triennial Cat. MSS., Madras,* 1916-19, R. No. 2342, we find 1-18 chapters of the eighth section or *Rahasya sthāna* and 1-9 chapters of *Unnaya sthāna.*

Relation of Sālihotra to Suśruta: Now in the *I. O. Cat. MS.*, and in the Śāstrī's MS., Suśruta is said to be the son of Śālihotra Muni who addressed his lectures to his son (putra). Suśruta also calls Śālihotra his father (verse 2). But in the *Suśruta Saṁhitā*, Suśruta is said to be the son of the celebrated sage Viśvāmitra: 'Brahmarṣi-puttra (S. S., 11, i), 'Viśvāmitrātmaja' (IV. ii), 'Viśvāmitrasūta' (VI. lxvi), 'Vaiśvāmitra' (VI, xviii). In the *Mahābhārata*, *Anuśāsanaparva* Ch. 139, vs. 8-11, Suśruta is described as a son of Viśvāmitra. In the genealogical table of sage Viśvāmitra (see my *History of Indian Medicine, Vol. II*, p. 282 (*a*), I have shown Suśruta to be one of the sons of Viśvāmitra. Thus there is an anomaly as regards the father of Suśruta. If Viśvāmitra was his father how could Śālihotra call Suśruta his son. Both the views can, however, be reconciled if we accept Viśvāmitra as Suśruta's father and Śālihotra as his *guru*. A *guru* can address his disciple as son, and a disciple can likewise call his preceptor father. Such a practice is sanctioned by sāstras, and also by usage. In the *Harīta Saṁhitā*, Ātreya addressed his disciple Hārīta as his son, शृणु पुत्र समासेन यथावत् सत्प्रकाश्यये । See also *Hārita Saṁhitā* II, i, ii, iii, vii ; III, iii, v, xi, xii, xiii, xxii ; IV, i ; V, i. In the Madras MS., we find, in the Rahasya sthāna, Śuśruta to be a disciple, and not a son, of Śālihotra.

Again we must consider whether besides the evidence of this manuscript, we possess any corroborative testimony that Śālihotra was Suśruta's preceptor. In Nakula's *Aśvacikitsā* and Jayadatta's *Aśvavaidyaka* we find no mention of Suśruta as a disciple of Śālihotra who is described as the source of the science. Jayadatta quotes from Śālihotra, Nakula, Śāraṅgadhara and Jayadeva. Gaṇa in his *Aśvāyurveda* (*Nepal Cat.* 765, p. 151) refers to Śālihotra as his source but does not mention Suśruta. In G.O. M.L. xxiii, 13319, Gaṇa in the colophon to his Aśvāyurveda, professes to summarise the treatises of Śālihotra,

Suśruta, Garga, etc. ये शालिहोत्रसुश्रुतगर्गः महर्षिभिः पूरा कथिता।
Śālihotra and Pālakāpya are quoted in later treatises on topics in relation to the veterinary science. As an instance I may mention that Śibodāsa Sena in his *Tattva Candrikā*, a commentary on Cakradatta's *Saṁgraha*, quotes Śālihotra and Pālakāpya, but not Suśruta. In the *Agni Purāṇa*, however, we find that Suśruta is said to have learned the science of horses, elephants and cattle from Dhanvantari, who is represented, in the *Suśruta Saṁhitā*, to have taught his disciple Suśruta Major Surgery only. In the *Bower MS.*, l. i. (p. 11) Suśruta is represented to have approached Muni Kāsirāja with the inquiry about the 'nature of a plant with leaves dark-blue like sapphire, and with bulbs white like jasmine, crystal, the white lotus, moon's rays, conch-shell or mica' or garlic plant. Kāśirāja addressed Suśruta and set forth its virtues (p. 15). Thus we find that Suśruta learned the different branches of Āyurveda, *viz.*, surgery, botany and veterinary science from Dhanvantari. Thus we find that Śālihotra is said to be Suśruta's father and teacher of veterinary science in this MS. of *Śālihotra* only.

Sālihotra, according to Nakula, expounded the science of medicine for horses for the benefit of the equine race. He wrote the Āyurveda for horses at the request of Indra, for whom the sage maimed them by cutting their wings. The original *Saṁhitā* of Śālihotra consisted of 12,000 slokas :—

सपचा वाजिनः सर्व्वे सञ्जाता व्योमचारिणः।
गन्धर्व्वैर्थ्यो यथा कामं गच्छन्ति स समन्ततः॥
तान् दृष्ट्वा जवसम्पन्नान् सद्यान्वाहनोचितान्।
शक्रः प्रोवाच पार्श्वस्थं शालिहोत्रं मुनीश्वरम्॥
नास्त्यसाध्यं मुने किञ्चिद्भवतो भूवनत्रये।
तस्मादाशु कुरुष्व त्वं वाहनार्हान् हयोत्तमान्॥

ये च मे युद्धकालेषु प्रवहन्ति रथं सदा ।
अशक्यं वारणेन्द्रैश्च दानवैर्बलवत्तरैः ॥
तेषां शस्त्रं समुत्सृज्य पक्षच्छेदं व्यधात्तदा ।
वाजिनां शक्रवाक्येन शालिहोत्रो महामुनिः ॥
छिन्नपक्षास्तु ते सर्व्वे गत्वा तमृषिमब्रुवन् ।
दीनाः सुदुःखसम्पन्ना रुधिरेण परिप्लुता ॥
भगवन् किं निमित्तं नः पक्षच्छेदः कृतस्त्वया
अपराधविहीनानां नेच्छन्ति पण्डिताः ॥
तस्माद्गतिर्भव प्राज्ञ सर्व्वेषामिह वाजिनाम् ।
तथा स्यात् सर्व्वदा सौख्यं पुष्टिश्च मुनिपुङ्गव ॥
अथासौ कृपयाविष्टस्तानुवाच सुदुःखितान् ।
इन्द्रादेशात्कृतं सर्व्वं भवतां पक्षपातनम् ॥
तस्मादहः प्रकरिष्यामि भविष्यति यथा सुखम्
पुष्टीरम्या यथा देहे गौरवं च जगत्त्रये ॥

*　　*　　*

एवं विसृज्य तानं स्वर्गान् शालिहोत्रस्तुरङ्गमान् ।
चक्रे द्वादशसाहस्रीं तदर्थे संहितां सुधीः ॥

*　　*　　*

Śālihotra is said to have lived in Śālatur, a country near Gāndhāra, the modern Kandahara. As such, he is identified with Pāṇiṇi by some, and with Dhanvantari by others (see Dr. Mitter's opinion in the *Proceedings of the A. S. B.*, July, 1835). Cunningham (*Ancient Geography of India*, pp. 57-58) identified Śālātur with modern Lahore (Śālātur, Halātur Aalātur, Lahore) but without sufficient evidence. Hiuen Tsiang's 'Śalatulo' which is situated at a distance of 20 li or about $3\frac{1}{2}$ miles in a north-western direction from the province of Ohinda corresponds to Śalātura, the birthplace of Pāṇiṇi (Śālāturīya), in which designation he is referred to in the copperplate inscription of the Vallabhis found in Kathiward (*Indian Antiquary*, Vol. I, pp. 16, 17 and 45). According to Nakula he was the son of Hayaghoṣa or Turâṅgaghoṣa, which are merely descriptive synonymous names. He lived in Srāvastī and was a Brāhmaṇa by caste.

येन ज्ञानवता हिमालयतरुच्छायासु विक्रीड़ितं ।
यः स्नातो हिमपुष्पवातशिशिरे गङ्गाजले पावने ॥
रेभे यस्तु तुरङ्गय यजनितैर्नानाविधैर्हेषितैः ।
पायद्वः स तुरङ्गघोषतनयः श्रीशालिहोत्रो मुनिः ॥

Nakula, Aśvacikitsita I. i.

He explained the science at his retreat in the forest of Campaka (the Campakābatī forest in Magadha Deśa) at the foot of the Himalaya mountain:

जाह्नव्या उत्तरे तीरे प्रालेयाद्रेस्तटान्तरे ।
स्वाश्रमे चम्पकारण्ये वेदिकायां कुशासने ॥
शालिहोत्रं सुखासीनं ऋषिभिः परिसेवितं ।
ब्रह्मसूर्य्याग्नितेजस्कं हयशास्त्रविशारदम् ॥

Burnell's Tanjore, Cat. of. S. MSS. 75.,

Hayaghoṣa or Turaṅgamaghoṣa is said to have been the father of Śālihotra. Hayaghoṣa has been identified with Aśvaghoṣa from the similarity in the names which are synonymous (Haya = Aśva, a horse). Hayaghoṣa may thus be identified with the celebrated Buddhist preacher and writer Aśvaghoṣa Bodhi-satva, the author of *Buddha-Carita* or 'Life of Buddha for the Northern Buddhists' (edited by Cowell) and *Saundarānanda Kāvya* (edited by H. P. Sastri, in the *Bibliotheca Indica*). He is also the author of many philosophical treatises (see Nanj

Catalogue of the Chinese Tripiṭhaka)—the total number being 7 (Nanjo), or 8 (Suzuki), or 9, if we include the *Vajrasūeī* in the list. There is evidence to connect Aśvaghoṣa to the court of the renowned Indo-Scythian monarch Kaniṣka of Peshawar and so he must have flourished towards the end of the first century A.D. His work *Buddha Carita* was translated by Dharmarakṣā into Chinese in the fourth century A.D. His other work (*Ka-coyam-yan-kim-lin*) was translated by Kumārajīva, a Chinese pilgrim, about the same time. His name appears as the twelfth patriarch of the Buddhists from the Venerable Budhha, third from Pārśva, the President of the Buddhist Council during the reign of Kaniṣka, and Nāgārjuna's name occurs as the third from Aśvaghoṣa in a descending line. He is described as an inhabitant of Sāketa, the ancient name of a city in the modern Province of Oudh, a Brāhmana by caste and as the son of Suvarṇākṣī :

आर्य्य-सुवर्णाक्षी पुत्रस्य साकेतस्य भिक्षोवाचार्य्य: ।
तद्स्ताश्वघोषस्य महाकवेर्हावादिन: कृतिरिममिति ॥

Hayaghoṣa is also described to be a Brāhmaṇa Muni who had hermitage in the Campaka forest at the foot of the Himalaya mountain. Thus the age of Śālihotra may be known, but neither Aṣvaghoṣa nor Śālihotra has given us any clue as to their identity. Again Suśruta, to whom Śālihotra addressed his lectures, flourished long before Kaniṣka, unless by Suśruta is meant Nāgārjuna, the celebrated Buddhiist chemist, the redactor of *Suśruta Saṁhitā*, who flourished during the second century A.D.

Translations of Śālihotra: "A work on veterinary medicine ascribed to Sālotar, said to have been the tutor of Suśruta, was translated from Sanskrit in the year 1381. A copy of it was preserved in the Royal Library of Lucknow" (Max Müller's *Science of Language*, Vol. I,

p. 167). In the footnote, he comments that "*Śālotar* is not known as the author of such a work. *Śālotarīya* occurs instead of *Śālāturīya* in *Rāja Rādhākṛnt*; but *Śālāturīya* is a name of *Paṇini*, and the teacher of *Suśruta* is said to have been *Divodāsa*. Professor Weber, in his *Cat. of Sanskrit MSS.*, (p. 298), has pointed out Śālihotra, who is mentioned in the *Pañcatantra* as a teacher of veterinary medicine, and who is quoted by Garga in the *Aśvāyurveda*. Śālotri is the every-day Urdu and Hindi word for a horse-doctor. Professor Aufrecht has discovered a work on medicine by *Sālihotra* in the Library of the East India House. A medical work by *Śālinātha* is mentioned in the *Catalogue of Sanskrit MSS. of the College of Fort William*, p. 24. An Arabic translation of a Sanskrit work on veterinary medicine by Cāṇakya is mentioned by Haji Chalfa, v, p. 59." The work of Śālinātha referred to above is called *Rasamañjarī*, which elaborates a system of treatment of diseases by mercurial preparations. It is not a book on veterinary science and has been printed by Kshemaraja Krishnaraja of Bombay. The Sūtra of Śālihotra exists in two recensions.

There is a similar work known in the Berlin Library, No. 944. "The information gathered in the *Berlin Cat.* by Prof. Weber regarding the adaptation of such works in Arabic and Persian may here be completed by the quotation of an English book published at Calcutta in 1788 under the following title: "A Treatise on horses, entitled Saloter, or, a complete system of Indian Farriery, in two parts: the first, containing a particular description of the different colours and marks of horses, etc., the second, a description of all the disorders they are subject to, etc. Compiled originally by a Society of learned Pundits, in the Sanskrit Language, translated thence into Persian, in the reign of Emperor Shah Jehan by Abdullah Khan Firoze Jung, an Emeer of his Court, which is now translated into English, by Joseph Earles."

Cf. also Garcin de Tassy, *Histoire de la Litterature Hindouie,* 2nd edi. iii. 294. (Gaikawar.)

Two Persian translations bearing the name of *Saluteri* have been noticed by Sir Henry Elliot, but it is not known if they are translations of Nakula or of any other author whose work he abridged.

Elliot informs us that the Persian rendering "*Kubrat-ul-Mulk*" of the Sanskrit original "*Śālotar*" was done during the reign of Ghiyasuddin, son of Mahammed Shah, in the year Hegira 784 or 1381 A.D. Then Feroze Shah Tughlak was the reigning emperor. He was distinguished for the enlightened spirit of his regulations, and the extent and utility of his public works. He ordered several Sanskrit works to be translated from Sanskrit. But Feroze was the nephew and not the son of Mahammad Tughlak whom he succeeded to the throne. Ghiyasuddin Tughlak, the founder of the House of Tughlak reigned from 1321-25 A.D., and Ghiyasuddin Tughlak II, the grandson of Feroze Tughlak, was raised to the throne in 1389 A.D. and after a short reign of five months was deposed and murdered.

The translator in the preface to his book thus remarks about the necessity of his translation: "The translation from the barbarous Hindi language to the refined Persian tongue is finished. This translation was attempted to avoid reference to the books of the un-believers." The Persian work has eleven chapters and thirty sections. A short analysis of its contents is given in the following table.

Chapters.	Subjects.	Sections.
I	Names and races of horses	4
II	On the smell, nursing and riding of horse.	4
III	On the management of horses. On wasp-hives in stables.	2
IV	On the colour and varieties of horses.	2
V	On defects of horses	3
VI	On anatomy of the different members of the body of horse.	2
VII	On diseases and their treatment.	4
VIII	On bleeding and hæmorrhage.	4
IX	On the food of horses.	4
X	On the fattening of the horse's body.	2
XI	On the determination of the ages of horses from their teeth.	1

Another work on the treatment of animals was translated in Arabic. It was done by Saiyad Abdulla Khan Bahadur Feroze Jung from a Sanskrit work which was secured from Chitor during an expedition to Mewar in the reign of Shah Jahan. The translated book is called "*Kitab-ul-Vaitart.*" It consisted of 16,000 slokas and was twice as big as the "*Kubrat-ul-Mulk,*" the Sanskrit original of which was known as "*Śālotari.*"

The work of Śālihotra was translated in the Tibetan tongue and it exists in its Tibetan garb in the celebrated encyclopædia, the *Tangyur,* and is mentioned in Cordier's list.

The Hindi work *Śālihotra* from which the Persian translation was made in the 14th century cannot be definitely identified but Mitra refers to a Hindi *Śālihotra* by Cetana as the possible original.

The book has been translated into Bengalee '*Śālihotra Aśva-cikitsā Sāra Saṁgraha*' or 'Epitome of the Treatment of Horses according to Śālihotra' by Nidhiram Mukerjee, Chandi Press, Calcutta, 1296 B.S. The author states in his Preface that he derived his materials from Śālihotra, Nakula, Bhojarāja and Jayadatta.

An analysis of the contents of the Śalihotra as given in the I. O. MS.

1. Āyurvedotpatti (fol. 5*a*)	On the origin of Āyurveda and of the science and treatment of horses.
2. Vidyādhyayanaṁ (7*a*, *b*)	Initiation of disciples.

I.—Unnaya sthāna.

1. Saṁbhavaḥ (20*a*)	On the origin of horses.
2. Garbhasaṁbhavaḥ (28*b*)	On pregnancy and uterine development.
3. Prakṛti (33*a*)	On the nature of horses.
4. Varṇavijnānaṁ (38*b*)	On the colour of horses.
5. Caturvarṇaṁ (41*b*)	On the four castes or classes of horses.
6. Sarvāṅga saṁparīkṣā (48*a*)	On examination of all parts of the body of horse.
7. Pradeśa (54*a*)	On description of different parts and their names.
8. Vyañjanāni (55*b*, 64*a*)	On signs and characteristics of horses.
9. Āvarta (76*b*)	On whirls of hairs on the body of horse.
10. Vayasa jñānaṁ (87*b*)	On the age of horses.
11. Śarīrotkarsanaṁ (91*b*)	On improvement of horse's body.

12. Gatih	(96*b*)	On motion of horse. His paces generally.
13. Gandhāh	(92*b*)	On the smell of the horse's body.
14. Puṣpāni	(94*b*)	On coloured spots which differ from the general colour of the body.
15. Puṁdrāni	(98*b*)	On marks and signs like sukti, conch-shell, etc., on the horse's body.
16. Satvāmakāni	(102*b*)	On the inherent qualities of the horse.
17. Sāradā	(107*b*)	On the four types of deasease called Sāradā in which there is difficulty in drinking fluids.
18. Mānasūtraṁ	(111*b*)	On measurement and size of the horse.
19. Kūlādhyāya	(121*b*)	On the pedigree of horses.
20. Vikṛtāvikṛtaṁ	(125*a*)	On horses in health and disease.
21. Daśāṅgāvijnānaṁ	(126*a*)	On the ten members of the horse's body.
22. Miśraṁ	(141*a*)	On miscellaneous topics.
23. Varṇalakṣaṇaṁ	(145*a*)	On the signs of the race of horses.
24. Mātrajñānaṁ	(149*a*)	On dosage of veterinary medicines.
25. Vidhāyogaḥ	(152*a*)	On appropriate remedies ?
26. Śobhā	(154*b*)	On the beauty of the horses.
27. Śūkala	(159*b*)	On the management of unruly horses.
28. Dhābitaṁ	(165*a*)	On running of horses.
29. Krayaḥ	(*to end of MS.*)	On the purchase of horses.
30. Rājopavāhyaḥ		On horses fit for kings.
31. Saugandhī		On good and auspicious smell ?

32.	Vedhanaṁ	... On puncture. Venesection?

II.—Utlarasthāna.

1.	Mahāpraśnaḥ	On questions.
2.	Aṇḍajasaṁbhavaḥ	On the origin from eggs!
3.	Trividhaṁ rogavijñānaṁ.	On the three methods of diagnosis of disease.
4.	Durmanojñānam	On the science of symptoms, such as moroseness, etc., indicating approaching death in healthy horses.
5.	Vartātisāra (vātatisāra?)	On colic pain with diarrhœa?
6.	Vartāh	On the varieties of colic pain.
7.	Praskanna	On some disease of the chest.
8.	Liṅgitāni	On lameness of horses.
9.	Catardoṣāḥ (caturdoṣaḥ?)	On the four kinds of defects in horses.
10.	Abhiṣyandam	On ophthalmia.
11.	Anuṣyanda	
12.	Ṣaḍartukaṁ	On the keeping and feeding of horses during the six seasons.
13.	Pādaroga	On diseases of the feet.
14.	Abhitāpaḥ	On heat? On fever of horses.
15.	Hikkā Svāsah	On hiccough and asthma.
16.	Jvaraḥ	On fevers.
17.	Hāridrakaṁ	On jaundice.
18.	Ajñānaṁ	On fainting and insensibility.

19.	Kṛmi	On worms.
20.	Śūlaṁ	On colic pain.
21.	Siṁghāṇakaḥ	On running from the nose.
22.	Kāsaḥ	On cough.
23.	Atisāraḥ	On diarrhœa and dysentery.
24.	Kṣīrasaṁvṛhaṇaṁ	On galactagogue medicines.
25.	Kaṭukapiṁcchikā (katukapindikā ?)	On bolus consisting of katukā (*Picrorrhiza kurroa*, Benth.)
26.	Vālādakī	
27.	Śudabhraṁśa (Gudabhraṁśa ?)	On prolapse of rectum.
28.	Śoṇitapittakaṁ	On . hæmorrhage from the internal organs.
29.	Adhidanta cikitsā	On the treatment of a tooth which grows upon another.
30.	Pādolūka cikitsitaṁ	On swelling in the leg in kūrcca (incurable).
31.	Vijñānaṁ sarpajātīnāṁ	On the different varieties of snake and its characteristics.
32.	Daṣṭavyāñjanabheṣajaṁ	On symptoms and treatment of snake-bite.
33.	Vigarhanīyaṁ	On the defects of horses.
34.	Vegavijñānaṁ	On the speed of a horse.
35.	Vyāñjanaṁ viṣapītasya	On the signs and symptoms of poisoning.
36.	Digdhaṁ viddhasya	On signs when pierced by a poisoned arrow.
37.	Grahaṇī	On chronic diarrhœa, Sprue.

38.	Vandhavidhah	On the method of securing or tying a horse?
39.	Viṣopaśama	On toxicology and treatment of poisons.

III.—Śārīrakṁ.

1.	Garbhotpattih	On the formation of the embryo.
2.	Sarīranicayah	On the anatomy of the different parts of body.
3.	Kāyotpattih	On the formation of the body. Development of parts of body in uterus.
4.	Sirovyūhah	On the vessels and nerves of the horse.
5.	Desapramanikā	On the habitat of the horses.
6.	Hināni	On horses belonging to a bad type.
7.	Riktamadhyātmyaṁ	
8.	Kāryākāryaṁ (krītyākṛtyam?)	On various measures.
	Nipānikaṁ (Nipanakaṁ?)	On the construction of stone reservoirs for drinking water.
9.	Adhikāra cikitsā	On treatment.
10.	Jaḍāndhavadhirāni	On the dumb, blind and deaf horses.
11.	Rasaskandhāh (Rasaskandāh)	On diseases of shoulder joint? Tetanus?
12.	Yavasānāṁ rasāh	On grasses as food for horses.
13.	Śvayathuḥ	On swelling or intumescence.

14. Dvivraṇīyaṁ	On two kinds of wounds caused by external and internal causes.
15. Mūtrakāvaraṇāni (Mūtrakavarodhani ?)	On urination and its retention.
16. Laṁghanaṁ	On fasting and other methods to make the horse light and nimble.
17. Vṛṁhanaṁ	On the methods of making a horse strong.
18. Mūḍhagarbha cikitsitaṁ	On the management of difficult labour due to malpresentations.
19. Praṇaṣṭaśalyodharanaṁ	On the extraction of dead or deep-seated śalya or splinters.
20. Śalyodharaṇaṁ	On the extraction of foreign bodies as arrow.
21. Nāḍībhagna cikitsā (Nāḍīvraṇa) ?	On the treatment of sinus and fistula ?
22. Arbuda cikitsitaṁ	On the treatment of tumours.
23. Vālārditā	On facial paralysis ?
24. Yonidoṣāḥ	On treatment of diseases of female organs of generation.
25. Vṛṣaśukra cikitsitaṁ	On treatment of diseases of semen of horse.
26. Laksaṇaṁ prasūkānāṁ	On signs of mares.

IV. *Cikitsita sthānaṁ* ... *On Treatmeut.*

1.	Vyānakaḥ	... On some nervous disease?
2.	Aśvanyonirānakaḥ (Niryānka)	... On some disease of corner of eyes?
3.	Avālukīravantakī (Alābuka, Reventaka?)	... On treatment of a disease of mouth; the horse suffers from swollen palate, and so cannot eat grass. On the influence of Revanta?
4.	Jihvāstambhaḥ	... On treatment of sores on tongue causing its paralysis.
5.	Ghṛṇiḥ	... On a treatment of sores within the nostrils, and running from the nose. Glanders?
6.	Śālukī (Galasāluki)?	... On treatment of tonsillitis? Ulcer in throat?
7.	Śirasāntāpaḥ	... On treatment of headache.

11 *slokas wanting, then ending* :

8.	Ādhmānaḥ	... On treatment of tympanitis or flatulence.
9.	Atisāraḥ	... On treatment of diarrhœa.

V. *Kiśoracikitsā* : *Treatment of a colt* :

1.	Miśrakaṁ	... On miscellaneous topics, as diseases of ears, etc.
2.	Grahabhūpaḥ	... On Planets and their influence on horses.
3.	Jarādhyāyaḥ (Jvrādhyāya ?)	... On the different varieties of fever.
4.	Pāmādhyāyaḥ	... On diseases of skin; scabies?
5.	Kṛmi koṣṭhe	... On Intestinal worms.

4 slokas ending :

6.	Bhagna cikitsā	... On fractures of bones.

VI. *Uttarottaraṁ: Supplement:*

1.	**Hayamāro Vāstuvidyā (Hayāgāro ?) :** ...	On the construction of stables ?
2.	**Revantasya pūjanaṁ** ...	Worship of Revanta.
3.	**Grahāṇāṁ śāntikaṁ** ...	Expiation for the evil influence of nine planets.
4.	**Śrīyaḥ Sāṁpūjanaṁ** ...	Worship of Lakṣmī.
5.	**Svātī sampāta** ...	On the influence of Svātī star ?
6.	**Nirājana kriyā** ...	On waving lights before an image. Sprinkling of water for bliss and peace and on the expiatory ceremonies for the cure of diseases and safety of horses and elephants.
7.	Lohābhiharaṇaṁ ...	After Nirājana of horse, the same ceremony was performed before the king in his arms.
8.	Aśvānāṁ Viceṣṭitaṁ ...	On measures for horses.

VII. *Siddhisthānaṁ : Complications of treatment.*

1.	Sneha vyāpat ...	On diseases caused by the use of oleaginous articles of diet.
2.	Kṣīra vyāpat ...	On diseases caused by the use of milk as article of diet.
3.	Surā vyāpat ...	On diseases caused by the use of wines as articles of diet.
4.	Dhānya vyāpat ...	On diseases caused by the use of rice as article of diet.
5.	Lavaṇādi vyāpat ...	On diseases caused by the use of salts, etc., as articles of diet.

6. Nāḍī vyāpat ... On dangers from the use of tubular instruments for enema, etc.

VIII. *Rahasya sthānaṁ* : *On some mysterious topics.*

1. Rekhāniryānakaḥ ... On lines, their positions and import.
2. Āyur Jñānaṁ ... On the duration of life.
3. Riṣṭikādhyāya ... On signs of death. Prognostications.
4. Kalpāriṣṭakaṁ ... On kalpas or various prescriptions of medicines.
5. Upaṣargāriṣṭakaṁ ... On complications foreboding death.
6. Nakṣatrahatariṣṭakaṁ On signs of death caused by the influence of stars.
7. Harītakīnāṁ kalpaḥ ... On the preparations of harītakī (myrobolana) or *Chebulic myrobolana.*
8. Rasoṇa kalpaḥ ... On the preparations of Rasona (garlic) or *Allium sativum.*
9. Gugguloḥ kalpaḥ ... On the preparations of Guggulu (*Balsamodrendron mukul,* Hooker).
10. Sarṣapānāṁ kalpaḥ ... On the preparations of sarṣapa (mustard) or *Brassica Campestris,* L.
11. Lākṣāyāḥ kalpaḥ ... On the preparations of lac.
12. Triphalāyāḥ kalpaḥ ... On the preparations of Triphalā.
13. Svarjjikā kalpaḥ ... On the preparations of resin.
14. Rasāyanāni ... On remedies to prolong life.

15.	Vājīkaraṇāṁ	... On remedies which stimulate sexual power.
16.	Śikṣā Aśvānāṁ	... On the training of horses.
17.	Vālānāṁ damanakriyā	On the management and nursing of foals.
18.	Bhārādānaṁ	... On weights to be carried by horses.
19.	Vividhā raṇakalpanā	On various arrangements of cavalry in war.
20.	Rathāvandaḥ	... On the methods of yolking horses to a chariot.
21.	Vāsasarakriyā (Vāsāgāra ?)	... On management of stables.
22.	Mantrayogaḥ	... On mantras, charms or incantations.
23.	Kriyāyogaḥ	... On remedial measures.
24.	Rahasyopaniṣad	... On the Rahasyopaniṣad.

I have attempted the following restorations in the contents :

	Words as they occur in the MS.	*Suggested alterations.*
1.	Vārtātisāra	Vātatisāra
2.	Catardoṣa	Caturdoṣa
3.	Katukapinchikā	Katukapindikā
4.	Sūdabhrāṁśa	Gudabhraṁśa
5.	Nipānikaṁ	Nipānakaṁ
6.	Mūtrakavaraṇāni	Mūtrakavarodhani
7.	Nāḍibhagna	Nāḍivraṇa
8.	Avālukīravantakī	Alābuka Revantaka
9.	Hayamārovāstuvidyā	Hayāgarovāstuvidyā
10.	Revaṁ (!) tasya	Revantasya
11.	Aśvanyonirānaka	Aśvanyoniryyānaka
12.	Jarādhyāya	Jvarādhyāya
13.	Vāsasarakriyā	Vāsāgārakriyā

MSS : *Tanjore Cat., LVII, Śālihotronnaya.* This seems to be a recent compilation. (12,302) D. ff. 302. Recent. Ends with Ch. xxviii avārtyādhyāya of Lakṣanasthāna, Gr. 1880. Begins :—

जाङ्गव्या * * * विश्वरदम् ।

see page 378.

They ask : Sambhavoḥ kathaṁ aśvanāṁ वाहनत्वं कथमगताः ?

It iṣ in the Paurānic form of a dialogue between Śālihotra and Suśruta. The first third is purely mythological ; then some chapters on age, colour, marks, castes, horses suitable for king, etc., āvarta, which is the last xxviii), but several chapters appear to be wanting.

Two other books are attributed to Śālihotra :

11. *Aśvapraśaṁsā* : A short essay on the importance of horses said to have been taught by Śālihotra to Suśruta.

MS. : G. O. M. L. 13317.

A short essay on the importance of horses said to have been taught by Sālihōtra to Suśruta

Beginning :

शालिहोत्रं मुनिश्रेष्टं सुश्रुतः परिपृच्छति ।
अश्वप्रशंसामाहात्म्यं न ज्ञातं तत्त्वतो मया ॥
तदहं श्रोतुमिच्छामि विस्तरेण वदस्व मे ।
साधु पृष्टं त्वया पुत्र नृपाणां हितकाम्यया ॥
शृणु सुश्रुत सर्वज्ञ तत्प्रभावं प्रचक्ष्महे ।
अश्वैर्हस्तगता पृथ्वी श्रीरश्वैर्विमलं यशः) ॥
विजयश्च भवेदश्वैः अश्वैर्हर्म्यादिभूषणम् ।
तस्य राज्यं यशो लक्ष्मीधर्मकामार्थसम्पदः ॥
वाजिनो यस्य तिष्ठन्ति सर्वलक्षणसंयुताः ।
अश्वेभ्यः परमं नास्ति राज्ञो विजयकारिणम् ॥
तैर्विना न जयस्तस्य वैरिणो वारणैरपि ।

End :

मोक्षात्परा गतिर्नास्ति नास्ति वेदात्परा श्रुतिः ।
नास्ति कृष्णात्परो देवो नास्ति यानं हयात्परम् ॥
वाजिनो यत्र तत्राहं यत्राहं तत्र वाजिनः ।
न ते यत्र न तत्राहं नाहं यत्र न तत्र ते ॥

Colophon :

इति अश्वप्रशंसाध्यायः ॥

Aśvapraśaṁsā is, however, a chapter of Gana's *Sāra-saṁgraha* ; see Burnell's *'anjore Cat.*, LVI, pp. 73, 74. (11,087) Te. 42. (*aśvaprasamsā* only).

111. *Aśvalakṣaṇaśāstraṁ* with Telugu meaning :

MS. : G. O. M. L. 13318 : A treatise on the different breeds of horses and their characteristics with hints for finding out the good specimens among them, the duration of their lives, the marks on their bodies, their vital parts, etc., and for feeding them, etc. The work is attributed to Śālihotra. Reference is also made to a big treatise on the subject by Siṁhadatta :

अश्वशास्त्रसमुद्रं तं सिंहदत्तेन भाषितम् ।

A Telugu rendering is added. The name of the Telugu translator is not given, but he gives introductory and concluding stanzas in Sanskrit.

Beginning :

श्रीहयग्रीवाय नमश्चन्द्रिकाकान्तकान्तये ।
उपासकजनाज्ञानतमिस्रासप्तसप्तये ॥
शुक्लाम्बरधरं विष्णुं शशिवर्णं चतुर्भुजम् ।
प्रसन्नवदनं ध्यायेत्सर्वविघ्नोपशान्तये ॥
अभङ्गुरकलादानस्थूललक्षल्मीयुषे ।
तुङ्गाय महसे तस्मै तुरङ्गाय सुखे नमः ॥

आरभ्याश्वद्रुमस्तां ध्यात्वाचार्यपरम्पराम् ।
अश्वलक्षणशास्त्रं तद्व्याकरोम्यान्ध्रभाषया ॥

पुस्तकान्तरदौर्लभ्याद्विशोध्येदं यथामति ।
क्रियतेऽयश्वशास्त्रस्य टीका प्रतिपदात्मिका ॥

*   *   *

शालिहोत्रमहं वन्दे वेदवेदाङ्गपारगम् ।
अश्वशास्त्रार्थतत्त्वज्ञं शिवध्यानपरायणम् ॥

*   *   *

अश्वशास्त्रसमुद्रं तं सिंहदत्तेन भाषितम् ।
वक्ष्यामि लक्षणं कृत्स्नमश्वानां च विशेषतः ॥

*   *   *

आदौ ब्रह्मण आनन्दाश्रुजातास्तु तुरगा मुखात् ।
तस्मादश्वसमुद्भूता इति ख्यातास्तथाभवन् ॥
ब्रह्मणो नाभिजातास्ते अतश्चैवाग्निसम्भवाः ।

*   *   *

देवैश्च राक्षसैश्चैव मिलित्वा मथिया ध्व(य)तः ।
जाताः समुद्रात्तत्ख्याता अश्वा अमृतसम्भवाः ॥

*   *   *

Colophon :

इति शालिहोत्रीये परीक्षा नाम प्रथमोऽध्यायः ॥

*   *   *

वातपित्तश्लेष्महरा सप्तधातुविवर्धनी ।
इन्द्रियाणां बलकरी गुप्तिशाला च वक्ष्यते ॥

*   *   *

निशापामार्गसिद्धार्थनिम्बलोध्रवराटिका ।
कुबेराक्षौ दारुनिशा कस्तूरी केसरं तथा ॥
मधूकारग्वधं मोहगुग्गलगरूलोचनम् ।

*   *

देवालयस्य मृत्स्ना च दन्तिवल्मीकमृत्तिका ।
एतानि पिष्ट्वा लेपं च शरीरे कारयेदनु ॥

End :

वदनं च पुरः पादौ पूर्वकाय इति स्मृतम् ।
तन्मध्यो मध्यकायः स्यात् तत्पश्चिम इति स्मृतः ॥
*   *   *

शिरोनेत्रमुखं कण्ठकर्णौ वृषणमेहनौ ।
चरणाश्च दश स्थानं तुरगाणां बलांस्मृतम् ॥
*   *   *

यानि स्थानानि वर्तन्ते तुरगाणां विशेषतः ।
सामान्यतः शास्त्रकारैरुक्तानि सुबहूनि च ॥
ज्ञातानि ज्ञायमानानि त्वज्ञातानि स्मृतानि च
तानि सर्वाणि विज्ञाय ह्युक्तानि च मयाधुना ॥
*   *   *

Colophon :

इति शालिहोत्रीये मर्मविभागो नामाष्टमोऽध्यायः ॥

अश्वलक्षणशास्त्रस्था शालिहोत्रर्षिभाषिता ।
विहृतीयं यथामूलमष्टाध्याय्यान्ध्रभाषया ॥
हयग्रीवः प्रसीदन्तां (दैत्त) व्याख्यामाख्यापयन्मया ।
विचिन्त्यैतां प्रसीदन्तु सन्तः सारस्य चिन्तकाः ॥
अश्वशास्त्रं सम्पूर्णम् ॥

Analysis: It is complete in eight chapters with the following topics :

1. Aśvaparīkṣā—On the examination of horse.

2. Varṇaparīkṣā—On the examination of colour of horse.

3. Puṇḍrapuṣpagandhādivarṇanam.—On the description of marks, spots and smell of the horse.

4. Subhāśubhāvartvicāraḥ—On the good and bad whirls of hairs.

5. Hayavayojñānaṁ—On the knowledge of the age of horse.

6. Rekhāyujñānādivarṇanaṁ—On the duration of life of the horse as indicated by lines, etc.

7. Aśvapoṣanavidhiḥ—On the nursing and feeding of a horse.

8. Garbhavibhāgaḥ—On pregnancy.

The MSS. 1321, 1322 and 1323, G. O. M. L. XXIII, treat of Aśvayurveda based mainly on Śalihotra's work.

Reference to Śalihotra.—In the *Liṅga Purāṇa* (Chs. vii and xxiv), a list of the different Avatāras of Śiva, the Vyāsas (Yogācāryas) and their disciples in the Varāha Kalpa of the (Vaivasvata) seventh Manvantara is given. In it we find the names of Śālihotra, Agniveśa, Yuvanāśva and Śāradvasu as the four disciples of Yogācārya Ṛkṣa or Rakṣa and Sūlī was the Avatāra of Śiva in the Naimiṣa land in the 24th yūga. The occurrence of the names of Sālīhotra and Agniveśa as disciples of the same teacher undoubtedly points to the remote age in which they flourished. In S. R. Bhāndarkar's *Collection of MSS.* 1899-1925 (*List of MSS. collected for the Govt. MSS. Library*, published by *Oriental Research Institute*, Poona, 1925, p. 54) we find a MS. called *Śālihotra*, No. 581, described as a Koṣagrantha or Dictionary by Vikramātmaja. We have no knowledge of Sālihotra as a writer of dictionary.

Śālihotra is quoted in *Tatta Candrika*: शालिहोत्रादावप्येरण्ड-मूलेषोवेति, p. 22, where the author says that "Suśruta and Śālihotra read 'Eraṇḍamūla' instead of 'Gokṣura' in the Daśamūla. Caraka however reads Goksura.

Śālihotra is quoted in *Ṭīkāsarvasva* a Commentary on the celebrated *Nāmaliṅgānuśāsana* of Amarsiṁha by

50

Sarvānanda, which was composed between 1417 and 1431 A.D. (P. of MS, 26, 187. See *Rep. Sans. Tamil. MSS.*, 1893-94, No. 2, p. 31).

The progress in veterinary medicine achieved by the ancient Indians may be compared with the knowledge possessed by the cultured European nations about a century back. The age of Śālihotra is unknown, but as Suśruta was his disciple or son, he must have flourished about 1000 B.C., the age of Suśruta. I have discussed about the probable age of Suśruta in my work '*Surgical Instruments of the Hindus*,' Vol. I, p. 11, and I would take the liberty to refer my readers to its pages. The reference in the *Aśva-cikitsā*, the treatise of Kuntī-sūta Nakula, undoubtedly lends support to a very early age, the age of the celebrated battle of Kurukṣetra. Animal hospitals or 'Piñjrāpoles' still exist in India. The early European travellers mention their existence in Surat and Broach for the support of old animals and cure of their diseases. I have described such institutions in Chapter II '*Hospitals and Dispensaries*' of the same book. In Europe, on the other hand, we have no trustworthy history of the art and science of farriery which can be traced to such a remote period of time. In France, veterinary schools were established at an earlier period than in any other country in Europe. Bourgelat was its first director and the principal projector; and he has been justly regarded as the founder of the veterinary art based on anatomico-physiological studies. His Anatomy appeared first in 1769. Attempts were made at a much earlier period, to diffuse a knowledge of veterinary anatomy, principally by Ruini, an Italian, in 1598. His book was the source of Sollysel's celebrated work which was published in 1698. The earliest English writer on Farriery is Mascal who flourished in the reign of Edward the Sixth. Gervase Markham, the most celebrated of ancient farriers, published his '*Masterpiece*' in 1666. The work of Snape, Farrier to King Charles the Second, based on Sollysel's book, appeared later, and a host of writers, Layard, Bracken, Bartlet, Osmar, Clark and Taplin wrote on the subject. In 1792 the Veterinary College was established with Sainthel as its Professor. He was succeeded by Coleman and Morecroft in the professorial chair. In 1807, Morecroft came out to India to superintend the breeding stud of the East India Company.

Now for the training of students in veterinary science, there are colleges, provided and maintained by the Government, at Calcutta, Madras, Bombay and Lahore and schools at Insein and Tunggyi in Burma. The scheme for establishing a college at Lucknow for the United Provinces is now receiving the attention of the Government. The Madras Veterinary Department publishes a bi-monthly magazine entitled the *Madras Veterinary Journal* which educates the public in veterinary matters. The Imperial Bacteriological Laboratory, Mukteswar, and the Research and Experimental Station at Badshabhag, U. P., are doing useful work for he observation and study of diseases and methods of research.

PĀLAKĀPYA.

In the Hasti-Āyurveda, Pālakāpya is described to be the son of Sāmagāyanākhya Muni by a female elephant which drank his urine containing his seminal discharges. He was invited by King Romapāda who wanted to subdue elephants for human use. Romapāda or Lomapāda was king of Campā, which has been identified by Cunningham with Pātharghātā, some 24 miles distant from the modern town of Bhagalpur. Romapāda was the father-in-law of Ṛṣyaśṛṅga Muni and was a contemporary of Daśaratha, father of Rāma. Fa Hian describes Campā to be a large town containing many Buddhist Stupas and Vihāras. Campā or Mālini, the capital of the country of Aṅga, was called after king Campa, son of Pṛthu-lākṣa.

The author of *Trikāndaśeṣa* identifies Pālakāpya with Dhanvantari, the founder of the Surgical School in India. Suśruta is said to have learned major surgery from Dhanvantari; but from other accounts we learn that Suśruta also learned the veterinary science from Dhanvantari. So if we accept them (Pālakāpya and Dhanvantari) to be identical persons, we get a solution of the difficulty. But the evidence of their identity is by no means complete, and is far from satisfactory.

Pālakāpya's work:

1. *Hasti-Āyurveda or Pālakāpya.*—It is a voluminous work on elephants, describing in detail their diseases and treatment, both medical and surgical.

MSS:

Bik. MSS.: 1395.

Tanjore Cat. MS.: IX., p. 75.

Editions:

1. The book has been edited and printed at the Anandāśram Press, Poona, in the Anandāśram Series.

Translations:

1. Hasti-Āyurveda: translated in Bengali. Only a few chapters have been translated by Mahārājā Soshikanta Ācharya Chaudhury of Mymensing.

An analysis of the contents of the Pālakāpya has never appeared in the English language. Burnell in his *Catalogue of the Tanjore MSS*. refers to the work as *Gajavaidya* and says: "This name appears to be not very certain; it consists of dialogues between a king of *Aṇga* and a *muni* called *Pālakāpya*, who is the offspring of a *Rishi* and a pious female elephant. There is a great deal of mythological matter about the creation, the origin of elephants, who were originally winged, and were deprived of these appendages by the curse of an angry saint, who was pestered by their tumbling down on him from the trees round his hermitage, on which they used to perch in order to graze on the leaves. The rest refers to the points of animals, as usual, very fanciful; their castes and dispositions; the way of taming them; their diseases and the way of treating and curing them. The number of their diseases appears to be put at 106. There can be no doubt that this is a very modern compilation, even later than the *Sārasaṁgraha* (on horses). Some of the verses, however, which are found here, occur in *Cāraṅgadhara* as by *Pālakāpya*. See Aufrecht's paper in the Z. d. D. M. G., Vol. XXVII., pp. 1-120."

No detailed analysis is given in any catalogue, and therefore I have attempted it in the following pages:

Analysis of Contents of Pālakāpya.

I. *Mahārogasthānaṁ* : *Major Diseases.*

1. Vanānucaritaṁ ... Salutation to Ganeśa. To subdue the wild elephants, King Romapāda of Campā holds a meeting of the sages, Gautama and others. They send a messenger to *Pālakāpya Muni* and the elephants. Romapāda's questions to Pālakāpya at Campā. The wings of the elephants were severed owing to the curse of Dīrghatapā. Origin of *Hasti-Āyurveda* by Brahmā. Birth of Pālakāpya : his mother was a female elephant who drank the seminal discharge of Sāmagāyanākhya *Muni*. The story of Ruci who was cursed by Brahmā. Mataṅga Muni's curse and the origin of the science. The cause of the appearance of diseases among elephants is said to be due to the change of environment : their freedom in the forest and their captivity under men. Pālakāpya promised to remain in the court of Romapāda and the Muni was ordered to teach the

Sages the science of *Hasti-Āyurveda.*

2. Annasamācāraḥ .. On the smearing of oil and ghee and bathing in water; time and measure of feeding elephants with rice and treacle; time of giving them solid and liquid food and their quantity.

3. Sātmyaviniścayaḥ ... Causes of 15 kinds of death of wild elephants, such as fall from a mountain, etc. Natural food of elephants: leaves of trees and grasses.

4. Śāstrasaṁgrahaḥ ... The 4 main sections of the book: (1) Major Diseases, (2) Minor Diseases, (3) Surgery, and (4) the Supplement The number of chapters are 18, 72, 34 and 36, respectively. The total number of ślokas would be about 20,000.

5. Gajarakṣaṇavinyāsaḥ .. Eulogy on elephants; their qualifications; their use in war, "the ornament of the army." The 8 characteristics of the owners of elephants.

6. Śiṣyopanayanaḥ ... Initiation of the disciples. The requisite qualifications of a good student; the ceremonial rites to be

		observed. Qualifications of a good teacher; the relation between the teacher and his disciples; their mutual responsibilities. Origin of the science from the *Atharvaveda*. The fitness of students belonging to the Brāhmaṇa, Kṣatriya and Vaiśya castes. The teachers are prohibited from teaching the atheists the science of elephants.
7.	Rogavibhaktiḥ	Two classes of diseases—inherent and accidental. 76 nervous diseases; 27 bile diseases; 32 phlegm diseases; 15 blood diseases; 22 sannipātic diseases; 14 nervous-bile diseases; 16 nervous-phlegm diseases, 7 nervous-blood diseases; names and number of mixed diseases; the total number of inherent diseases; names and number of the accidental diseases. Classification of diseases: curable, incurable and curable with difficulty.
8.	Jvarotpattiḥ ...	On the origin of fever; its signs and symptoms. War between the gods and demons; the Devas approach

	the higher gods Śiva and Viṣṇu who created fevers. The demons being oppressed with fever prayed Brahmā to cure them. He then sent away fevers to the House of Death.
9. Pākalaḥ Jvarahetuniścayah	On the different names of Fever in different animals; Pākala is the name of the fever of elephants. The different classes of fever or pākala; their origin, signs, symptoms and pathology.
10. Skandādhyāyaḥ ...	On Tetanus? Three kinds:—Antarāyāma (Emprosthotonos), Vahirāyāma (Opisthotonos) and Vyaviddhaskandā; the first variety is curable, the latter two incurable.
11. Purānakṛsarogaḥ (Pāṇḍurogaḥ) ...	Anaemia or chlorosis? Origin and treatment of the varieties of the disease as caused by vāta, pitta and śleṣma.
12. Ānāhan ...	On flatulence. The different varieties of the disease according to different causes: excessive eating, rice-eating, earth-eating, etc.
13. Murcchāḥ ...	On swooning or fainting. 12 kinds of the disease: caused

		by excessive food, eating of rice and incompatible food stuffs, water, wine, grasses, vāyu, pitta, śleṣma, etc.
14.	Śirabhitāpaḥ Śirorogaḥ	... On the diseases of the head, 27 kinds ; caused by vāta, pitta, śleṣma and their combinations and by worms.
15.	Pādarogaḥ	... On diseases of the foot, 30 kinds; diseases of the foot of the wild and domesticated elephants. 9 kinds of accidental diseases. Aetiology, pathology and treatment of the different varieties.
16.	Aṣtavyāpadrogāḥ	... 8 kinds of dangers from oil, ghee, fat, milk, wine, rice, water and irregular administration of diet; their origin and treatment.
17.	Śophaḥ	... On anasarca; its 7 kinds; their origin and treatment.
18.	Svedaḥ	... On the different modes of sweating.
	Śāntirakṣāḥ	... Religious rites to be performed at the beginning of treatment.
	Akṣirogādhyāyaḥ	... On the various forms of eye diseases; their origin and treatment.

II *Kṣudrarogasthānaṁ : On Minor diseases.*

1.	Vamathurogaḥ	... On Vomiting; its two kinds: (1) doṣaja:—due to defect of

humours; (2) āgantuka :— external or accidental : their origin and treatment.

2. Atisāracikitsitaṁ ... On the treatment of Diarrhœa; its two kinds—gastric and intestinal; their prognosis and treatment.

3. Madanajagdhakaḥ ... On swooning caused by the use of Madana plant (Randia dumetorum. *Lamk.*). Its pathology and treatment.

4. Tṛṇaśoṣī ... On wasting caused by the excessive eating of unwholesome diet: diseased grass, poisonous plants and fruits.

5. Karmātinītacikitsitaṁ On diseases caused by excessive work, their pathology and treatment.

6. Viṣaparikṣādhyāyaḥ On poisons. Protection of the elephants from poisons administered by enemies in the stables. Signs of the poisoner; methods of detecting poisons by the cats, crows, and other birds, water, fire, oil and milk. 3 classes of poisons; symptoms and treatment of poisoned elephants.

7. Dūṣīviṣaḥ (incomplete) On poisons which derange the system of the elephant; their origin and action.

8. Viṣalakśmaṇaṁ ... On the signs and symptoms of poisoning. The symptoms

vary according as one or more of the ten essential structures of the body are involved, *viz.*, skin, flesh, bones, etc. The elephants suffer from 3 stages (*Vega*) of the poison, but the other animals suffer from 7 stages; the treatment by medicines and mantras or charms.

9. **Digdhaviddhah** ... On signs and symptoms when elephants are pierced by poisoned arrows.

10. **Sarpadaṣtah** ... On snake-bite and its treatment: 3 methods of biting; 4 kinds of snakes; treatment varies accordingly.

11. Sphotikādhyāyah ... On boils; their origin, prognosis and treatment; Vasiṣṭha's curse on the animals; origin of the spiders.

12. Apavādavaddhaḥ ... On the influence of the planets.

13. Pūrvāvaddhah ... On elephants which were not restrained or trained properly when young. It is an incurable mental disease; forest-life in the company of the female elephants,—its charms and beauties.

14. Visarpādhyāyaḥ ... On erysipelas: its 5 kinds; their pathology and treatment.

15.	Hṛdayasphālī	... On nervous and anxious heart caused by fear.
16.	Vālaksānīrogah	... 2 varieties; Doṣaja and Āgantuka.
17.	Meḍrakṣāni	... 2 varieties; external and internal; their treatment.
	Hastagrahanarogaḥ	Its prognosis and treatment.
18.	Hastonmathitaḥ	... On elephants agitated by mental disorder; its origin and treatment. Prediction of the time of death from the study of its pathology.
19.	Udāvartah	... On the stoppage of urination, defaecation and flatus; its origin and treatment.
20.	Utkarṇakarogaḥ	... On Farcy. Its 3 kinds due to 3 humours, and their treatment.
21.	Vātagati	... On unnatural movements due to the derangement of vāta.
22.	Manyāgrahah	... On wryneck; accidental pain in the shoulder and neck.
23.	Madakṣīṇa	... On weakness due to undue stimulation of the animal during rut or by intoxication.
24.	Kṛśādhyāyaḥ	... On the thinning of elephants and its treatment.
25.	Valaksīnah	... On loss of strength; on weakness of elephants.
26.	Ślesmābhisanna	... On the phlegmatic appearance of elephants due to a diet which causes an increase of phlegm.

27.	Mukhodvāraviśodhanaḥ Vanasātmyanulomika	On the purification of mouth of elephants by the natural food of the forest.
28.	Tālakāśīrogaḥ	... On the wounds of the plantar surfaces of the feet of elephants.
29.	„ cikitsitaṁ	... On the treatment of plantar wounds.
30.	Galagrahaḥ	... On inflammation and pain in the throat.
31.	Tṛṣṇārditaḥ	... On the signs of a thirsty elephant.
	Siddhārthakarogaḥ	On the prickly tongue of elephants.
32.	Bhūtagrahaḥ	... On the signs and symptoms of possession by supernatural beings such as Kämakhyā, etc., and their treatment.
33.	Unmādaḥ	... On Insanity; its origin and treatment.
34.	Apasmāraḥ	... On Hysteria or Epilepsy. Adoration of 9 planets to rectify their evil influences.
35.	Vātakuṇḍalikāḥ	... Acute rheumatism ?—Its origin and treatment.
36.	Bhāronmathitaḥ	... On the excitement of elephants due to heavy weight.
37.	Luptacikitsitaṁ	... On the wasting of muscles; its origin and treatment.
38.	Patrakṛmiḥ	... On the signs, symptoms, pathology and treatment of the disease caused by eating

		worms which live on the leaves of trees.
39.	Uraḥkṣataḥ / Urastambhaḥ	On chronic inflammation of the lungs. Its origin and treatment.
40.	Śonitāṇdaḥ	... On inflammation of the scrotum; Haematocele? Its origin and treatment.
41.	Yavagandaśirah	.. A variety of disease of foot; severe inflammation of foot and nails.
42.	Carmakīlah	... On warts; their causation and treatment.
43.	Vṛddhacikitsitaṁ	... On the treatment of old age.
44.	Avasanna	... On tired elephants; on lassitude.
45.	Jatharakah	... On diseases of the digestive tract; dyspepsia? Its origin and treatment.
46.	Vālacikitsāḥ	... On the care and treatment of the young elephants.
47.	Rātrikṣiptaḥ	... On insanity during the night? Its cause and treatment. Influence of Rakṣograha and its remedy.
48.	Mūtrasaṅgaḥ	... On retention of urine; dysuria, strangury; bloody urine; its treatment; incurability of rupture of the urinary bladder.
49.	Sūtikāh	... On puerperal fever; its pathology and treatment.

50.	Dantarogaḥ ...	On the diseases of the teeth. 4 different classes; the number and treatment of the diseases.
51.	Cetovhramśaḥ ...	On mental derangement caused by fear; shyness; oppression with fear.
52.	Śūlādhyāyaḥ ...	On colic pain; its 2 varieties; its primary origin from Siva's anger towards Madana.
53.	Śāradāḥ ...	On the 4 types of the Śāradā disease; its main cause :—want of exercise; its prominent symptom :—difficulty in drinking fluids.
54.	Madhumakṣikādaṣṭaḥ	On the bites of the honey-bee and their treatment.
55.	Cchavidoṣaḥ ...	On the 11 kinds of defects of the body of elephants, such as ringworm, vitiligo, psoriasis ? etc.; their origin and treatment.
56.	Mṛttikāḥ ...	On soils and on the habit of earth-eating; the diseases caused thereby with their treatment.
57.	Grahaṇīcikitsitaṁ	On the treatment of the 3 kinds of chronic diarrhœa; Sprue.
58.	Āmādhyāyaḥ ...	On the treatment of dysentery; its causation and pathology.
59.	Kṛmikoṣṭhīḥ ..	On the intestinal worms; their origin and treatment.
60.	Kṣayādhyāyaḥ ...	On the 4 kinds of weakness, 10 kinds of wasting; pathology and treatment of phthisis pulmonalis.

61	Prabhinnaḥ Madasrāvaḥ.	On the discharge of mada of elephants; mada is the juice which flows from the temples of an elephant in rut. 14 causes and 5 kinds of the disease.
62.	Karṇavālakṛmiḥ...	On the worms which frequent the hairs and the ears, their cause and treatment.
63.	Karṇarogaḥ ...	On the diseases of the ears; their cause and treatment.
64.	Abhaktacchandīḥ	On anorexia and loss of appetite and its treatment.
65.	Bhaktagrāsoparuddhaḥ.	On the digestive fire; its seat and functions.
66.	Droṇikaśophaḥ ...	On the 5 kinds of inflammation in the chest and abdomen.
67.	Atiyātaḥ ...	On animals which have been unreasonably worked out; an animal whose strength is spent up.
68.	Gulmaḥ ...	On tumours; its 5 kinds and their treatment.
69.	Hṛdrogacikitsitaṁ.	On the diseases of the heart; their 3 kinds and treatment.
70.	Gātrarogaḥ ...	On the diseases of the skin; their 4 classes and treatment.
71.	Āgantukagātrarogaḥ.	On skin diseases caused by external causes, or accidental skin diseases.
72.	Gātrarogaḥ ...	On the 12 kinds of skin diseases and their treatment.

III. Śalyasthānaṁ : Surgery.

1. **Dvivraṇīyaḥ** ... On two kinds of wounds caused by external and internal causes. The subject is dealt with in detail and the author describes it under the following heads: signs and symptoms of 3 kinds of Yoṇi (cause), 8 kinds of Adhiṣṭhāna (seat), 2 kinds of Srāva (discharge), pure and impure; 24 varieties of Wounds according to Vastu (substance), 3 kinds of Ātmanaḥ (nature), curability or incurability, 2 kinds of Śalya (splinters), 5 kinds of Upakrama (treatment), 6 kinds of Doṣa (defects), and medicines for ointments, steam, granulation, etc.

2. **Sadyakṣata-lakṣaṇaṁ** Symptoms of fresh wounds inflicted by lions, tigers, etc.

3. **Sadyakṣata-cikitsitaṁ.** On the treatment of fresh wounds; signs indicating death; prognosis from the messenger; auspicious time for the attendance of the Vaidyas; action of digestive fire.

4. **Saḍatyayopacāraḥ** On the 6 kinds of surgical procedures.

5. **Vraṇopakrama-lakṣaṇaḥ.** On the origin and symptoms of ulcers; 21 kinds of ulcers; suppurating and non-suppurating ulcers. 44 methods of treatment.

6. Dvādaśopakramaḥ On 5 elements. 7 dhātus, 4 kinds of animals, 5 prāṇas, 4 minds. On the functions of the body and digestion of food; treatment of animals.

7. Garbhasambhavah On pregnancy; on the formation of the fœtus: its growth by months; the structures derived from the father and the mother.

8. Garbhāvakrāntiḥ On the pregnant woman; menstruation; signs of pregnancy; formation of the fœtus; its development; the sex of the fœtus; white and black spots on the skin; the 3 types of elephants.

9. Śarīravicayah ... On Anatomy: the number and descriptions of teeth, nails, vital parts, vessels, nerves, bones, ligaments and joints; the seat of the 3 humours.

10. Śāstrāgnipraṇidhiḥ On the sharp instruments and actual cautery; their uses; the modes of their application.

11. Yantrabidhiḥ ... On the blunt instruments; their uses; their manufacture; the trees and pillars to be used with them; prayer to gods.

12. Śalyopaharaṇaḥ On the extraction of foreign bodies, splinters, arrows, etc. Teachers of medicine from Brahmā downwards; symptoms of injuries caused by śalyas

		which pierce the external and internal structures respectively; extraction of arrows from special regions; incurability of wounds on the vital parts.
13.	Vidradhirogaḥ	On abscess; its 4 kinds; their origin and treatment.
14.	Vraṇacikitsitaṁ	On the treatment of ulcer; its two kinds and prognosis.
15.	Nāḍīvraṇacīkitsitaṁ.	On the fistula and sinus; their origin, prognosis and treatment by knife, cautery and caustics.
16.	Śirāvyūhavyadhaḥ	On vessels and venesection; 700 vessels; their location; vessels conveying 7 dhātus and 3 humours; venesection in special cases and their treatment.
17.	Dantanāḍicikitsitaṁ.	On the treatment of sinus caused by disease of the tooth.
18.	Adhikadantacikitsitāṁ.	On the treatment of extra tooth; the normal number of teeth is 16; 2 extra teeth are found sometimes.
19.	Śirācchedaḥ ...	On venesection; 107 vital parts; their descriptions; the number of vital parts, which, when injured, cause immediate death and death after some time respectively.
20.	Marmapramāṇaḥ	On the vital parts; their description; 107 in number.

21.	Erandakaḥ	... On the bite of dogs; 4 races of dogs; the cause of their poisonous nature; the 3 stages of action of the poison and their treatment.
22.	Marmasthāna-viddhaḥ.	Description of wounds of vital parts in detail and their treatment.
23.	"	The same subject continued.
24.	Doṣavicayaḥ	... On defects. On the origin of pākala or fever in young elephants; description of the seats of the humours.
25.	Agnidagdhacikitsitaṁ.	On the treatment of burns by means of fomentation, unguents, etc.
26.	Lūtādhāyaḥ	... On the spiders; their classification;—21 kinds, names, their poison and treatment.
27.	Visakīṭacikitsāḥ	... On the treatment of bites of poisonous insects; their names, number, etc.
28.	Vyāladaṣṭaḥ	... On snake-bite; classes of snakes, their bites, pathology and treatment; symptoms in an incurable case.
29.	Pradeśajnānaṁ	... On the different members of the elephant's body; their number is 15; names, parts, etc.
30.	Śāstravidhih	... On the method of using 10 different kinds of sharp

instruments, knife, bistouri, etc.; extraction of arrows.

31. Kṣārādhyāyaḥ ... On the preparation and use of caustics or potential cautery.

32. Bhagnacikitsitaṁ ... On fractures and their treatment; their causes, classes, descriptions, prognosis and treatment.

33. Muḍhagarbhapanayanaṁ. On difficult labour and its treatment; signs of a dead fœtus, methods of its extraction by excision of obstructing parts, etc., favourable and unfavourable cases and their treatment.

34. Dantoddharaṇaṁ ... On the extraction of tooth of elephants; the rite to be observed; the difference in structure of the different teeth.

IV. Uttarasthānaṁ: the Supplement.

1. Snehapānaḥ ... On drinking of oleaginous medicines; 2 kinds of fat, animal and vegetable, and their differences; ghee and oil, time of their administration, their measure and dosage.

2. Snehapānvidhikathanaṁ. On the modes of drinking the oils and fats in detail, the proper and improper times of their administration; the

		good and bad results of their daily use.
3.	Annapānavidhikathanaṁ.	On the methods of taking food and drink. 3 kinds of animals,—good, intermediate, and bad; the difference of ages; 4 kinds of food-stuffs; (1). to be chewed, (2). to be swallowed, (3). to be drunk and (4). to be sucked; 3 divisions of the food to be sucked up; measure of rice and treacle as food; defects and merits of wine as a drink; milk and dadhi as articles of food; śāli rice, barley, pulses and wheat as articles of diet; on washing of the body, cleaning of the head and washing of the teeth and eyes.
4.	Snehavidhikathanaṁ	On snehas; their 9 kinds; Gargya's opinion; time for drinking oils; on fat and marrow; influence of seasons; on the administration of fresh oleaginous medicines: enemas and their use; oils and their use.
5.	Vastidānakathanaṁ	On the administration of 9 kinds of enemas.
6.	Śālāvidhānaṁ ...	On stables; their size, construction, soil, planetary

		influence, seasons, fitness for the 3 kinds of elephants, ceremonial rites to be observed, etc.
7.	Nasyadānavidhikathanaṁ.	On snuffs; their use and abuse; consequences of its use in sufficient, insufficient and excessive doses.
8.	Yavasādhyāyaḥ ...	On the use of grass as food; use of green and dry grass according to the season and month.
9.	Ariṣṭajñānakaṭhanaṁ	On prognostications; signs of death; symptoms which predict unfavourable results.
10.	Dantakalpanādyhāyah	On the modes of artificial preparations of the elephant's teeth to fit them for use in war, fight with animals, for self-protection and beauty, etc.; the teeth fit for such operations are modelled by the artists; different classes of the teeth, their measure, etc.
11.	Rasavīryavipākādhyāyaḥ. (*Incomplete.*)	On the derangements of the *rasas* of the body,—the chyle, semen, etc., and their defects.
12.	Ikṣudānavidhikathanaṁ.	On the mode of feeding elephants with sugar-cane.
13.	Nasyakarmavidhiḥ...	On the modes of giving snuffs to elephants in detail.

14. Añjanāvidhiḥ ... On the various methods of using collyrium to elephant's eyes; Vijayā guṭikā its preparation and uses; different kinds of collyrium and prescriptions for eye diseases.

15. Rtucaryādhyāyah ... On the nursing of elephants during the six seasons; their food and drink in different seasons; on baths and fomentation, etc.

16. Kāryākāryavidhih ... On the reason why the drinking of water during a meal is not recommended.

17. Apānagunādhikāra ... On the use of salts for digestion of food-stuffs and the use of condensed milk for increase of muscles.

18. Souvīrakapānavidhiḥ On the use of sour gruel as a drink.

19. Surāpratipānavidhiḥ On the good and bad effects of wine for drinking by the three classes of elephants; on some counter-drink after the drink of wine; on the mixture of salt and treacle with wines; on the good effects of wine when churned with five kinds of salts, lac, etc.

20. Gugguluvidhih ... On the method of administering guggulu (*Balsamodendron mukul* Hooker) accord-

		ing to season; on the mixture of guggulu with oil.
21.	Kṣıradānavidhiḥ	... On the use of condensed milk; quality of the milk of cows and buffaloes.
22.	Gajasaṁbhavaḥ	... On the origin of elephants; war between Devas and Dānavas; Siva's boon to the son of Rāvaṇa; on the mounting of an elephant.
23.	Kimarthakināmādhyāyaḥ.	On the reasons of giving oil, ghee, etc., in detail.
24.	Paricārakahetujñānaṁ.	On servants to look after the elephants; how to know if the elephant has been sufficiently oiled, medicated and sweated.
25.	Trividhiḥ	... On the 3 kinds of means; (1) two kinds of grasses as food; (2) three kinds of eating; (3) three kinds of country.
26.	Pathyāpathyavicāraḥ	On good and bad food according to the three humours; duration of life of the three types of elephants.
27.	Karīṣamūtrādhyāyaḥ	On the urine and fæces of animals, as cow, buffalo, elephant, etc.
28.	Laśunakalpaḥ	... On the origin of Laśuna (garlic, *Allium sativum*, Linn.); on sweet and bitter tastes of the various parts of the plant, *viz.*, root, seeds, etc.

29.	Lavaṇayogaḥ	... On the use of salts with medicines, such as, pippalī (*Piper longum*, Linn.) and śṛṅgavera (*Zingiber officinale*, Rose).
30.	Pāṁsudānaṁ	... On the use of ashes for elephants; 4 kinds of elephants.
31.	Madāvasthā	... On elephants in rut and excitement; 7 stages due to 7 dhātus.
32.	Nāgatantukagrāhah	On the two kinds of grāha :—nāgagrāha and tantukagrāha; their origin and treatment.
33.	Jalahastilakṣaṇaṁ	... On water elephants; gifts of food on auspicious days.
34.	Jalaukādhyāyah	... On the leeches, 12 varieties of leeches; 2 classes :—poisonous and non-poisonous; their origin and characteristics.
35.	Upasarganirupaṇaṁ	On some complications. The Bhūtas frequent the stables as diseases; on fever or pākala; fear of the elephant; worship of Śiva and Viṣṇu to cure fever.
36.	Gajaśāntih	... On expiatory ceremonies. Nirājanavidhi, or sprinkling of water for bliss and peace. On auspicious moments for the rite. Worship of Viṣṇu for protection of elephants.

In the introductory chapter the names of the sages who were invited by Romapāda in an assembly to learn the science of treatment of elephant are given as follows :—

Gautama.	Mataṅga.
Agniveśa.	Urmimālī.
Prince Vāṣkali.	Sārasvata.
Kāśyapa.	Cyavana.
Mṛgaśarmaṇa.	Pulastya.
Bharadvāja.	Pulaha.
Souvala.	Kratu.
Kāṅkāyaṇa.	Viśvāmitra.
Gārgya.	Vaśiṣṭha.
Raivya.	Yamadagni.
Vṛhaṣpati.	Bhārgava.
Arimeda.	Agastya.
Māṇḍavya.	Triśaṅku.
Kumuda.	Marīci.
Yājñavalkya.	Atri.
Hiraṇya.	Suparvaṇa.
Bhṛgu.	Dīrgha.
Aṅgirasa.	Parikara.
Parāśara.	Kāpya.
Acūḍa.	Nārada.

RĀVAṆA.

Rāvaṇa, the son of Viśravā, a Brāhmaṇa, by his wife Nikaṣā, daughter of Rākṣasa Sumāli, and the grandson of Ṛṣi Pulastya, expelled his half-brother Kuvera and became King of Ceylon. By his penance he received the boon from Brahmā, by which he became invulnerable against gods and demons.

In the *Rāmāyaṇa* he is described as a supernatural being with ten mouths (*Daśānana, Daśāsya*), ten necks (*Daśakaṇṭha and Paṅktigrīva*), twenty hands :— epithets derived from his prowess in wars and conquests. He was defeated by Vālī and Māndhātā and once he was taken prisoner by Kārtavīrya. Even the natural forces, sun, moon, lightning, oceans and winds obeyed him through terror. He carried off Sītā Debī, wife of Rāma from Daṇḍakāraṇya, in retaliation of his wars against the Rākṣasas. Rāma with the help of Sugrīva and Hanumāna built Rama's bridge and after many battles, defeated and killed Rāvaṇa and rescued Sītā Debī. His chief wife was Mandodarī, daughter of Maya Dānava. His sons were Meghanāda or Indrajit, Rāvaṇī, Akṣa, Triśīrā, Devāntaka, Narāntaka and Atikāya. Kumbhakarṇa and Bibhīṣaṇa were his brothers and Śūrpanakhā his sister He was cursed by Vedavatī who burnt herself to death to avoid his immoral proposal. He tried to oppress Apsarā Rambhā for which he was cursed by Nala Kuvera to meet with death if he would try to insult any other lady against her will. So Sītā Devī was saved from dishonour.

Rāvaṇa. the famous king of Ceylon, whose wars with Rāma are celebrated in the *Rāmāyaṇa* of Vālmīki is said to have written works on medicine.

His works :

1. *Kumāra Tantra :* He is said to have written a medical treatise on the diseases of children.

Rāvaṇa's *Kumāra Tantra* is quoted by many medical authors :—

1. ओँ नमो रावणाय अमूकस्य व्याधिं हन् हन् मुञ्च मुञ्च ह्रौं फट् स्वाहा।

Cakradatta, p. 338.

इदानीं प्रसिद्धफलं रावणकृतकुमारतन्त्रमाह ओं नारायणाय नमः।

Tattva Chaṇdrikā, p. 338.

2. It is quoted in Trimalla's *Yogataraṅginī*, MSS. :—I. O. 2705, 2706.

3. In the *Vaṅgasena*, a *Kumāratantra* is ascribed to Pārvatī in one place, while in another, we have reference to a *Kumāratantra* attributed to the son of Rāvaṇa. The section, in which these quotations and references occur, seems to be an extract from the *Kaumāra Tantra*, if not the *Kumāra Tantra* itself. MSS. :—I. O. 2698-2700.

4. The *Kumāra Tantra* is perhaps given entire in Vindyarāja's *Sukhobodha*. MSS. :—I. O. 2679. fol. 242-245*a*.

5. In the *Yogasaṁgraha* by Jagannātha, "we notice that the particular method of healing children's maladies by the recitation of magic spells, referred to in other works as "Ravanakṛtaṁ Kumāratantraṁ" is here mentioned (fol. 124*b*) under the title of "Rāvanakṛtir Vālatantram." MSS. :—I. O. 2682.

6. It is also mentioned by Gayadāsa in the *Nāya Candrikā*.

See Cambridge University Library MSS. :—2491.

7. In the *Vālacikitsā* G.O.M.L. (Madras), MS. No. 13175, the treatment of children is described according to Rāvaṇa. रावण मते वालचिकित्सा कथ्यते।

II. *Arka Prakāśa* :—It is also called *Arka Cikitsā*,—a book written by a physician named Rāvaṇa. He expounds a new system of treatment by means of tinctures and extracts.

Begins :—

द्रव्यकल्पः पञ्चधा स्यात् कल्क चूर्ण रसस्तथा ।
तैलमर्कः क्रमाज्ज्ञेयं यथोत्तरगुणं प्रिये ॥

Ends :—

केतक्यर्कोबहुशो गन्धपाषाणा धूपितोदशधा ।
तद्युक्तलिङ्गभोगाद योनिर्लिङ्गं सुगन्धि स्यात् ॥

But in the end of the printed Bengali edition where the translator has added a supplement containing other prescriptions from various books, we find.

कृशानां पुष्टिजननो बन्ध्यानां पुत्रदं परम् ।
अरिष्टोदशमूलाख्यस्तेजः-शुक्र-बलप्रदः ॥

The book is also called *Rājmārtaṅda* in MS. L. xi, p. 96. There, it is said that "Rāvana, king of Lankā, recounted it for the edification of his wife Maṇdodari, soon after her confinement." It begins and ends differently as follows :—

Beginning :—

औषधपतिनेत्राय पद्मिनीपतिमूर्त्तये ।
कालकालाय नीलाय पार्व्वतीपतये नमः ॥
गर्भभारपरिक्लान्ता कान्या मन्दोदरी शुभा ।
रावणं पारिप्रपच्छ पूजान्ते तुष्टमानसः ॥

End :—

एवमुक्त्वा तु भैषज्यरहस्यं स दशाननः ।
सायंसन्ध्याविधिं कर्त्तुमुत्थितो मन्दिरं ययौ ॥

Colophon :—

इति श्रीलङ्केश्वररावणकृतेऽर्कप्रकाशे धातुशुद्धिशतकं पूर्णं ।

The book treats of opium, and so cannot be very old. Mercury with Samkhadrāvaka is prescribed as the remedy for Phiraṅga-roga ; the term Yasada is used to indicate zinc. A tinned copper-vessel is recommended for the operation of distillation. The title of the book is the Saṅscritised form of the Persian Arrak (essence). So the probable age of the book is 16th century.

MSS : L. ii. 27, xi, p. 96.
Ul. 1614.
Weber., p. 291.
E. 409.

Editions :—

1. *Arka Prakāśa* by Rāvaṇa with a Bengali translation by Kavirāja Sures Chandra Gupta Śāstrī B. S. 1300, Calcutta.

III. *Nāḍī Parīkṣā* : Rāvaṇa is said to have written a treatise on Pulse. The book has been edited by Vināyaka Padmākara Jośī and published by Jādavji Tricumji Ācārya in the *Āyurvedīya Granthamālā* in 1912. The editor quotes a couplet from Janārdana, the author of *Sadvaidya Kaustubha* to show that Rāvaṇa was an authority on pulse :

नार्य्याः सव्यकरे परीक्षणविधिः पुंसः शये दक्षिणे
लङ्केशादिविपश्चितां मतमिदं लब्धं स्वभावादतेत् ॥ स० वै० कौ० १.१५

Rāvaṇa refers to authorities on the subject (पूर्वाचार्यैः सुभाषिता) and especially to Nandi (प्रोक्ता नन्दिना तत्त्ववेदिना). At the end of the book, the author, curiously enough, refers to the name of Rāma, his mortal foe, as the best medicine for patients in a moribund condition.

रामनामौषधं तत्र कारयेत्पारलौकिकम् ।

IV. *Uḍḍīśatantraṁ* : This medical work in ten chapters is also attributed to Rāvaṇa.

CHAPTER XII

ATRI.

Atri is one of the seven sages (*Saptarṣi*), the mind-born sons of Brahmā (mānasputra). Dowson, in his *Dictionary of Hindu Mythology*, p. 32, describes his life thus:

"Atri. 'An eater.' A Rishi, and author of many Vedic hymns. 'A Maharshi or great saint, who in the Vedas occurs especially in hymns composed for the praise of Agni, Indra, the Aswins, and the Viswa-devas. In the epic period, he is considered as one of the ten Prajāpatis or lords of creation engendered by Manu for the purpose of creating the universe; at a later period he appears as a mind-born son of Brahmā, and as one of the seven Rishis who preside over the reign of Swāyambhuva, the first Manu, or according to others, of Swarochisha, the second, or of Vaivaswata, the seventh. He married Anasūyā, daughter of Daksha, and their son was Durvāsas.' —*Goldstücker*. In the Rāmāyaṇa an account is given of the visit paid by Rāma and Sītā to Atri and Anasūyā in their hermitage south of Chitrakūṭa. In the Purāṇas he was also father of Soma, the moon, and the ascetic Dattātreya by his wife Anasūyā. As a Rishi he is one of the stars of the Great Bear."

His works:

1. *Atri Saṁhitā*: A treatise on medicine ascribed to Ṛṣi Atri is well-known in the Punjab and is said to be as old as the *Caraka Saṁhitā*.

2. *Atri Saṁhitā*: Atri is also a famous author of law book, *Atri Saṁhitā*.

ĀTREYA PUNARVASU.

Ātreya or the son of the sage Atri, is also called Punarvasu. We find three Ātreyas mentioned in the *Caraka Saṁhitā*—Ātreya Punarvasu, Kṛṣṇa Ātreya and Bhikṣu Ātreya. Punarvasu Ātreya is the speaker in the *Agniveśa Tantra* which was edited by Caraka.

Ātreya learned the science of medicine from Indra. He composed several works bearing his name, among which is the book called *Ātreya Saṁhitā*, in five parts, containing 46,500 verses in all. He is one of the oldest authorities on Hindu medicine, and several later writers have based their works on his treatise. His six disciples were Agniveśa, Bhela, Jatukarṇa, Parāśara, Kṣārapāṇi and Hārīta, all of whom distinguished themselves as authors of medical works. The *Agniveśa Tantra* as redacted by Caraka and Dṛḍhavala is the well-known *Caraka Saṁhitā*. The *Bhela Saṁhitā* is mentioned in the *Tanjore Catalogue*; it has been published by the University of Calcutta. The *Hārīta Saṁhitā* has also been printed. The works of Jatukarṇa, Parāśara and Ksārapāṇi are not available now.

Analysis of Ātreya Saṁhitā :

" Chapters 1 to 3 may be considered as a general introduction. Ch. 1 relates the meeting of Ātreya with some of his pupils on the northern face of the Himalaya. Hârîta, one of these pupils, asks questions on the origin and treatment of disease. Ātreya explains that the Āyurveda, meaning medical science, could not be fully communicated within the limits of human life, and that his pupils must therefore content themselves with a brief account of the smallest of his own compositions, which is composed within 1,500 slokas (or verses).

Chapter 2 shows the general division of his work into 6 books, and gives their names. In conclusion, it states the 8 constituent parts of the Āyur-Veda.

Chapter 3 classifies diseases, as: 1st, curable; 2nd, incurable; 3rd, curable by charms; 4th, scarcely possible to cure. This chapter also distinguishes the patients to whom physicians must attend, and on what terms, and signifies to what persons they must refuse assistance.

Ch. 4 treats on the physical influence of soil and season; on age and temper, and on the influence of the winds.

Ch. 5 enumerates the 6 tastes: as sweet, astringent, bitter, sour, salt, and pungent; and enumerates the influence of each on the human body.

Ch. 6 treats of the medical qualities of different kinds of water: as the water of the Ganges, which comes from heaven; water which comes from the sea; water which comes from clouds in general; and water which comes from thunder-clouds, snow, or ice.

This chapter concludes with prescriptions for the use of hot water or cold water in specified diseases.

Ch. 7 discusses the physical and medical properties of milks,—distinguishing the milk of kine, goats, ewes, buffaloes, camels, women. It states the cases in which the drinking of milk, of either kind, is beneficent; and concludes by discoursing on the medical properties of butter-milk.

Ch. 8 continues this subject.

Ch. 9 treats on the medicinal qualities of sugar-cane, and of preparations from it.

Ch. 10 on sour gruel.

Chs. 11 and 12 on infusions prepared from rice, barley, and other grains.

Ch. 13 on oils prepared from tila, flax, the castor-oil plant, and others.

Chs. 14, 15 and 16, also treat on the medical properties of rice, and various kinds of grain.

Ch. 17 discusses 4 kinds of pot-herbs, according to their leaves, flowers, fruits, and bulbous roots.

Ch. 18 is on sweet fruits,—as mangoes, rose-apples, pomegranates, myrobalans, citrons, grapes, and the fruits of carissa-coriander, and of the Mimusops Elengi.

Ch. 19 treats on 4 kinds of spirituous liquor as made from molasses, honey, meal and nogweed.

Ch. 20 describes animals, as hoofed or horned beasts of prey, birds, fishes, snakes living in the water or in arid tracts. Many species are given under each division, and the medical properties of their flesh are described.

Ch. 21 gives dietetical rules and prescriptions, and discusses the properties of food prepared from various combinations of the materials previously described.

The second main division of Ātreya's work, called Arishtaka consists of 8 Chapters.

Chapter 1 treats on the moral causes of disease. All diseases are said to spring from men's actions. All resemble hell, the curable as well as the incurable. And to some crimes fantastic punishments are assigned; as, if a man kills a Brâhman, he will be afflicted with jaundice; one who kills a king, with consumption.

Chapter 2 is on dreams

The subject of the 6 remaining chapters appears to be lucky and unlucky symptoms and forebodings.

The third division of this work is called Chikitsá, which means, we observed, medical treatment. This portion treats of diseases in detail. It appears to display much accurate observation, which can only be glanced at in these pages. Intermittent fevers are distinguished as of 4 kinds, returning at an interval of 1 day, 3 days, 4 days, or at some longer interval.

Much is said of diarrhœa, dysentery and allied diseases. Indigestion is described as flatulency, caused apparently by over-eating; and accompanied by sleeplessness, pains in the limbs, burning of the throat, etc. The 8th chapter is devoted to the sound and unsound condition of the digestive fire (Agni) of the stomach. The 10th treats of sharp pains, especially in the stomach, produced by excessive fatigue, night-walking, sorrow, cold food, etc.

The remaining chapters continue the subject of diseases, touching also on consumption and various kinds of hæmorrhage.

The last division treats of antidotes."

Mrs. Manning: *Ancient and Mediæval India, Vol. I*, pp. 340-42.

Books :—

1. *Ātreya Saṁhtiā*: In the *Hārīta Saṁhitā*, Ātreya is said to have written five treatises on medicine, for an account of which see Pseudo-Hārīta. A very old copy of the *Ātreya Saṁhitā* is mentioned in Dr. Bhāndārkar's *Second Report for the Search of Sanskrit Mss.*—p. 46. There is another Ms. noted in L. 2633 which resembles Ul. 1618.

Reference :—Muni Ātreya is quoted in Gada Nigraha Vol. I, pages 168.

आसवानां विकल्पसंस्कारगुणाः ।

विकल्पा बहुधा ज्ञेयाः संस्कारश्च यथाविधिः ॥ ३२ ॥

स्वयोनिसंस्कृता ह्येते स्वं स्वं कर्म प्रकुर्वते ।

संयोगसंस्कृतैर्देशकालमात्रस्वभावतः ॥ ३३ ॥

पृथक्तेषां स्वभावांस्तु ज्ञात्वा कार्यं प्रयोजयेत् ।

श्लोकद्वयमिदाय तु मुनिरात्रेय उक्तवान् ॥ ३४ ॥

Formulæ :		*Author*	*Books*	*Page*
1.	The Agni-clarified Butter	Ātreya	Bower Ms.	187.
2.	Rājavallabha Taila Ghṛtaṁ	„	V.M.	479.
3.	Ardhamātrika Vasti	„	„	575.
4.	Viṁśati Sārāsavā	„	G.N.,I.	167.
5.	Dādhika Ghṛta	„	„	197.
6.	Mahāmāyūra Ghṛta {	„	„	207.
		„	C.S.	570.
7.	Vṛhat Guḍucī Taila	„	A.R.	259.

1. Agni-clarified Butter.

अग्निघृतम् ।

* * * पाठानाम् तेजोवत्यास्तथैव च ।

पिप्पलीनाञ्च मूलस्य भागान् कुर्याच्चतुष्पलान् ॥ २५ ॥

* * * *

f * तायाः प्रवाड़ानाम् मालतीकरवीरयोः ॥ २६ ॥

त्वक्च सप्त पलाग्रस्य तथा श्राकोटक (स्य च ।

* * * *निधा) पचेत् ॥ २७ ॥

अग्निना चैव युक्तेन सम्यक्तु ब्रवीत साधनम् ।

चतुर्भागावशिष्टाम् तु चयेनमवतारयेत् ॥ २८ ॥

* * * म।

अथैदतिविषायास्तु तुल्या कटुकरोहिणी ॥ २९ ॥

पिप्पलीनाञ्च कुड़वम् विड़ङ्गानाम् तथैव च।

कु(टजस्य च) * * * ॥ ३० ॥

* * यवोयाच दद्यात् द्वे पले धृते।

क्षारस्य यावशूकस्य स्वर्ज्जिकायास्तथैव च ॥ ३१ ॥

अनेन च का * * * * ।

क्षाराभ्याम् लवणाभ्याञ्च पचेद्वैद्यो घृताढ़कम् ॥ ३२ ॥

कार्ष्णजीर्णे तु पातव्यो विष्टम्भेर * * ।

* * * सर्व्वे शाम्यन्ते देहिनाम् ॥ ३३ ॥

रक्तपित्ताश्रयाण्व्याधिल्गुमाम् येष पृथग्विधाम्।

* * * * * * ॥ ३४ ॥

स्निग्धं भुञ्जीत चात्यर्थं स्वादिष्मांसं,च पिवरम्।

अत्यग्निप्रतिघातार्थं कामच * * ॥ ३५ ॥

* * न्व्याधिग्निष्टन्यात्प्रकीर्त्तिताम्।

एतदग्निघृतं नामा आत्रेयविहितं पुरेति ॥ ३६ ॥

The Agni-clarified Butter of Ātrêya.

(25-36a). Take four pala each of—Pâṭhâ (*Stephanos hernandifolia*), Têjôvatî (*Piper Chaba*) and roots of long pepper, (26)......of coral. Mâlatî (*Jasminium grandiflorum*) and oleander, (27) and add seven *pala* of cinnamon-bark, Palâśa (*Butea frondosa*), Sâkôṭaka (*Trophis aspera*). ......(28) Now boil *the whole* thoroughly with the addition of some plumbago-root, and take it off *the fire* when it is reduced to one-fourth *of its original quantity*. (29) *Now throw in*......of Ativishâ (*Aconitum heterophyllum*), and an equal quantity of Kaṭukârôhinî (*Picrorrhiza Kurroa*), (30) also one kuḍava each of long pepper and baberang, and of Kuṭaja (*Holarrhena antidysenterica*)......(31) and add two pala each of...and...also of the carbonates of potash and soda. (32) With *the whole* of this...and with various kinds of alkaline ashes and salts, the physician should boil one aḍhaka of clarified butter. (33) At the time of digesting, one karsha of *this preparation* may be taken to relieve constipation and all...of mankind. (34) *It also relieves* disorders connected with hæmorrhagia, and the different kinds of abdominal tumours. The patient should partake of oleaginous substances in great abundance, and eat fat meat. (35) In cases of obstructed digestion *this preparation* is very desirable, it cures...well-known diseases. (36) It is called the Agni (or 'plumbago-root') clarified butter, and was devised by Âtrêya of old.

Bower Ms., Part III, p. 187.

2. Rājballabha Taila Ghṛta.

राजवल्लभं तैलं घृतम् ।

जीवकर्षभकमेदा द्राक्षांऽशुमती निदिग्धिका बृहती ॥
मधुकं बला विडङ्गं मञ्जिष्ठा शर्करा रास्ना ॥ २१३ ॥
नीलोत्पलं श्वदंष्ट्रा प्रपौण्डरीकं पुनर्नवा लवणम् ॥
पिप्पल्यः सर्वेषां भागैस्त्वांशकैः पिष्टैः ॥ २१४ ॥
तैलं वा यदि वा सर्पिर्दत्त्वा क्षीरं चतुर्गुणं पक्वम् ॥
आत्रेयनिर्मितमिदं तैलं नृपवल्लभं सिद्धम् ॥ २१५ ॥

तिमिरं पटलं काचं नक्तान्ध्यं चार्बुदं तथाऽन्यांश्च ॥
स्रेदं च लिङ्गनाशं नाशयति नीलिकाव्यङ्गम् ॥ २१६ ॥
मुखनासादौर्गन्ध्यं पलितं चाकालजं हनुस्तम्भम् ।
श्वासं कासं शोषं हिक्कां स्तम्भं तथाऽत्ययं नेत्रे ॥२१७ ॥
मुखजाड्यमर्धभेदं रोगं बाहुग्रहं शिरस्तम्भम् ॥
रोगानथोर्ध्वजत्रोः सर्वानचिरेण नाशयति ॥ २१८ ॥

3. Ardhamātrika Vasti.

अर्धमात्रिकं बस्तिम् ।

दशमूलीकषायेण शताह्वाद्यं प्रपेषयेत् ॥
तत्समं सैन्धवं दद्यान्मधुतैलं चतुष्पलम् ॥
मदनस्य फलं चैकं यथायोगेन दापयेत् ॥ १ ॥
आस्थापनप्रयोगेण भुक्त्वा बस्तिं विचक्षणः ॥
न चाभ्यङ्गो न च स्वेदः परिहारविधिर्न च ॥ २ ॥
आत्रेयस्यानुमतो ह्येष सर्वरोगनिबर्हणः ॥

यक्ष्मघ्नश्च कृमिघ्नश्च शूलघ्नश्च विशेषतः ॥ ३ ॥
शुक्रसंजननो ह्येष वातशोणितनाशनः ॥
बलवर्णकरो ह्येषोऽर्धमात्रिकसंज्ञितः ॥ ४ ॥

4. Vimśati Sārāsavā.

विंशतिः सारासवाः ।

शालप्रियङ्गुस्यन्दनचन्दनखदिरार्जुनैश्च कदरयुतैः ।
असनाश्वकर्णसप्तपर्णशमीशिंशिपासहितैः ॥ २७ ॥
अरिमेदतिन्दुकिंशुकशाकशिरीषैश्च वञ्जुलसमेतैः ।
धन्वनमधुकसारैर्विंशतिरात्रेयमुनिनोक्ताः ॥ २८ ॥

5. Dādhika Ghṛta.

दाधिकं घृतम् ।

द्वे पञ्चमूल्यौ सुषवी साश्वगन्धा पुनर्नवा ।
काला छिन्नरुहा चैव रास्ना गोक्षुरको बला ॥ ४ ॥
शठी पुष्करमूलं च देवदारुस्तथैव च ।
एषां द्विपलिकान् भागान् जलद्रोणे विपाचयेत् ॥ ५ ॥
कोलकानां कुलत्थानां माषाणां च यवैः सह ।
प्रस्थं प्रस्थं ततः कृत्वा तस्मिन्नेव समावपेत् ॥ ६ ॥

तेन पादावशेषेण घृतप्रस्थं विपाचयेत् ।
दद्यादेभिः समं शुक्तमारनालं तुषोदकम् ॥ ७ ॥
दाडिमाम्रातकरसं मातुलुङ्गरसं तथा ।
चतुर्गुणं चात्र दधि गर्भमेषां समावपेत् ॥ ८ ॥
पुनर्नवौषधं दन्ती चीव्येव लवणानि च ।
हिंस्रा रास्ना बला चैव यवानी चाम्लवेतसम् ॥ ९ ॥
विडङ्गं दाडिमं हिङ्गु ग्रन्थिकं विडता तथा ।
द्वौ क्षारावजमोदा च पाठा पाषाणभेदकम् ॥ १० ॥
ऊषकं वृषको भार्गी श्वदंष्ट्रा हपुषा तथा ।
त्रपुषैर्वारुबीजानि शतावर्युपकुञ्चिका ॥ ११ ॥
अजाजी चित्रकं मूर्वा तुम्बरु गजपिप्पली ।
धान्यकं सुरसं चैतान् दद्यादक्षसमान् भिषक् ॥ १२ ॥
गर्भेणानेन तत्सिद्धं पाययेत्सर्पिरुत्तमम् ।
पित्तगुल्मं तथा सर्वान् गुल्मानन्यान्व्यपोहति ॥ १३ ॥
एकाङ्गे पक्षवधे तथा दुष्टे च रेतसि ।
हृद्रोगे ग्रहणीरोगे सर्पिरेतद्यथामृतम् ॥ १४ ॥
यक्ष्माणं नाशयत्येतदपस्मारं च नाशयेत् ।
दाधिकं नाम विख्यातमात्रेयानुमतं शृतम् ॥ १५ ।

6. Mahāmāyūra Ghṛta.

महामायूरं घृतम् ।

एतेनैव कषायेण घृतप्रस्थं विपाचयेत् ।
चतुर्गुणेन पयसा कल्कैरेभिश्च कार्षिकैः ॥ १०३ ॥
जीवन्तीत्रिफलामेदामृद्वीकर्द्धिपरूषकैः
समङ्गाचविकाभार्गीकाश्मरीसुरदारुभिः ॥ १०४ ॥
आत्मगुप्तामहामेदातालखर्जूरमस्तकैः ।
मधुरःपिण्डखर्जूरशृङ्गीजीवकपद्मकैः ॥ १०५ ॥
शतावरीविदारीक्षुबृहतीसारिवायुतैः ।
पुनर्नवातुगाक्षीरीकाकोलीधन्वयासकैः ॥ १०६ ॥

मधुकाचोटवातामसुञ्जाताभिषुकैरपि ।
द्रव्यैरेभिर्यथालाभं घृतं मम्यग्विपाचयेत् ॥ १०७ ॥
तत्पक्वं नावनेऽभ्यङ्गे पाने बस्तौ च योजयेत् ।
शिरोरोगेषु सर्वेषु कासे श्वासे च दारुणे । १०८ ॥
मन्यापृष्ठग्रहे शोषे स्वरभेदे तथाऽर्दिते ।
योनिशुक्रप्रदोषेषु शस्तं वन्ध्यासुतप्रदम् ॥ १०९ ॥
ऋतुस्नाता तथा नारी पीत्वा पुत्रं प्रसूयते ।
महामायूरमित्येतद्घृतमात्रेयपूजितम् ॥ ११० ॥

7. Vṛhat Guḍucī Taila.

बृहद्गुडूची तैलं ।

शतं छिन्नरुहायाश्च जलद्रोणे विपाचयेत् ।
तेनपादावशेषेण तैलप्रस्थं विपाचयेत् ॥
क्षीरं चतुर्गुणं दद्यात् कल्कानेतान् प्रयत्नत ।
अश्वगन्धा विदारी च काकोलीहरिचन्दनम् ॥
शतावरी चातिवला श्वदंष्ट्राबृहतीद्वयम् ।
क्रिमिघ्नं त्रिफलारास्ना त्रायमाणा च शारिवा ॥
जीवन्तीग्रन्थिकं वोध्यं वागुजीभेकपर्निका ।
विशाला ग्रन्थिपर्णश्चमञ्जिष्टा चन्दनं निशा ॥
शताह्वसप्तपर्णौ च कार्षिकाण्यपकल्पयेत् ।
पानाभ्यञ्जननस्येषु वातरक्ते प्रयोजयेत् ॥
वातरक्तमुदावर्त्तं कुष्टान्यष्टादशैव तु ।
हनुस्तम्भं प्रमेहश्चकामलां पाण्डुतां जयेत् ॥
विस्फोटश्च विसर्पश्च नाडीव्रणभगन्दरम् ।
विचाचिकां गात्रकण्डूपाददाहं विशेषत: ॥
एतत्तैलवरं श्रेष्टं वलीपलित नाशनम् ।
आत्रेयनिर्म्मितं चैववलवर्णकरं स्मृतं ॥

KṚṢṆA ĀTREYA.

In the medical literature of the Hindus we find references to four different Ātreyas: Punarvasu Ātreya, Kṛṣṇa Ātreya, Dattātreya and Bhiksu Ātreya. In the *Caraka Saṁhitā* Punarvasu Ātreya appears to have taught the six disciples, Agniveśa and others ; and in that book, his name is always written as Punarvasu Ātreya and never as Kṛṣṇa Ātreya. Bhikṣu Ātreya is the reputed teacher of Jīvaka, the famous physician of Buddha. We find from quotations from Kṛṣṇa Ātreya that he belonged to the surgical school and could not have been the same as the Punarvasu Ātreya, the speaker in the Agniveśa Tantra. Śrīkaṇṭha Datta in commenting on Kavalādhikāra (Vṛnda's *Siddhayoga*) says :—

ननूच च तन्त्रान्तरीये: षड्विध: कदल: पठित:। तथा च कृष्णात्रेय:। &c. ; again शालाकिभिस्तु प्रतिदोषं पठितानि द्रव्यानि। तथा च कृष्णात्रेय: &c. (p. 600) and again in the Unmādādhikāra, षोड़शगुणं चाम्ब: कृष्णात्रेय परिभाषायां मन्तव्यं। (p. 191). From these quotations we learn that Kṛṣṇa Ātreya was a surgeon.

In the *Tattva Candrikā*, Śivadāsa while commenting on Daśamūlaśaṭpala ghṛta quoted from ज्वराधिकार of Cakradatta 'पञ्च प्रभृतिभ्य यत्नस्य' cites the names of Gopura Rakṣita, Jatukarṇa, Caraka, Suśruta and Kṛṣṇa Ātreya. This proves that Kṛṣṇa Atreya's work was quite different from that of Caraka.

But there is a difficulty to be solved. Dṛḍhavala mentions नागवाद्यचूर्णं in the treatment of Grahaṇī or Diarrhœa. This formula occurs also in *Cakaradatta* and *Siddhayoga*. Both Śrīkanṭha Datta and Śivadāsa, from whose comments we have tried to prove before that Krsna

Ātreya was a surgeon and was a different author from Punarvasu Ātreya, in commenting on the line "नागराद्यमिदं चूर्णं कृष्णात्रेयेन पूजितम्" distinctly states: "कृष्णात्रेयः पुनर्वसुः" "Kṛṣṇa Ātreyaḥ Punarvasuḥ." We cannot explain this identity satisfactorily. Kavirāja B. C. Gupta thinks that it is a mistake of the writers! Kavirāja Umes Chandra Gupta, the author of *Vaidyaka Śavda Sindhu*, however, makes Kṛṣṇa Ātreya the teacher of Agniveśa: अस्यां भगवान कृष्णात्रेयो वक्ता, अग्निवेश श्रोता, चरकमुनि -प्रतिसंस्कर्त्ता च। But Agniveśa was one of the six pupils of Punarvasu Ātreya.

Pandit Jogindranāth Sen Vaidyaratna in his highly meritorious commentary in Sanskrit '*Carakopaskāra*' on the *Caraka Saṁhitā* tries to tide over the difficulty by assuming the name of Atri to be Kṛṣṇa Atri. Thus he explains Ātreya in I. i, as आत्रेयः कृष्णात्रिपुत्र पुनर्वसुः। 'Ātreya, the son of Kṛṣṇa Atri.' This no doubt reconciles the conflicting statements of commentators but makes Kṛṣṇa Ātreya and Ātreya Punarvasu to be the same Ṛṣi. But this conclusion is open to objections. No where has he been so styled in the *Caraka saṁhitā*. He has been quoted as an authority in surgery. In *Cakradatta*, the formula Kuṭaja Puṭapāka is, however, attributed to Kṛṣṇātri-putra or 'son of Kṛṣṇa Atri.' Moreover the assumption that Kṛṣṇa Atri is the projenitor of the Ātreyas requires proof which is not forthcoming.

Ātreya Punarvasu has been identified by some with Bharadvāja, but Cakrapāṇi in his *Āyurvedadīpikā* distinctly states that that this theory of some commentators is untenable as Ātreya has never been styled Bharadvāja anywhere is the medical texts: अत्र केचिद्भरद्वाजात्रेययोरैक्यं वदन्ते। तन्न। भरद्वाजसंज्ञया आत्रेयस्य क्वचिदपि तन्त्रप्रदेशेऽकीर्त्तनात। p. 7, I. i. In the list of the sages who met to learn Āyurveda, Ātreya and Bharadvāja are seperately mentioned. This theory perhaps had its origin in the deversity of opinion as regards the relation of the two sages. In the *Caraka Saṁhitā* I. i., Bharadvāja, the desciple of Indra, is the teacher of Ātreya Punarvasu. Cakrapāṇi notes that Hārita was of the same opinion (हारीते आत्रेयादिगुरुतया भरद्वाजः उक्तः) Vāgbhaṭa on the other hand describes Ātreya as the desciple of Indra : सहस्राक्षं सोऽश्विपुत्रादिकान् मुनीन Bhāva Miśra describes both Ātreya (गतवानात्रेयस्त्रिदशालयम्) and Bharadvāja (भरद्वाजो मुनिश्रेष्ठो जगाम त्रिदशालयम्) as desciples of Indra.

Quotations from Kṛṣṇa Ātreya occur in the following books :—

Kṛṣṇa Ātreya in *Vyākhyā Kusumāvalī*—

1. द्रव्यमापोथितं क्वाथं दत्वा षोड़शिकं जलम् ।
   पादशिष्टः कषायः स्यादेष क्वाथविधिः स्मृतः ॥ p. 145, 191.
2. नतकुष्ठ स्रावयतो धूमवर्तिंप्रयोजिते ।
   मस्तुलुङ्गं प्रभावेन तस्मात्ते न प्रयोजयेत् ॥ p. 586.
3. मनु च तन्त्रान्तरीयैः षड़्विधः कवलः पठितः । तथा च कृष्णात्रेयः । तत्र कवलग्रहः स्नैहिको रोपणीयो वैरेचनः स्तम्भनः शोधनो निर्वापनश्च । p. 600.
4. शालाकिभिस्तु प्रतिदोषं पठितानि द्रव्याणि । तथा च कृष्णात्रेयः । अथ द्रव्यप्रविभाग एष वातघ्नैर्भेषजैः सिद्धः स्नेहः क्षीरं वलीसु(ऽनु)र्णां क्षीरं चाम्ललवणौ वाते पटोलमधूकशर्करानीलोत्पलक्षीरेक्षुरसशर्करोदकघृतादीनि पैत्तिके त्रिकटुसर्षपसैन्धवतैलयुक्तं किराततिक्तकतेजोवतीहरिद्रागोमूत्रलवणोष्णोदकानि श्लेष्मिके । एतान्येवोत्कर्षापकर्षतः संसर्गे संनिपाते वा कवलग्रह इति ॥
   p. 600-1.
5, कवलग्रहादिषु च विशेषः कृष्णात्रेयेण दर्शितस्तथा:—
   सप्तवर्षमुपदाय नस्त(स्य) कर्म चतुर्विधम् ॥
   प्रतिमर्शोऽथ वमनं जन्मप्रभृति शस्यते ॥
   धूमो द्वादशवर्षस्य कवलः पञ्चमे ततः ॥
   दोषव्याधिवलावस्थां वीक्ष्य चैतान्प्रयोजयेत् ॥ p. 602.

Kṛṣṇa Ātreya in *Nivandha Saṁgraha*—

1. सप्तवर्षमुपादेयं नस्यकर्म चतुर्विधम् ।
   प्रतिमर्शश्च वमनं गुल्म प्रभृति शस्यते ॥ p. 1202

Kṛṣṇa Ātreya in *Sarvāṅga Sundarī*—

1. निष्पावा मधुरा रूक्षाः सकषाया विदाहिनः ।
   उदावर्त्ते प्रशस्यन्ते गुरवो वातपित्तलाः ॥ I. p. 128

Kṛṣṇa Ātıeya in *Tattva Candrikā*—

1. स्नेहपाकविधौ यत्र प्रमाणं नोदितं क्वचित् ।
स्नेहस्य कुडवं तत्र पचेत् कल्कपलेन तु ॥ p. 30.

2. See 1. V.K.V.
3. See 1. Ni. S.

Formulae attributed to Kṛṣṇa Ātreya :

Name.		*Author.*	*Book.*	*Page.*
1. Kuṭaja Puṭapāka		Kṛṣna Ātreya	V K.V. C.D.	77. 43.
2. Nāgarādya cūrṇa		,,	V.K.V. C.D. A.R.	84. 47. 52.
3. Vijaya cūrṇa		,,	C.D. A.R.	60. 72.
4. Śatāvarī oil		,,	Sa.S.	174.
5. Caturmukha		,,	R.C. ix, A.R.	64. 251-2.
6. Kaduka	ghṛta	,,	G.N.,I.	4.
7. Mahāygouıādya	,,	,,	,,	12.
8. Rohitaka	,,	,,	,,	18.
9. Gauryādya	,,	,,	,,	19.
10. Vindu	,,	,,	,,	22.
11. Mahāvindu	,,	,,	,,	,,
12. Abhayādya Vaṭaka		,,	,,	122.
13. Aṣṭacatvāriṁśa guggula			,,	136.
14. Guḍa Kuṣmāṇḍa		,, Aśvins	,,	141.
15. Khadirāsava		,,	,,	175.
16. Dvātriṁśaka Kvātha or Rāsnādi Kvātha		,,	G.N.II.	224.
17. Candanādya powder		,,	H.S.	232.
18. Nārāyana oil		,,	,,	244.
19. Oil for diseases of head		,,	C.S., vı (Gaṅgādhara)	596.
20. Jogendra Rasa		,,	A.R.	252.

1. Kūṭaja Puṭapāka.

कूटजपुटपाकः ।

स्निग्धं घनं कुटजवल्कमजन्तुजग्ध-
मादाय तत्क्षणमतीव च पोथयित्वा ।
जम्बुपलाशपुटतण्डुलतोयसिक्तं
बद्धं कुशेन च बहिर्घनपङ्कलिप्तम् ॥
सुस्विन्नमेतदवपीड्य रसं गृहीत्वा
क्षौद्रेण युक्तमतिसारवते प्रदद्यात् ।
कृष्णात्रिपुत्रमतपूजित एष योगः
सर्व्वातिसारहरणे स्वयमेव राजा ॥

स्वरसस्य गुरुत्वेन पुटपाकपलं पिबेत् ।
पुटपाकस्य पाकोऽयं बहिरारक्तवर्णता ॥

2. Nāgarādya Cūrṇa.

नागराद्यं चूर्णम् ।

नागरातिविषामुस्तं धातकीं सरसाञ्जनाम् ।
वत्सकत्वक्फलं बिल्वं पाठां कटुकरोहिणीम् ॥
पिबेत् समांशं तच्चूर्णं सक्षौद्रं तण्डुलाम्बुना ।
पैत्तिके ग्रहणीदोषे रक्तं यश्चोपवेश्यते ॥
अर्शांस्यथ गुदे शूलं जयेच्चैव प्रवाहिकाम् ।
नागराद्यमिदं चूर्णं कृष्णात्रेयेण पूजितम् ॥

शीतकषायमानेन तण्डुलोदककल्पना ।
केऽप्यष्टगुणतोयेन प्राहुस्तण्डुलभावनाम् ॥

3. Vijaya Curṇa.

विजयचूर्णम् ।

त्रिकत्रयवचाहिङ्गुपाठाक्षारनिशाद्वयम् ।
चव्यतिक्ताकलिङ्गाग्नि-शताह्वालवणानि च ॥
ग्रन्थिबिल्वाजमोदा च गणोऽष्टाविंशतिर्मतः ।
एतानि समभागानि श्लक्ष्णचूर्णानि कारयेत् ॥

ततो विड़ालपदकं पिबेदुष्णेन वारिणा ।
एरण्डतैलयुक्तन्तु सदा लिह्यात् ततो नरः ॥
कासं हन्यात् तथा शोथमर्शांसि च भगन्दरम् ।
हृच्छूलं पार्श्वशूलञ्च वातगुल्मं तथोदरम् ॥
हिक्काश्वासप्रमेहांश्च कामलां पाण्डुरोगताम् ।
आमान्वयमुदावर्त्तमन्त्रवृद्धिं गुदं क्रिमीन् ॥
अन्ये च ग्रहणीदोषो ये मया परिकीर्त्तिताः ॥
महाज्वरोपसृष्टानां भूतोपहतचेतसाम् ।
अप्रजानान्तु नारीणां प्रजावर्द्धनमेव च ।
विजयो नाम चूर्णोऽयं कृष्णात्रेयेण पूजितः ॥

---

4. Śatāvarī Taila.

शतावरीतैलम् ।

शतावरी बलायुग्मं पर्ण्यौ गन्धर्व्वहस्तकः ।
अश्वगन्धा श्वदंष्ट्रा च विल्वः काशः कुरण्टकः ॥
एषां सार्द्धपलान् भागान् कल्पयेच्च विपाचयेत् ।
चतुर्गुणेन नीरेण पादशेषं शृतं नयेत् ॥
नियोज्य प्रस्थतैलेन क्षीरप्रस्थं विनिर्क्षिपेत् ।
शतावरीरसप्रस्थं जलप्रस्थञ्च योजयेत् ॥
शतावरीदेवदारुमांसीतगरचन्दनम् ।
शतपुष्पाबलाकुष्ठमेलाशैलेयमुत्पलम् ॥
ऋद्धिर्मेदा च मधुकं काकोली जीवकस्तथा ।
एषां कर्षसमैः कल्कैस्तैलं गोमयवह्निना ॥
पचदनेन सिद्धतैलेन नरः स्त्रीषु वृषायते ।
नारी च लभते पुत्रं योनिशूलञ्च नश्यति ॥
अङ्गशूलं शिरःशूलं कामलां पाण्डुतां तथा ।
गृध्रसीं प्लीहशोषञ्च मेहान् दण्डापतानकम् ॥
सदाहं वातरक्तञ्च वातपित्तगदार्द्दितम् ।
असृग्दरं तथाध्मानं रक्तपित्तं नियच्छति
शतावरीतैलमिदं कृष्णात्रेयेन भाषितम् ॥

---

5. Catūrmmukha.

चतुर्म्मुखः।

रसगन्धकलौहाभ्रं समं सूताद्धि हेम च।
सर्व्वं खल्लतले क्षिप्ता कन्यारसविमर्द्दितम्।
एरण्डपत्रैरावेष्ट्य धान्यराशौ दिनत्रयम्।
संस्थाप्य च तदोद्धृत्य सर्व्वरोगेषु योजयेत्।
एतद्रसायनवरं त्रिफलामधुसंयुतम्।
क्षयमेकादशविधं पाण्डुरोगान् प्रमेहकान्।
शूलं श्वासञ्च हिक्काञ्च मन्दाग्निं चाम्लपित्तकम्।
व्रणान् सर्व्वानामवातं विसर्पं विद्रधिं तथा।
अपस्मारं महोन्मादं सर्व्वार्शांसि त्वगामयान्।
क्रमेण शीलितं हन्ति वृक्षमिन्द्राशनि र्यथा।
पौष्टिकं बल्यमायुष्यं पुत्रप्रसवकारणम्।
चतुर्मुखेन देवेन कृष्णात्रेयस्य सूचितम्॥

6. Kaṭūka Ghṛta.

हारीतात्कटुकं घृतम्।

त्रिफलां पञ्चमूल्यौ द्वे कुलत्थान् बदरान् यवान्॥
द्विपलिकान् जलद्रोणे त्वष्टभागावशेषितम्।
निःस्राव्य विपचेत्कल्क दत्वा प्रस्थं च सर्पिषः॥
पिप्पली पिप्पलीमूलं चव्यचित्रकनागरम्।
पुष्करातिविषे भार्गी शठी सप्तच्छदं वचा॥
रजन्यौ नक्तमालं च पाठे द्वे शिग्रुतुम्बरु।
सोमवल्कोऽर्कमूलानि मदनं कटुरोहिणी॥
तेजस्विनी सगोजिह्वा चन्दनं कण्टकारिका।
किराततिक्तकं मुस्तं पटोलं सदुरालभम्॥
वयस्थां पिचुमन्दं च कटुकं हिङ्गुना सह।
एतानक्षसमान् दत्वा चारौ च्चार्धपलोन्मितौ॥
लवणानां च पञ्चानां कर्षं कर्षं प्रदापयेत्।
सिद्धं तन्मात्रया पीतं सर्वजीर्णज्वरापहम्॥

हृत्प्लीहग्रहणीदोषश्वासकासार्शसां हितम् ।
गुल्मघ्नं कटुकं नाम कृष्णात्रेयेण पूजितम् ॥

दीर्घकालप्रयुक्तानां ज्वराणाममृतोपमम् ।

7. Mahāgouryādya Ghṛta.

कृष्णात्रेयाद्युक्ते महागौर्याद्यं घृतम् ।

गौरी हरिद्रा मञ्जिष्ठा मांसी कटुकरोहिणी ॥
प्रपौण्डरीकं मधुकं भद्रमुस्तं सचन्दनम् ।
जातीनिम्बपटोलं च कारञ्जं बीजमेव च ॥
कटुफलं समधूच्छिष्टं समभागानि कारयेत् ।
पञ्चवल्ककषायेण घृतप्रस्थं विपाचयेत् ॥
क्षीरद्विप्रस्थसंयुक्तं शनैर्मृद्वग्निना पचेत् ।
एतद्गौरं महावीर्यं सर्वव्रणविशोधनम् ॥
आगन्तुसहजा श्चिष्टाश्च ये व्रणाः ।
विषमामपि न हयेच्छीघ्रमेव च ॥

8. Rohītaka Ghṛta.

कृष्णात्रेयात् प्रोक्तं रोहीतकं घृतम् ।

रोहीतकात् पलशतं संक्षुद्य मदराढके ।
पाचयित्वा जलद्रोणे चतुर्भागावशेषिते ॥
घृतप्रस्थं समावाप्य छागं क्षीरं चतुर्गुणम् ।
तस्मिन् द्रव्यानिमांश्चैव सर्वान् कर्षसमन्वितान् ॥
व्योषं फलत्रयं हिङ्गु यवानीं तुम्बुरुं बिडम् ।
अजाजीकुष्ठलवणं दाडिमं देवदारु च ॥
पुनर्नवां विशालां च यवक्षारं सपुष्करम् ।
विडङ्गं चित्रकं चैव हपुषां चविकां वचाम् ॥
एभिर्द्रव्यैर्घृतप्रस्थं स्थापयेद्भाजने शुभे ।
पाययेच्च पलं मात्रां व्याधीन् शमयते हठात् ॥
प्लीहं प्लीहोदरं चैव प्लीहशूलं तथैव च ।
हृच्छूलं पार्श्वशूलं च कुक्षिशूलमरोचकम् ॥

विबन्धशूलं शमयेत् पाण्डुरोगं सकामलम्।
हृद्यं तीसारशूलघ्नं तन्द्राज्वरविनाशनम्॥
रोहीतघृतं ह्येतत् प्लीहानं शमयेतद्द्रुतम्।

9. Gauryādya Ghṛta.

कृष्णात्रेयाद्गुणे गौर्याद्यं घृतम्।

गौर्यारिष्टपटोलरोध्रफलिनीयष्ट्याह्वनीलोत्पलै-
र्मञ्जिष्ठाकटुकेन्द्रवारुणिजपामूर्वानिशाचन्दनैः।
जातीचीरकपद्मकेशरदलैः पूतीकचोटाफलै-
स्तुल्यैः सिक्थकसारिवाद्वययुतैर्गव्यं घृतं पाचयेत्॥
यष्टिचीरसपञ्चकोलजलदक्वाथैश्च गौर्यादिभिः
सिद्धं सर्पिरिदं हितं विषु भवेत्सद्यःचतेषु ध्रुवम्।
ये गूढाश्चिरकालजातगतयः प्रोच्छिन्नमांसा व्रणा
सस्रावाः सरुजः सदाहपिडिकाः शुष्यन्ति रोहन्ति च॥

10. Vindu Ghṛta.

कृष्णात्रेयाद्बिन्दुघृतम्।

त्रिवृता त्रिफला पाठा दन्ती कटुकरोहिणी॥
चतुरङ्गुलमज्जा च तथा च कटुकत्रयम्।
चित्रकं च बृहत्यौ च तथा च गजपिप्पली॥
स्नुहीचीरपलं दद्यात् घृतस्याष्टौ प्रदापयेत्।
यावन्तः स पिबेद्बिन्दून् तावद्वेगान् विरिच्यते॥
एतद्बिन्दुघृतं सिद्धमृषिभिः परिकीर्तितम्।

11. Mahāvindu Ghṛta.

कृष्णात्रेयाद्गुणे महाबिन्दुघृतम्।

स्नुहीचीरपले द्वे च प्रस्थार्धं चैव सर्पिषः॥
कम्पिल्लकपलं चैव शाणार्धं सैन्धवस्य च।
त्रिवृतायाः पलं चैव कुडवं धात्रिजाद्रसात्॥
तोयप्रस्थेन संयुक्तं शनैर्मृद्वग्निना पचेत्।
वर्षप्रमाणं दातव्यं जठरे शैलगुल्मयोः॥

तथा कर्णोत्थरोगेषु युञ्जीत कुशलो भिषक् ।
एतद्ध्याद्विनिचयान्समूलान् सपरिग्रहान् ॥
निहन्त्येष प्रयोगो हि वायुर्जलधरानिव ।
पञ्चगुल्मवधार्थाय सर्पिरेतत् प्रकीर्तितम् ॥
सर्वासुरवधार्थाय यथा वज्रं बिडौजसा ।
महाबिन्दुघृतं सिद्धं सर्वोदरहरं परम् ॥

---

12. Abhayādya Vaṭaka.

गुल्मेऽभयाद्या वटकाः ।

हरीतकीनां द्विपलं ग्रन्थिकं वेतसं तथा ।
पलाध चार्धकर्षांशा व्योषञ्चाम्लवाष्पिकाः ॥
यवानी चाजमोदा च कारवीशठिपौष्करम् ।
चव्यसौवर्चलबिडं हपुषाजाजिधान्यकम् ॥
कोलाम्लं दाडिमं चेति चातुर्जातं च कार्षिकम् ।
चूर्णं गुडद्विगुणितं कृत्वा तु वटकान्भजेत् ॥
गुल्मानाहोदरप्लीहपाण्डुर्शोग्रहणीगदान् ।
कासातीसारपार्श्वार्तिश्वासरोगं च कामलाम् ॥
मदात्ययवमीमेहहिक्कापीनसपित्तजान् ।
शूलं ज्वरं च शमयेदग्निदीप्तिकराः परम् ॥
कृष्णाविस्मृतियुक्तास्तु नित्यं जीवेत्समा शतम् ।

---

13. Aṣṭacatvāriṁśa Guggulu Guṭikā.

गरुडमालायामष्टाचत्वारिंशत्संज्ञा गुग्गुलुगुटिका ।

त्रिकटुत्रिफलामुस्तं कुटजं गजपिप्पलीम् ।
त्वगेलापत्रहपुषाग्रन्थिकं जीरकद्वयम् ॥
विडङ्गं चित्रकं पाठां त्रायमाणां दुरालभाम् ।
पटोलेन्द्रयवान् दारु पञ्चैव लवणानि च ॥
यवानीं बाष्पिकां भार्गीं हरिद्रे सारिवाद्वयम् ।
दाडिमं पौष्करं धान्यं वचां चारद्वयं तथा ॥

पिप्पलीं चाजमोदं च तिन्तिडीकाम्लवेतसम् ।
तुम्बुरूणि च सर्वाणि कार्षिकाण्युपकल्पयेत् ॥

सूक्ष्मचूर्णीकृतेष्वेषु पलानि दश पञ्च च ।
महिषाक्षस्य मतिमान् तत्पादेन च माक्षिकम् ॥

अष्टचत्वारिंशत्संज्ञः कृष्णात्रेयेण भाषितः ।

गण्डमालापचीग्रन्थिमूकसुप्तिश्च गद्गदान् ॥

क्षयाढ्यवातशोफांश्च मन्यास्तम्भं तथार्दितम् ।
अर्शांसि च प्रमेहांश्च स्थौल्यदोषगुदामयान् ॥

अर्बुदं घ्राणरोगं च बाधिर्यं गृध्रसीं तथा ।
पूतिनासं प्रतिश्यायां पिटकं चलविद्रधम् ॥
सोदरामन्त्रवृद्धिं च जयेदग्निं च दीपयेत् ॥

14. Guḍa Kuṣmāṇḍakāvaleha.

गुडकूष्माण्डकावलेहः ।

कूष्माण्डकात्पलशतं सुखिन्नं निष्कुलीकृतम् ।
प्रस्थं तैलघृताद्देयं तस्मिंस्तप्ते प्रदापयेत् ॥

त्वक्पत्रधान्यकं व्योषं जीरकैलाद्वयानलम् ।
ग्रन्थिकं चव्यमातङ्गपिप्पलीशृङ्गवेरकम् ॥

शृङ्गाटकं कसेरुं च पेलवं तालमस्तकम् ।
चूर्णीकृत्य पलांशेन गुडस्य तुलया पचेत् ॥

शीतीभूते पलान्यष्टौ मधुनः संप्रदापयेत् ।
कफपित्तानिलहरं मन्दाग्नीनां च दीपनम् ॥

कृशानां बृंहणं श्रेष्ठं वाजीकरणमुत्तमम् ।
प्रमदासु प्रसक्तानां ये चान्ये क्षीणरेतसः ॥

क्षयेणैव गृहीतानां परमुक्तं भिषग्जितम् ।
कासं श्वासं ज्वरं हिक्कां हन्ति छर्दिमरोचकम् ॥
गुडकूष्माण्डकं ख्यातं कृष्णात्रेयेण पूजितम् ।

---

15. Khadirāsava.

कुष्ठे खदिरासवः।

खदिरस्य तुलार्धं तु तत्तुल्यं देवदार्वपि ॥
वराया विंशतिर्दार्व्याः पलानां पञ्चविंशतिः ।
बाकुच्या द्वादशपलान्यष्टद्रोणेऽम्भसः पचेत् ॥
द्रोणशेषे कषाये तु पूते शीते विनिक्षिपेत् ।
धातक्या विंशतिपलं माक्षिकस्य शतद्वयम् ॥
शर्करायास्तुलामेकां चूर्णानीमानि दापयेत् ।
कङ्कोलकं लवङ्गं च एला जातीफलं त्वचम् ॥
केसरं मरिचं पत्रं पलिकान्युपकल्पयेत् ॥
पिप्पलीनां तु कुडवं स्थापयेद्घृतभाजने ॥
मासार्धं पिबेन्मात्रामपेक्ष्याग्निबलाबलम् ।
सर्वकुष्ठहरो ह्येष पाण्डुहृद्रोगकासनुत् ॥
कृमिग्रन्थ्यर्बुदग्रन्थिगुल्मप्लीहोदरान्तकृत् ।
एष वै खदिरारिष्टः कृष्णात्रेयेण पूजितः ॥

---

16. Dvātriṁśaka Kvātha
Rāsnādi Kvatha.

सर्ववातरोगे रास्नादिक्वाथः।

रास्ना गुडूची देवाह्वमेरण्डमभया शठी ।
बला चारग्वधः शुण्ठी शतपुष्पा पुनर्नवा ॥
पञ्चमूली विषा मुस्ती सैरेयकदुरालभे ।
यवानी पौष्करं मूलं वाजिगन्धा प्रसारणी ॥
गोक्षुरश्चाटरूषश्च हपुषा वृद्धदारुकम् ।
शतावरी समङ्गा च गुग्गुलुर्गिरिजं तथा ॥
समभागैरिमैः सर्वैः कषायमुपकल्पयेत् ।
पिबेत्सर्वाङ्गगे वाते सामे सन्ध्यस्थिमज्जगे ॥
वातरोगेषु सर्वेषु कम्पे शोफेऽपतानके ।
मन्यास्तम्भे च हृद्रोगे पक्षाघातेऽपतन्त्रके ॥

अर्दितापेक्षके कुब्जे हनुग्रहशिरोग्रहे ।
गृध्रस्यां जानुरोगे च गुल्मे शूले कटिग्रहे ॥
सामे चैव निरामे च सप्तधातुगतेऽनिले ।
आवृतेऽनावृते चैव वातरक्ते विशेषतः ।
एष द्वाविंशकः क्वाथः कृष्णात्रेयेण पूजितः ॥

17. Candananda Cūrṇa.
चन्दनाद्य चूर्णं ।

चन्दनं तगरं कुष्ठं शटीत्रिगन्धवासकं ।
मञ्जीष्ठाभीरुमृद्वीकापाठाश्यामाप्रियङ्गुभिः ।
स्वयंगुप्ता पीलुपर्णी विषा रास्ना मदादनी ।
काकोल्यौ जीवकं मेदे पुष्करं घनवालुकं ।
विदारी चैव वासन्ती च उडं दन्ती विडङ्गकं ।
पद्मकश्चैन्द्रवचश्च तथाऽम्लतचित्रकं ।
धान्यकं पञ्चजीरेण तथा तालीशपत्रकं ।
खादिरं तगरञ्चैव कालीयकञ्च कैकतं ।
नागकेशरकञ्चैव पद्मवञ्च समांशिकं ।
सखर्ज्जुरं भिषक् सम्यक् सर्व्वमेकत्र भर्द्दयेत् ।
भावितं पुनरेवञ्च मधुना सघृतेन च ।
लेह्योऽयञ्च सदा मलश्चापस्मारेऽतिदारुणे ।
उन्मादे कामलारोगे पाण्डुरोगे हलीमके
राजयक्ष्मे रक्तपित्ते पित्तातिसारपीड़िते ।
रक्तातिसारे शोषे च शिरोरोगे सदाज्वरे ।
तमकभ्रमके च्छर्द्दिदाहे च समदात्यये ।
अश्मर्य्याञ्च प्रमेहेषु कासे श्वासे च पीनसे ।
एतेषाञ्च प्रयोक्तव्यो सर्व्वरोगनिवारणः ।
वन्ध्यानाञ्च प्रयोक्तव्यो वृद्धानाञ्च विशेषतः ।
बालानाञ्च हितश्चैव प्रणु चास्य प्रमाणकं ।
उत्तमे चोरमात्रञ्च पादहीनन्तु मध्यमे ।
दद्यात् चीरयुतं स्त्रीणां वाल नाचीरसंयुतं ।

एवं प्रयोजितो रोगी महाकल्को मतो बुधैः ।
बलवान् गुणवांश्चैव भवतीह फलप्रदः ।
वरकुञ्जरवाहानामुपयुक्तो हितो मतः ।
भिषग्भिः कथ्यते चेह कृष्णात्रेयेण पूजितः ।

इति चन्दनाद्यं चूर्णं ।

18. Nārāyaṇa Taila.

नारायणं तैलम् ।

सपित्तानिलश्वासः पक्वामः पतति लघः ।
न वस्तिशूलो भवति वामवाते भ्रमः क्लमः ।
आमपाकोऽग्नि विज्ञेयो न कुर्य्यात् तस्य पाचनम् ।
विरेचनं न कर्त्तव्यं स्तम्भनं तस्य कारयेत् ।
कटिपृष्ठे वक्षोदेशे तोदनं वस्तिशूलता ।
गुल्मवज्जठरं गर्ज्जेत् तथान्ते शोफमेव च ।
शिरोगुरुत्वं भवति वामि च पतते भ्रमम् ।
सर्व्वाङ्गगो भवेत् सोऽपि विज्ञेयः सुविजानता ।
तस्य वै पाचनं कुर्य्याद्विरेचनमतः परम् ।
विष्टम्भो गुल्मपाको च सर्व्वाङ्गगोऽन्यः कीर्त्तितः ।
विज्ञेयस्तत्र यः साध्यस्तान्यौ द्वौ कष्टसाध्यकौ ।
स्नेहो चामय कथितः कल्पाप्यआरनिग्रहम् ।
श्योणाकः पाटला विल्वं तर्क्कारी पारिभद्रकः ।
अश्वगन्धा कण्टकारी शोथघ्नी च प्रसारिणी ।
श्वदंष्ट्रा च वला चैवातिबला समभागिका ।
पादशेषं जलद्रोणे क्वथितं स्रावयेत्ततः ।
वक्ष्यमाणानि योज्यानि भेषजानि भिषग्वरैः ।
शतपुष्पा वचा मांसी दारु शैलेयकं वरा ।
पतङ्गं चन्दनं कुष्ठं तथान्यं रक्तचन्दनम् ।
करञ्जबीजांशुमती विसुगन्धि पुनर्नवा ।
रास्ना तुरङ्गगन्धा च सैन्धवं च दुरालभा ।
मिश्री च सुरसा चैतत् प्रत्येकन्तु पलद्वयम् ।

चूर्ण कृत्वा क्षिपेत् तत्र क्षिपेल्लाक्षारसाढ़कम्।
शतावरीरसं चैव अजाक्षीरं चतुर्गुणम्।
दधि तक्राढ़कं गव्यं तिलतैलं प्रयोजयेत्।
सिद्धं तत्र प्रदृश्येत ततो मङ्गलवाचनम्।
प्रतिच्छेनं प्रतिष्ठाप्य नारायणमिदं स्मृतम्।

हन्ति वातविकारांश्च अपस्मारग्रहांस्तथा।
शिरोरोगान् कर्णरोगान् कुष्ठान्यष्टादशान्यपि।
वन्ध्या च लभते पुत्रं षण्डोऽपि पुरुषायते।
क्रशो युवायते मूर्खो विद्याराधनतत्पर:।
नारायणमिदं तैलं कृष्णात्रेयेण भावितम्।

इति नारायणं नाम तैलम्।

19. Mahāmayūra Ghṛta.

महामायूर घृतम्।

See pages 438-39.

20. Jogendra Rasa.

योगेन्द्ररस:।

विशुद्धंरससिन्दुरं तदर्द्धं शुद्धहाटकम्।
तत्समंकान्तलौहञ्च तत्समं चाभ्रमेवच॥
विशुद्धं मौक्तिकञ्चैव वङ्गञ्चतत्समंमतम्।
कुमारिका रसैर्भाव्यं धान्यराशौदिनत्रयम्॥
तयोरक्तिद्वयमितांवटीं कुर्य्याद्विचक्षण:।
योगवाहीरसोह्येष सर्व्वरोग कुलान्तक:॥
वातपित्तभवान रोगान् प्रमेहान् वहुमूत्रताम्।
मूत्राघात सपस्मारं भगन्दर गुदामयम्।
उन्मादमूर्च्छां यक्ष्माणं पक्षाघातं हतेन्द्रियम्।
शूलाम्लपित्तकं हन्तिभास्करस्तिमिरं यथा॥
त्रिफलारसयोगेन शुभय शीतयापि वा।
भक्षयित्वाभवेद्रोगी कामरूपी सुदर्शन:॥
रात्रौसेव्यं गवां क्षीरं कृशाणाञ्च विशेषत:।
योगेन्द्राख्योरसोनाम्ना कृष्णात्रेय विनिर्म्मितम्॥

DATTĀTREYA.

Dattātreya was the son of Maharṣi Atri and Anasūyā. It is said that he was an incarnation of Viṣṇu. He taught Prahlāda, the pious dānava prince, the science of Ātma Vidyā or knowledge of soul. He had three sons, Nimi, Somadatta and Durvāsā. He favoured Kārtavīrya with a thousand hands.

His works: *Nāḍītatvavidhi*—

Mss: G.O.M.L. No. 13158. Vol. xxiii.

दत्तात्रेय मतम् अन्ध्रटीका सहितम :—A treatise dealing with the symptoms, diagnosis and treatment of diseases and also the preparation of various medicines, etc., according to Dattātreya with Telugu meaning :

Beginning :

नारायणं गुणवासं वन्दे षटत्रिंशकं विभुम् ।
नरं च जन्तुस्थानां तदांशं पञ्चविंशकम् ॥
नाडीनां लक्षणं वक्ष्ये दत्तात्रेयमतानुगम् ।
यदभ्यासं न जनाति चिरं प्राणगतिं सुधी: ।
पञ्चभूतात्मको देहस्त्रिदोषश्च सप्तधातुक: ।
त्रिगुणोऽनेकविकृतिरनेकमलसञ्चय: ॥

* * * *

स्पर्शनात् पीडनात् घातात् खेदनान्मर्दनादपि ।
तासु(च) प्राणसञ्चोरं प्रयत्नेन विशोधयेत् ॥
विज्ञेयनाडिका वक्ष्य सामान्येन मतक्रमात् ।
पादयोर्हस्तयो: कण्ठमूलयोर्घ्राणमूलयो: ॥
पादयोर्नाडिकास्थानात् गुल्फस्य द्व्यङ्गुलित्रयम् ॥

* * * *

Colophon

इति नाडीतत्त्वविधौ दत्तात्रेयमते प्रथमोऽध्याय: ॥

End :

आढकं यूषपक्व(क्कं) च ताम्बूलं सेवितं नरः।
स्त्रीणां च रोगसंहारं नानारोगहरं परम् ॥
सूतसूतं देवदारु त्रिकटुश्चेन्द्रवारुणी।
शर्करासहितं खादेच्छासकासहरं परम् ॥

* * * *

देवदानवगन्धर्वयक्षराक्षसपन्नगाः।
पिशाचादितरं चेति भूतग्रहगणोऽष्टधा ॥

MS: G.O.M.L. Vol. xiii. 6400-6411, 14548 = दत्तात्रेयवज्रकवच etc.

There are numerous charms, hymns and stotras addressed to Dattātreya to destroy one's enemies, to make one wise, etc.

HIRAṆYĀKṢA.

He is referred to in the *Caraka Saṁhitā* I. xxv. as having refuted the arguments of Vāryovid on the origin of diseases. He says that men and diseases owe their origin to the five elements, and cites the opinion of the Sāṁkhya philosophers in support of his arguments:

हिरण्याक्षस्तु नेत्याह न ह्यात्मा रसजः स्मृतः।
नातीन्द्रियं मनः सन्ति रोगाः शब्दादिजास्तथा॥
षड्धातुजस्तु पुरुषो रोगाः षड्धातुजास्तथा।
राशिः षड्धातुजो ह्येष सांख्यैराद्यैः परीक्षितः॥
तथा ब्रुवाणं कुशिकमाह Caraka Saṁhitā, I. xxv.

He is described there as Kuśika also. But Kuśika occurs as the name of another physician in the list of sages who wanted to learn the Science of Medicine.

* * * कुशिको बादरायणः।
शर्कराक्षो हिरण्याक्षः * * *॥ Caraka Saṁhitā, I. i.

But he is again called Kauśika Hiraṇyākṣa हिरण्याक्षश्च कौशिकः। in the *Caraka Saṁhitā I. xxxi* where he is referred to as holding a discourse on Taste रस, with the other sages:—

चत्वारो रसा इति हिरण्याक्षः कौशिकः स्वादुर्हितश्च स्वादुरहितश्चास्वादुर्हितश्च अस्वादुरहितश्च॥ Caraka Saṁhitā, I. xxvi.

Hiraṇyākṣa is quoted in Vyākhya Madhukoṣa where his name is written as Hiraṇākhya हिरणाख्य:—

हिरण्याख्येऽप्युक्तं—
संस्रावदाह-पाकाद्यैश्चितः स्फोटैर्भयान्वितः।
स्रस्ताङ्गो मिश्रगन्धिः स्यात् शकुन्या पीड़ितः शिशुः॥
Vyākhyā Madhu Koṣa, Vālaroga Nidāna p. 391.

Cakrapānidatta in his *Ayurvedadīpikā* or *Commentary* on *Caraka Saṁhitā* I. xxv identifies Kuśika and Hirṇyākṣa कुशिक इति हिरण्याक्षस्य नाम। "Kuāśika is the name of Hirṇyākṣa."

VAḌISA.

He is surnamed Dhāmārgava (*i.e.*, Vaḍisa Dhāmārgava in the *Caraka Saṁhitā I. xii*). There he supports Kumāraśirā Bharadvāja in the discussion on the qualities of the Vāyu, and says :

तच्छ्रुत्वा वाक्यं वड़िशो धामार्गव उवाच। एवमेतद्यथा भगवानाह। एतान्येव वातप्रकोपनप्रशमनानि भवन्ति। यथा ह्येनमसङ्घातवन्तमनवस्थितमनासाद्य प्रकोपन प्रशमनानि प्रकोपयन्ति प्रशमयन्ति वा तदनुव्याख्यास्यामः। वातप्रकोपनानि खलु रूक्षलघु-शीतदारुणखरविषदशुषिरकराणि शरीराणां। तथाविधेषु हि शरीरेषु वायुराश्रयं लब्ध्वा आप्याय्यमानः प्रकोपमापद्यते। वातप्रशमनानि पुनः स्निग्धगुरूष्णश्लक्ष्णमृदुपिच्छिल-घनकराणि शरीराणां। तथाविधेषु शरीरेषु वायुरासज्ज्य मानश्चरन प्रशान्तिमापद्यते॥

Caraka Saṁhitā, I. xii.

He appears again in the discourse on Taste or "Rasa" where he says: The tastes are of 8 kinds :

अष्टौ रसा इति वड़िशो धामार्गवो मधराम्ललवणकटुतिक्तकषायक्षाराव्यक्ताः॥

Caraka Saṁhitā, I. xxvi.

In the discussion, as regards the part of the fœtus which appears first, he holds the opinion that the upper and lower extremities are the members which are formed before any other structures :

हस्तपादमिति वड़िशस्तत्करणत्वात् पुरुषस्य इन्द्रियाणीति।

Caraka Saṁhitā, IV vi.

SĀṄKṚTYĀYANA.

In the *Caraka Saṁhitā, I. xii* there is recorded a conversation between the sages as to the qualities of the Vāyu. There Sāṅkṛtayana is referred to as Kṛśa or lean. He mentions six qualities of Vāyu:

1. Rūkṣa = Dryness.
2. Laghu = Lightness.
3. Sīta = Coldness.
4. Dāruna = Motion or causing hardness by absorption.
5. Khara = Roughness.
6. Viṣadā = Plain or Smoothness.

He was supported by Kumārasira Bharadvāja, Vaḍiśa Dhāmārgava and others.

तत्रोवाच कृशः साङ्कृत्यायनः। रूक्षलघुशीतदारुणखरविषदाः षड़िमे वातगुणा इति।

Caraka Saṁhitā, I. xii.

ŚARALOMĀ.

Śaralomā Ṛṣi is said to have expressed his view as regards the question of origin of diseases, raised by Rājarsi Vāmaka. He appears to have contradicted the view of Maudgalya in the *Caraka Saṁhitā*.

"Then Śarolomā Ṛṣi said, "No, that cannot be; Soul cannot be the cause of disease. The soul naturally avoids sorrow; it will never try to plague itself with diseases. The Mind, being under the influence of Raja and Tama qualities, originates the body and the diseases."

शरलोमा तु नेत्याह न ह्यात्मात्मानमात्मना ।
योजयेद्व्याधिभिर्दुःखैर्दुःखद्वेषी कदाचन ॥
रजस्तमोभ्यान्तु मनः परीतं सत्वसंज्ञकम् ।
शरीरस्य समुत्पत्तौ विकाराणाञ्च कारणम् ॥

Caraka Saṁhitā I. xxv.

KĀPYA.

In the *Caraka Saṁhitā* he is styled as Bhadra Kāpya or Kāpya the Noble. He refutes the arguments of Śanuaka that the diseases are caused by hereditary transmission and says:

"No that nnot be; the offspring of a blind father is not necessarily blind, so the parents cannot be said to have originated the body and its diseases. The man and his diseases owe their origin to his own works in a previous birth."

भद्रकाप्यस्तु नेत्याह न ह्यन्धोऽन्धात् प्रजायते ।
मातापित्रोश्च ते पूर्व्वमुत्पत्तिर्नोपपद्यते ॥
कर्म्मजस्तु मतो जन्तुः कर्म्मजास्तस्य चामयाः ।
न ह्यृते कर्म्मणो जन्म रोगाणां पुरुषस्य च ॥

Caraka Saṁhitā, I. xxv.

He is mentioned as one of the sages present at a meeting of the Ṛṣis as narrated in the *Caraka Saṁhitā I. xxvi*; the chapter is called *Ātreya Bhadra Kāpīya*. A discussion about Taste and Food was the result. Bhadra Kāpya says: "There is surely a single taste or *rasa* only. This *rasa* is only recognisable by tongue, and the wise consider it to be one of the objects,—*rupa*, *rasa* etc. This *rasa* or taste is nothing but water."

एक एव रस इत्युवाच भद्रकाप्यो यं पञ्चानामिन्द्रियार्थानामन्यतमं जिह्वावैषयिकं भावमाचक्षते कुशलाः । स पुनरुदकादनन्य ॥

Caraka Saṁhitā, I. xxvi.

In the same chapter he expresses himself again on the incompatiblity of fish and milk as articles of dietary; he allows all the fishes except the Cilcima, which, he says, if eaten with milk, may cause diseases, and sometimes even death.

तदनन्तरमात्रेयवचनमनुनिशम्य भद्रकाप्योऽग्निवेशमुवाच। सर्व्वानेव मत्स्यान् पयसा सहाभ्यवहरेत् अन्यत्रैकस्माच्चिलिचिमात्। स पुन: शकली, स्थूलवती लोहितराजी रोहिताकार: प्रायो भूमौ चरति तच्चेत् पयसा सहाभ्यवहरेन्नि:संशयं शोणितजानां विबन्धजानां वा व्याधीनामन्यतमम् अथवा मरणं प्राप्नुयादिति ॥

Caraka Saṁhitā, I. xxvi.

As regards the question of the part of the fœtus first formed, he says: "The navel is the part which appears first, for this is the part where nutriment from the mother enters the body of the fœtus:

नाभिरिति भद्रकाप्य आहारगम इति।

Caraka Saṁhitā IV. vi.

This opinion has been ascribed to Parāśara in the *Suśruta Saṁhitā, IV, iii*:—

नाभिरिति पाराशर्य्यस्ततो हि वर्द्धते देहो देहिन:।

KĀṄKĀYANA.

Kāṅkāyana is the name of an ancient physician who is referred to in the *Caraka Saṁhitā I. xxvi* as the foremost among the Vaidays of Vālhika or Balkh : काङ्कायनश्च वाह्लीको वाह्लीकभिषजां वरः॥ He is there represented as having held with Nimi and other physicians a discussion on the number of "*rasa*" or tastes. He was of opinion that the tastes were innumerable and that they could only be described according to their seat, quantity, and mode of action :

अपरिसंख्येया रसा इति काङ्कायनो वाह्लीकभिषगाश्रयगुणकर्म्मसंस्कारविशेषाणामपरिमेयत्वात् ।

He is also referred to in the *Caraka Saṁhitā I. xxv* as contradicting the opinion of Kumāraśirā Bharadrāja about the origin of diseases and as having held the view that Brahmā, the creator, is the cause of ease and disease.

काङ्कायनस्तु नेत्याह न ह्यारम्भः फलं भवेत् ।
भवेत् स्वभावाद्भावानामसिद्धिः सिद्धिरेव वा ।
स्रष्टा त्वामतिसङ्कल्पो ब्रह्मापत्यं प्रजापतिः ।
चेतनाचेतनास्यास्य जगतः सुखदुःखयोः ॥

He is named in the *Caraka Saṁhitā* I. I in a list which contains the names of a number of other ancient physicians. His opinion is also quoted in the same book IV. vi as regards the part of the fœtus formed first. His opinion is : "The heart being the seat of life and consciousness is the part formed first :

हृदयमिति काङ्कायनो वाह्लीकभिषक् चेतनाधिष्ठानत्वात् ।

But in the *Suśruta Saṁhitā III. iii*, the same view is asclibed to Kṛtabīrya

हृदयमिति कृतवीर्य्यो बुद्धेर्मनसश्च स्थानत्वात् ।

The ancient physician Kāṅkāyana is probably the Kankah or Katka of the Arabs (see *Reinaud, Mem. Sur l'Inde, p. 314 ff*), who is expressly termed Vāhlika-bhiṣaja. His name appears amongst the teachers of the Atharva-pariśiṣṭhas.

Formulæ attributed to Kāṅkāyana :—

Formula	*Author*	*Book*	*Page.*
1. Prescription of a purgative for bilious subjects	Kāṅkāyana	Bower Ms. xi. ...	166
2. Kāṅkāyana Modaka	„	V. K. V. ...	95
		C. D. ...	57
3. Kāṅkāyana Guṭikā	„	H. S. ...	203
		C. D. ...	180
		Sā. S. ...	133
		Śa. Sl. ...	17
		G. N., I. ...	103
4. Kāṅkāyana Vaṭaka	„	G. N., I. ...	103

1. Kāṅkāyana's Purgative.

काङ्कायन-विरेचनम् ।

गुड़म् द्राचारसम् चौद्रं तथैव च हरितकी ।
एतत्काङ्कायनप्रोक्तं पैत्तिकानां विरेचनम् ॥

(935) Molasses, juice of raisins, small bee's honey, and chebulic myrobalans (Haritakī) :—these make Kaṅkāyana's prescription of a purgative for bilious subjects.

Bower Ms. xi. p. 166.

2. Kāṅkāyana Modaka.

काङ्कायनमोदकः ।

पथ्या पञ्चपलान्यं कमजाज्या मरिचस्य च ।
पिप्पलीपिप्पलीमूल-चव्यचित्रकनागराः ॥

पलाभिहङ्गा: क्रमशो यवक्षारपलद्वयम् ।
भल्लातकपलान्यष्टौ कन्दस्तु द्विगुणो मतः ॥
द्विगुणेन गुडेनैषां वटकान सम्मितान् ।
कृत्वैनं भक्षयेत् प्रातस्तक्रमम्भोऽनु वा पिवेत् ॥
मन्दाग्निं दीपयत्येष ग्रहणीपाण्डुरोगनुत् ॥
कङ्कायनेन शिष्येभः शस्त्रक्षाराग्निभिर्विना ।

भिषग्जितमिति प्रोक्त श्रेष्ठमर्शविकारिणाम् ॥

3. Kāṅkāyana Guṭikā.

गुल्मे काङ्कायनगुटिका ।

सठीं पुष्करमूलं च वह्निं लवणपञ्चकम् ।
शृङ्गवेरं वचां चैव पलिकानि समाहरेत् ॥
त्रिवृतायाः पलं कुर्यात्त्रीन् कर्षानथ हिङ्गुतः ।
यवक्षारपले द्वे च द्वे पले चाम्लवेतसात् ॥
यवान्यजाजिमरिचं धान्याकं शीतपुष्पकम् ।
उपकुञ्च्याजमोदाभ्यां तथैवाष्टमिकामपि ॥
मातुलुङ्गरसेनैता गुटिकाः कारयेद्भिषक् ।
तासामेकां पिबेद्द्वे वा तिस्रोऽथ च सुखाम्बुना ॥
अम्लैश्च मद्यैः पातव्या घृतेन पयसा तथा ।
एषा काङ्कायनेनोक्ता गुटिका गुल्मनाशिनी ॥

अर्शोहृद्रोगशमनी कृमीणां च विनाशनी ।
गोमूत्रयुक्ता शमयेत्कफगुल्मं चिरोत्थितम् ॥
क्षीरेण पित्तगुल्मं च मद्यैरम्लैश्च वातिकम् ।
त्रिफलारसमूत्रैश्च नियच्छेत्सान्निपातिकम् ॥
रक्तगुल्मे च नारीणामुष्ट्रीक्षीरेण पाययेत् ।

Gada Nigraha.

Kāṅkāyana Guṭikā.

काङ्कायनगुटिका ।

यमानी जीरकं धान्यं मरिचं गिरिकर्णिका ।
अजमोदोपकुञ्ची च चतुःशाणा पृथक् पृथक् ॥

हिङ्गु षट्शाणिकं कार्य्यं क्षारौ लवणपञ्चकम् ।
विड्चाष्टमितैः शाणैः प्रत्येकं कल्पयेत् सुधीः ॥
दन्ती शटी पौष्करञ्च विड़ङ्गं दाड़िमं शिवा ।
चित्रोऽम्लवेतसः शुण्ठी शाणैः षोड़शभिः पृथक् ॥
बीजपूररसेनैव गु टिकां कारयेद् बुधः ।
घृतेन पयसा मद्यैरम्लैरुष्णोदकेन वा ।
पिबेत् काङ्कायनप्रोक्तां गुटिकां गुल्मनाशिनीम् ॥

मद्येन वातिकं गुल्मं गोक्षीरेण च पैत्तिकं ।
मूत्रेण कफगुल्मञ्च दशमूलैस्त्रिदोषजम् ॥
उष्ट्रीदुग्धेन नारीणां रक्तगुल्मं विनाशयेत् ।
हृद्रोगं ग्रहणीं शूलं क्रिमीनर्शांसि नाशयेत् ॥

Śāraṅgadhara.

Kāṅkayana Guṭika.

काङ्कायनगुटिका ।

तद्वत्काङ्कायनीऽप्येकपलचयकणाग्रन्थिचव्याग्निविश्वे ।

द्रोणकप्रस्थाष्टपञ्चैकयवजमरिचार्शोऽर्यैरु पथ्यजारम् ॥

4. Kāṅkāyana Vaṭaka.

अर्शसि काङ्कायनवटकः ।

पथ्या पञ्चपलान्येकमजाज्या जीरकस्य च ।
पिप्पलीपिप्पलीमूलचव्यचित्रकनागरम् ॥
पलाभिवृद्ध्या क्रमशो यवक्षारपलद्वयम् ।
भल्लातकफलान्यष्टौ कन्दस्तद्द्विगुणो मतः ॥
द्विगुणेन गुडेनैषां वटकानक्षसंमितान् ।
एकैकं भक्षयेत्प्रातस्तक्रमम्लं पिबेदनु ॥
वह्निं संदीपयत्याशु ग्रहणीपाण्डुरोगजित् ।
काङ्कायनेन शिष्येभ्यः शस्त्रक्षाराग्निभिर्विना ॥

कथितो वटको ह्येष गुदजानां विनाशनः ।

JĀVĀLA

Sage **Jāvāla** is said in the *Bramhavaivarta Purāṇa* to have written a work on medicine called *Tantra Sāraka* (*Epitome of the Science*). No such work however is known to us and he is not quoted by the later writers.

His opinion as to the true cause of living beings, is quoted in the *Ramāyaṇa* as follows :—

" Father is the remote cause of birth ; the true source of life is in the combination of the sperm and ovule." His name appears there as Jāvāli.

वीजमात्रं पिता जन्तोः शुक्रं शोणितमेव च ।
संयुक्तमृतुमन्मात्रा पुरुषस्येह जन्म तत् ॥

Rāmāyaṇa, Ayodhyākāṇḍa, Ch. 108. v. 11.

Jāvāla is known to us as the author of :—

1. *Vṛhat Jāvāla Upaniṣad*. G.O.M.L. MSS. 629. 14117.
2. *Rudrākṣa Jāvāla Upaniṣad*. G.O.M.L. 770, 14422.
3. *Jāvāla Upaniṣad*. G.O.M.L. MS : no 14424.

KUMARAŚIRĀ BHARADVĀJA.

He was a different physician from Bharadvāja Ṛṣi who was selected by the conclave of physicians to learn the science and art of medicine from Indra. He is a disciple of Ātreya Punarvasu. He is said to have held conversation about the qualities of Vāyu in the *Caraka Saṁhitā I. xii.* He supported what Kṛṣa Sāṅkṛāyayana said and explained his views :

तच्छुत्वा वाक्यं कुमारशिरा भरद्वाज उवाच। एवमेतद् यथा भगवानाह ; एत एव वातगुणा भवन्ति। स त्वेवंगुणै र्द्रव्यैरेवं प्रभावैश्च कर्म्मभिरभ्यास्यमानैर्वायुः प्रकोपमापद्यते समानगुणाभ्यासो हि धातूनां वृद्धिकारणमिति।

As to the origin of diseases he held the view (*Caraka Saṁhitā I. xxv*) that diseases are caused by Nature and thus refuted Bhadra Kāpy's opinion that diseases are the result of man's works in his previous births :

भरद्वाजस्तु नेत्याह कर्त्ता पूर्व्वं हि कर्म्मणः।
दृष्टं न चाकृतं कर्म्म यस्य स्यात् पुरुषः फलम्॥
भावहेतुः स्वभावस्तु व्याधीनां पुरुषस्य च।
खरद्रवचलोष्णत्वं तेजोऽन्तानां यथैव हि॥

His name again appears in the *Caraka Saṁhitā I. xxvi* where he expressed his view about rasa or tastes : there are five kinds of tastes, *i.e.*, of earth, water, fire, air and ether :—

पञ्च रसा इति कुमारशिरा भरद्वाजो भौमोदकाग्नेयवायव्यान्तरीक्षाः।

Again in the *Caraka Saṁhitā IV. vi.* his opinion is quoted as regards the part of the fœtus formed first :

The head of the fœtus is formed first as it is the seat of all the senses :

शिरः पूर्व्वमभिनिवर्त्तते कुचाविति कुमारशिरा भरद्वाजः पश्यति सर्व्वेन्द्रियाणां तदधिष्ठानमिति ।

But in the *Suśruta Saṁhitā* III. iii, this view is ascribed to Śaunaka

गर्भस्य हि सम्भवतः पूर्व्वं शिरः सम्भवतीत्याह शौनकः शिरोमूलत्वाद्देहेन्द्रियाणां ॥

RĀJARṢI VĀMAKA

Vāmaka was the King of Kāśī or Benares. He first raised the question about the origin of diseases in a meeting of the sages. He requested the sages to answer his question.—Whether the human being and the diseases to which he is liable have originated from the same cause?

तदनन्तरं काशिपतिर्वामको वाक्यमर्थवत्।
व्याजहारर्षिसमितिमभिसृत्याभिवाद्य च ॥
किं नु भोः पुरुषो यज्जस्तज्जास्तस्यामयाः स्मृताः।

Caraka Saṁhitā, I. xxv.

RĀJARṢI VĀRYOVID

Vāryovid is the name of an ancient physician mentioned in the *Caraka Saṁhitā* I. xii. He appears to support what is said by Vaḍiśa Dhāmārgava and then explains the actions of Vāyu, both in and on the human system, in its natural and deranged conditions. Then hearing the supernatural manifestations of Vāyu, Mārīci questioned the utility of this knowledge in connection with the science of medicine. Vāryovid replied: "The actions of Vāyu are mentioned here for the physicians having knowledge of the actions of Vāyu in its deranged state will try to keep it in its normal condition by medicines."

तच्छ्रुत्वा वड़िशवचनमवितथमृषिगणबहुमतमुवाच वार्य्योविदो राजर्षिरेवमेतत्, सर्व्वमनपवादं यथा भगवानाह। यानि तु खलु वायोः कुपिताकुपितस्य शरीराशरीरचरस्य च शरीरेषु चरतः कर्म्माणि बहिः शरीरेभ्यो वा भवन्ति तेषामवयवान् प्रत्यक्षानुमानोपदेशैः साधयित्वा नमस्कृत्य वायवे यथाशक्ति प्रवक्ष्यामः।

वायुस्तन्त्रयन्त्रधरः, प्राणोदानसमानव्यानापानात्मा, प्रवर्त्तकश्चेष्टानामुच्चावचानां नियन्ता प्रणेता च मनसः। सर्व्वेन्द्रियाणामुद्योगकरः। सर्व्वेन्द्रियार्थानामभिवोढ़ा, सर्व्वशरीरधातुव्यूहकरः, सन्धानकरः शरीरस्य, प्रवर्त्तकोवाचः, प्रकृतिः स्पर्शशब्दयोः, श्रोत्रस्पर्शनयोर्मूलं, हर्षोत्साहयोर्योनिः। समीरणोऽग्नेर्दोषसंशोषणः, क्षेप्ता बहिर्म्मलानां, स्थूलाणुस्रोतसां भेत्ता, कर्त्ता गर्भाकृतीनामायुषोऽनुवृत्तिप्रत्ययभूतो, भवत्यकुपितः।

प्रकुपितस्तु खलु शरीरे शरीरं नानाविधैर्विकारैरुपतपति। बलवर्णसुखायुषामुपघाताय मनो व्यावर्त्तयति, सर्व्वेन्द्रियाण्युपहन्ति, विनिहन्ति गर्भान् विकृतिमापादयत्यतिकालं धारयति, भयशोकमोहदैन्यातिप्रलापान् जनयति प्राणांश्चोपरुणद्धि।

प्रकृतिभूतस्य खल्वस्य लोकेषु चरतः कर्म्माणीमानि भवन्ति। तद्यथा—धरणीधारणं, ज्वलनोज्ज्वालनम्, आदित्यचन्द्रनक्षत्रग्रहगणानां सन्तानगतिविधानं, सृष्टिश्च मेघानाम्, अपाञ्च विसर्गः, प्रवर्त्तनं स्रोतसां, पुष्पफलानाञ्चाभिनिर्व्वर्त्तनमुद्भिदनञ्चोद्भिदानामृतुनां प्रविभागः, प्रविभागो धातूनां, धातुमानसंस्थानव्यक्तिः, वीजाभिसंस्कारः, शस्याभिवर्द्धनम्, अविक्लेदोपशोषणमवैकारिकविकारश्चेति।

प्रकुपितस्य खल्वस्य लोकेषु चरतः कर्म्माणीमानि भवन्ति। तद्यथा—शिखरिशिखरावमन्थनमुन्मथनमनोकहानामुत्पीड़नं सागराणामुद्वर्त्तनं सरसां प्रतिसरणमापगानामाकम्पनञ्च भूमेरवधूननमम्बुदानां नीहारनिर्ह्रादपांशुसिकतामत्स्यभेकोरगक्षाररुधिराश्मवज्राशनिविसर्गों व्यापादनञ्च षण्णामृतूनां शस्यानामसङ्घातो भूतानाञ्चोपसर्गों भावानाञ्चाभावकरणं चतुर्युगान्तकराणां मेघसूर्य्यानलानिलानां विसर्गः। स हि भगवान् प्रभवश्चाव्ययश्च भूतानां भावाभावकरः सुखासुखयोर्विधाता मृत्युर्यमो नियन्ता, प्रजापतिरदितिर्विश्वकर्म्मा विश्वरूपः सर्व्वगः सर्व्वतन्त्राणां विधाता भावानामणुर्विभुर्विष्णुःक्रान्ता लोकानां वायुरेव भगवानिति।

तच्छ्रुत्वा वार्य्योविदवचो मारीचिरुवाच। यद्यप्येवमेतत् किमर्थस्यास्य वचने विज्ञाने वा सामर्थ्यमस्ति भिषग्विद्यायां, भिषग्विद्यां वाधिकृत्येयं कथा प्रवृत्तेति।

वार्य्योविद उवाच। भिषक् पवनमतिबलमतिपरुषमतिशीघ्रकारिणमात्ययिकञ्चानुनिशम्य सहसा प्रकुपितमतिप्रयतः कथमग्रेऽभिसंरक्षितुमभिधास्यति, प्रागेवैनमत्ययभयादिति। वायोर्यथार्था स्तुतिरपि भवत्यारोग्याय बलवर्णविवृद्धये वर्च्चस्वित्वाय पचयाय च। ज्ञानोपपत्तये परमायुषः प्रकर्षाय चेति।

Again in I. xxvi, Vāryovid, the royal sage, held a hexade of tastes, "but its component parts were different from those of the usual hexade. They were rather related to the sense of touch and were the following: guru (heavy), laghu (light), śīta (cold), uṣṇa (hot), snigdha (greasy), rukṣa (dry). The established hexade was that taught by Ātreya," and they are sweet, sour, saline, bitter, acrid and astringent. (*Footnote* to *Bower MSS.* p. 165).

षड्रसा इति वार्य्योविदो राजर्षिगुरुलघुशीतोष्णस्निग्धरुक्षाः।

In I. xxv he is also referred to as contradicting the sage Śaralomā as regards the origin of diseases. He held the view that human body was the seat of disease and not the mind as put forward by Śoralomā; and that the diseases were caused by the "rasa," and thus remotely by water.

वार्य्योविदस्तु नेत्याह न ह्येकं कारणं मनः।
नर्त्ते शरीराच्छारीरा रोगाणां मनसः स्थितिः॥
रसजानि तु भूतानि व्याधयश्च पृथग्विधाः।
आपोहि रसवत्यस्ताः स्मृता निर्व्वृति हेतवः॥

SAUNAKA.

We do not know anything about the personal history of Bhadra Śaunaka. There are references to a sage Śaunaka by name. He is described to be "the son of Sunaka and grandson of Gritsa-mada. He was the author of the Brīhad-devatā, an Anukramani, and other works, and he was a teacher of the Atharva-veda. His pupil was Āśwalāyana. There was a family of the name, and the works attributed to Saunaka are probably the productions of more than one person" (Dowson. *Classical Dictionary*, p. 290). Śaunaka Muni is also known to us as a Law-giver of the Hindus and as such he is quoted in the *Tithyāditatva*.

Śaunaka is the name of an ancient physician mentioned as a member of the society of sages referred to in *Caraka Saṁhitā I. i.* Again in I. xxv he appears to have refuted the argument of Hiranyākṣya as to the origin of diseases. His view was that diseases originated from the father and the mother. He said : " How is it possible for men to be born simply from the six elements in the absence of a father and a mother ? For a cow is born of a cow, horse from a mare and man from woman ; and we know also tnat the hereditary transmission of diseases as Meha occurs from father to son. So diseases and our body owe their origin to our parents." Here we find that the hereditary transmission of diseases was well known to the ancient sages.

तथा ब्रुवाणं कुशिकमाह तन्नेति शौनकः ।
कस्मान्मातापितृभ्यां हि विना षड्धातुजो भवेत् ॥
पुरुषः पुरुषाद्गौर्गोरश्वादश्वः प्रजायते ।
पैत्र्या मेहादयश्चोक्ता रोगास्ता एव कारणम् ॥

His opinion is also quoted in the *Caraka Saṁhitā IV. vi*, as regards the organ first formed in the fœtus: "The Large Intestine is the seat of Vāyu and so this is the part formed first":

पक्कगुदमिति भद्रशौनको मारुताधिष्ठानात् ।

He is called भद्रशौनकः Bhadra Śaunaka but once in *Vivandha Saṁgraha* as मदशौनकः Mada Śaunaka.

Quotations from Śaunaka.

I. In the *Nivandha Saṁgraha.*

1. तथा च मदशौनकः। Mada Śaunaka.

तङ्मांससंश्रितो वायुस्तद्दाहेनैव शाम्यति ।
मांसे दग्धे हि शाम्यन्ति शिरास्नायुस्थिसन्धिजाः ॥

Nivandha Saṁgraha, I. xii, p. 108.

2. सामान्यं लेपजन्तु भद्रशौनकः प्राह। Bhadra Śaunaka.

स्नेहासिद्धातिशुद्धाम्बु निःक्वाथ्य च रसैः क्रमात् ।
कल्कस्य योजयेदंशं चतुर्थं षष्ठमंशकम् ॥

Nivandha Saṁgraha, IV. xxxi, p. 1097.

II. In the *Vyākhyā Kusumā Vali.*

1. तथा च भद्रशौनकः—

अल्पाभिष्यन्दि मधूरं वल्यं संवत्सरोषितं ।
अल्पक्लेदं च दोषाणां पुराणं सर्पिरुच्यते ॥
दशवर्षस्थितं प्रायः कटुकानुरसं स्मृतम् ।
स्थितं वर्षशतं श्रेष्ठं कुम्भसर्पिरुदाहृतम् ॥

Vṛnda Mādhava, LXII, p. 488.

2. भद्रशौनकेनापि—

संसृष्टभक्तः सुमनाः स्नेहपीतो दृढानलः ।
संशुद्धः परतो मासादनुवास्यस्ततो नरः ॥

Ibid, LXXV, p. 558.

3. शौनकमानमाह—

स्नेहपाके त्वमानोक्तौ चतुर्गुणविवर्धितम् ।
कल्क स्नेहद्रव्यं योज्यमधीते शौनकः पुनः ॥
स्नेहे सिध्यति शुद्धाम्बु निष्काथस्वरसैः क्रमात् ।
कल्कस्य योजयेदंशं चतुर्थं षष्ठमष्टमं ॥
पृथक् स्नेहसमं दद्यात्पञ्चप्रभृति तु द्रवम् ।
नाङ्गुलिग्राहिता कल्के न स्नेहेऽग्नौ सशब्दता ॥
वर्णादिसंपच्च यदा तदैनं शीघ्रमाहरेत् ।
घृतस्य फेनोपशमस्तैलस्य तु तदुद्भवः ॥
लेहस्य तन्तुमत्ताऽप्सु मज्जनं शरणं न च ।
पाकस्तु त्रिविधो मन्दचिक्कणः खरचिक्कणः ॥
मन्दः कल्कसमे किट्टे चिक्कणो मदनोपमे ।
किञ्चित्सीदति कृष्णे च वर्त्यमाने च पश्चिमः ॥
दग्धोऽत ऊर्ध्वं निष्कार्यः स्यादामस्त्वग्निसादकृतः ।
मृदुर्नस्ये खरोऽभ्यङ्गे पाने बस्तौ च चिक्कणः ॥

Ibid, LXXXII, p. 664.

Śaunaka's opinion is quoted by Suśruta (see p. 469). Bhadra Śaunaka is also quoted by Cakrapāṇi. In *Todarānanda*, Śaunaka is mentioned as an authority in Medicine. See *Ṛadh*, 32.

Books :—

1. *Śaunaka Tantra*—No books of Śaunaka are mentioned in the commentaries. That he was a medical author we know from the following remarks in the *Sarvāṅga Sundarī*, V. vi.

शौनक प्रस्तुत तन्त्रकृदधीते एवं पठति ।

Muller's reference to a book on Poison by Sānāq the Indian may be the *Śaunaka Tantra*. It was translated by the Arabians. Dr. Ray cites some parallel passages on the Examination of Poisoned Food and Drink from Sānāq, Caraka and Suśruta (*Hist. Hindu Chemistry, Intro.*, p. xviii.

2. In the *MS.* G.O.M.L. No. 14440 *Jamalajanana Śānti* यमलजननशान्ति which deals with the Śānti to be performed for overcoming the evil effects supposed to arise when the mother gives birth to twins, we find the work described to be a chapter from the Śaunaka's treatise :

Beginning :

वरुणं पाशहस्तं च मकरस्थं जलाधिपं ।
ग्रहदोषोपशान्त्यर्थं वरुणं पूजयाम्यहम् ॥
गोमहिष्यश्वनारीणां यमलौ यदि जायते ।
सिनिवाल्यां प्रसूतिश्च हयादद्भि प्रजायते ॥
* * * वित्तनाशाश्वग्रहाहनानां च सचय: ।
सम्पद्विनाशनं कर्त्तुर्भवेद्राष्ट्रविनाशनम् ॥
अतस्सर्वं विचार्याथ पश्चाच्छान्ति समाचरेत् ।

End :

ब्राह्मणान् भोजयेश्चैव शतं च मधुसर्पिषा ।
ताम्बुलं विप्रवचनात्कुर्य्यादेव प्रपूजयेत् ॥

Colophon :

इति शौनकीये यमलजननशान्ति: ॥

3. In the MS. 14442 कृष्णचतुर्दशीजननशान्ति: *Kṛṣṇachaturdaśī jananaśāntiḥ*, we find Śaunaka asking Garga Muni about the expiation 'Sānti' to be performed when a child is born on the 14th day of dark moon कृष्णचतुर्दशी: ।

मन्दरस्थं सुखासीनं गर्गं मुनिगणावृतम् ।
नम: कृत्वा तु प्रपच्छ शौनको मुनिसत्तम: ॥

4. Śaunaka is said to be the author of *MSS.* G.O.M.L. 14479 and 3297 :

इति शौनककृते ग्रहजननशान्ति: समाप्त ॥

5. The *Śaunaka Saṁhitā* of the *Atharva Veda* is ascribed to Ṛṣi Śaunaka. He is also the author of *Vṛhaddevatā* He is a Ṛṣi, and so seems to be a different individual from Bhadra or Mada Śaunaka.

Śaunaka seems to be a name borne by many sages in ancient days. The epithets applied to him, *e.g.*, Ṛṣi, Bhadra and Mada or Madra refer to different authors. Mada is possibly a corruption of Madra which may allude to Śaunaka of Madra country (Madras). In this way, the different views as regards the formation and development of the fœtal members, ascribed to Śaunaka in the *Caraka* and *Śuśruta Saṁhitās* may be explained. But Madra may again be a corrupted reading of 'Bhadra,' for in Sanskrit language the letters म and भ may easily be mistaken by the copyists.

KAṆĀDA

Kanāda, the famous sage who propounded the Vaiśeṣiki system of philosophy, is said to have written a treatise on *Pulse* consisting of 63 stanzas. It is known as *Naḍī Vijñāna*. He is said to have written a more comprehensive work the *Kanāda Saṁhitā*—a treatise on pathology and medicine, of which the chapter on pulse—the *Naḍī Vijñāna* only is extant. It forms the first chapter and is also called *Paribhāsā* (see *L.* 570). The pulse is treated as an index to disease and its indications may imply approaching death (see *L.* 2295). The Vaidyas rely principally on pulse and they diagnose diseases by the character of the pulse.

MSS. L. 570 ; 2295.

The book has been printed with *Naḍī Prakāśa* of Śaṅkara Sena by Nandalal Vidyāratnā Kaviranjana, Calcutta, 1887.

Begins :

नमः शिवाय ।

यद्वक्त्रेभ्यः पञ्चसंख्या गतेभ्यो

वेदा जाता ऋग्यजुः साम वेदाः ।

आयुर्व्वेदाश्चार्थवेदाश्च तस्मिन्

आस्तां शम्भौ श्रीकणादस्य भक्तिः ॥

End :

रक्तं वमति सूक्ष्मत्वं स्वस्थानस्य विमोचणं ॥

स्थैमित्यं गतिकौटिल्यं सर्व्वासां दुष्टलक्षणं ॥

इति महामुनि कणादविरचितं नाड़ीप्रकाशं समाप्तं ॥

In *MSS.*, *L.* 570 :

Begins :

अव्यक्तानुक्तलेशोक्त सन्दिग्धार्थ प्रकाशिकाः ।

परिभाषाः प्रवक्ष्यन्ते दीपीभूता सुनिश्चिताः ।

End :

इत्युक्तं नाड़ीकाज्ञानं निदानं कथ्यतेऽधुना।

Colophon :

इति श्रीकणादि संहितायां प्रथमं नाड़ीप्रकरणं

In *MSS. L.* 2295, we find an index of *Kaṇāda Saṁhitā* :—

प्रथमे नाड़िकाज्ञानं—द्वितीये रोगनिर्णयः।

तृतीये च कषायौधश्चतुर्थे पारदादिकं।

पञ्चमे तु महाविद्यारसजारणमारणं॥

End :

दिनैकं जीवितं तस्य द्वितीये मरणं ध्रुवं।

इति नाड़ीपरीक्षा—

Colophon :

इति कणादसंहितायां नाड़ीपरीक्ष प्रकरणं।

It is followed by a chapter on the tongue, but it not complete.

" But little is known of the reputed author of the Vaiśeshika system beyond his bearing the name of Kanâda. which native authorities derive from *kaná*, minute, and *áda*, eating, and sometimes change into *Kanábhuj* or *Kanábhaksha*, *bhuj* and *bhaksha* being synonyms of *áda*. These Sûtras, like the Nyáya Sûtras, have been commented by a triple set of commentaries, and popularised in several elementary treatises. The text, with the commentary of Sankar Misra, edited in Calcutta in 1861, by Jayanârâyana Tarka Panchânana, is the best edition for those who read Sanskrit; and even those who do not will find some portion translated by the late Dr. Ballantyne. Amongst the later works on the same subject, the most important is the Bhâsâ-Parichcheda (Trans. of Bhâsâ-Parichcheda, Intro. xxiv), to which we have already referred. The author is Viswanâtha Panchânan Bhatta, son of Vidyânivesa Bhatta. This is accompanied by a commentary, entitled "Siddhânta-Muktâvalî" ("The Pearl-Wreath of Truth"). Viswanâtha is known also by a commentary on the Nyáya-Sûtras. Pandits believe him to have lived about two hundred years ago. His Bhâsâ-Parichcheda is a text book in the present schools of Bengal. There is no Pandit of any repute who does not know it well, and many know the whole of it by heart. It is written in metre, although making no attempt to possess the merits of poetical composition. The Commentary by which he accompanies this work, called Siddhânta-Muktâvalî, "The Pearl-Wreath of Truth" is altogether different. It is written to support the views of the author and his school in controversy, and enters into discussion, and uses 'the whole armoury of the sometimes very abstruse technical language of the Nyaya." (Manning's *Ancient and Mediæval India*, Vol. I, p. 186-7.)

Kaṇāda distributes the contents of the universe under 6 categories or padarthas, to which the later writers of this school adds a seventh. These padarthas are Substance (Dravya), Quality (Guṇa), Action or motion (karman), Generality or community (Samanya), Atomic individuality or difference (Viśeṣa), co-inherence or intimate relation (Samavāya) and seventh non-existance (Abhāva). Roer pronounces the *Doctrine of Atoms* (Anuvāda) as elaborated by Kaṇāda to be vastly superior to that of Democritus because in the former "atoms are considered in their real motion as units of matter without any extent; and secondly, because the theory of atoms forms only a subordinate part of Hindu research."

Nāḍīvigñāna Editions:

1. Bombay Edition: It contains explanatory notes in Hindi.

2. By Devendranath Sen, Calcutta.

3. By Gangadhar Kavirāja, Calcutta: It contains exhaustive explanatory notes and quotations from Suśruta, Gautama, Vasiṣṭha and other authors.

Translations: The *Science of Sphygmica* or Sage Kaṇāda on Pulse: An English translation with Sanskrit passages, By Kavirāj Russick Lall Gupta. It is not a reliable work. The text is *Nādi-Prakāsa* of Śankara Sen and the English translation is copied from Wise's *Hindu Medicine*.

MAITREYA.

He is mentioned in the *Caraka Saṁhitā I. x.* as holding a conversation with Ātreya as to the efficacy of medicines in the cure of diseases. His contention is that men often die, even when treated by qualified physicians with good medicines; and that often they become cured of serious diseases even when they do not get skilful physicians and efficacious drugs.

Ātreya in reply said: "Diseases are either curable or incurable. Of course for the incurable diseases, medicines may be thought useless, but for the curable diseases, they are highly useful. A man may be cured of his diseases sometimes without medicines, but surely if medicines are used, they help him in getting out of the disease. A man who falls down on the ground may rise by his own exertion, but any help rendered by a friend saves him a great deal of trouble, and the man rises easily; so do medicines act as helpers, and thus they are really useful. He classifies diseases as साध्य *sādhya* or diseases amenable to treatment; याप्य *Jāpya* or diseases which cannot be cured but in which the life may be prolonged by judicious medication and असाध्य *Asādhaya* or incurable diseases in which medicines are useless.

चतुष्पादं षोड़शकलं भेषजमिति भिषजो भाषन्ते। यदुक्तं पूर्व्वाध्याये षोड़शगुणमिति तद्भेषजम्। युक्तियुक्तमलमारोग्यायेति भगवान् पुनर्व्वसुरात्रेयः। नेति मैत्रेयः। किं कारणं दृश्यन्ते ह्यातुराः केचिदुपकरणवन्तश्च परिचारकसम्पन्नाश्चात्मवन्तश्च कुशलैश्च भिषग्भिरनुष्ठिताः समुत्तिष्ठमानास्तथा युक्ताश्चापरे म्रियमाणास्तस्माद्भेषजमकिञ्चित्करं भवति।

तद्यथा—श्वभ्रे सरसि च प्रसिक्तमल्पमुदकम्। नद्यां स्यन्दमानायां पांशुधाने पांशुमुष्टिप्रकीर्णं इति। तथा परे दृश्यन्ते अनुपकरणाश्चापरिचारकाश्चानात्मवन्तश्च कुशलैश्च भिषग्भिरनुष्ठिताः समुत्तिष्ठमानाः। तथा युक्ता म्रियमाणाश्चापरे। यतश्च

प्रतिकुर्व्वन् सिध्यति प्रतिकुर्व्वन् म्रियते ; अप्रतिकुर्व्वन् सिध्यति अप्रतिकुर्व्वन् म्रियते ततश्चिन्त्यते भेषजमभेषजेनाविशिष्टमिति ।

मैत्रेय मिथ्या चिन्तत इत्यात्रेयः । किं कारणं ? ये ह्यातुराः षोड़शगुणसमुदितेनानेन भेषजेनोपपद्यमाना इत्युक्तं तदनुपपन्नम् । न हि भेषजसाध्यानां व्याधीनां भेषजमकरणं भवति । ये पुनरातुराः केवलाद्भेषजादृते समुत्तिष्ठन्ते, न तेषां सम्पूर्णभेषजोपपादनाय समुत्थान विशेषोऽस्ति । यथा हि पतितं पुरुषं समर्थमुत्थानायोत्थापयन् पुरुषो बलमस्योपादध्यात् । स च क्षिप्रतरमपरिक्लिष्ट एवोत्तिष्ठेत् । तद्वत् सम्पूर्णभेषजोपलम्भादातुराः । ये चातुराः केवलाद्भेषजादपि म्रियन्ते, न च सर्व्व एव ते भेषजोपपन्नाः समुत्तिष्ठेरन्, न हि सर्व्वे व्याधयो भवन्त्युपायसाध्याः । न चोपाय साध्यानां व्याधीनामनुपायेन सिद्धिरस्ति, न चासाध्यानां व्याधीनां भेषजसमुदायोऽस्ति, न ह्यलं ज्ञानवान् भिषक्मुमूर्षुमातुरमुत्थापयितुम् परीक्ष्यकारिणो हि कुशला भवन्ति । यथा हि योगज्ञोऽभ्यासनित्य इष्वासो धनुरादायेषुमपास्यन् नाति विप्रकृष्टेनातिकायेनापवाधी भवति, सम्पादयति चेष्टकार्य्यम् ; तथा भिषग् स्वगुणसम्पन्न उपकरणवान् वीक्ष्य कर्म्मारभमाणः साध्यरोगमनपवाधः सम्पादयत्येवातुरमारोग्येण न तस्मान्न भेषजमभेषजेनाविशिष्टं भवति ।

SĀKUNTEYA AND SĀKUNEYA.

Do the two names, Śākunteya and Śākuneya refer to the same individual? Śākuneya is the name of a sage who was present in the conclave of physicians assembled to learn the science of medicine.

शौनकः शाकुनेयश्च मैत्रेयो मैमतायनिः ।

Caraka Saṁhitā, I. i.

But in the *Caraka Saṁhitā I. xxvi*, Śākunteya is referred to in the discourse on taste or *rasa*. He was a Brahmana by caste. He says that tastes are of two kinds, corrective and calmative :—

द्वौ रसाविति शाकुन्तेयो ब्राह्मणश्छेदनीयश्चोपशमनीयश्चेति ।

Caraka Saṁhitā, I. xxvi.

PAILA.

He is mentioned in the *Brahmavaivarta Purāṇa* to have been the author of a treatise on *Nidāna* or *Pathology*. He is said to be one of the six disciples of Vedavyāsa whose name is mentioned in *Caraka Saṁhitā I. i*, as Vādarāyana. Of the six disciples, we find the names of Ātreya, Āśvarathy, Paila, connected with the science of medicine.

Paila is said to be " a learned man who was appointed in ancient days to collect the hymns of the *Rig*-veda. He arranged it in two parts, and must have been a coadjutor of Veda Vyāsa " (Dowson, p. 226)

KARATHA.

Karatha is mentioned in the *Brahma vaivarta Purāṇa* as the author of a medical work called *Sarvadhara Tantra* (see Vol. I, p. 7).

Reference :

Oxf. Cat. 226.

JĀJALI.

He is also mentioned in the *Brahma vaivarta Purāṇa* as the author of a medical work called *Vedāṅga-sāra* (*Epitome of the Auxiliary Branches of the Vedas*).

He is said to be "a Brahman mentioned in the Mahābhārata as having by asceticism acquired a supernatural power of locomotion, of which he was so proud that he deemed himself perfect in virtue and superior to all men. A voice from the sky told him that he was inferior to Tulādhāra, a Vaiśya and a trader. He went to this Tulādhāra and learnt wisdom from him." (Dowson—*Classical Dictionary of Hindu Mythology*, p. 130).

Reference :

Oxf. Cat. 226.

CHAPTER XIII

KING NALA.

Nala was the King of Niṣadha. He was handsome in appearance, heroic, pious, and a lover of sports. His special gift was his knowledge of horsemanship which he possessed to an extraordinary degree. He married princess Damayantī, the exquisitely beautiful daughter of Bhīma, King of Vidarbha. In a svayambara ceremony she chose Nala as her lord in preference to gods,—Agni, Indra, Varuṇa and Yama, who blessed the pair for their mutual love. They lived for a time in happiness and had a son and a daughter, Indrasena and Indrasenā by name. Kali, a malevolent god, resolved to ruin Nala, and instigated his brother Puṣkara to a game of dice in which Nala lost his kingdom. Nala with Damayantī left his city, suffered much for want of food and went to the forest. Some birds flew away with his only garment. He requested his wife to go to her father but she refused to leave him alone in the forest. Bereft of his senses, he forsook Damayantī alone in her sleep, leaving her to the protection of the gods and to her womanly honour. For three years she suffered great distress and at length she obtained the protection and company of the Princess of Chedi, whence she was brought to her own people. Nala wandering on his way in the forest saved the serpent king Karkoṭaka from forest-fire. The serpent bit him. His form was changed and he could not be now recognised. According to the advice of the snake, Nala went to Ṛtuparṇa, king of Ayodhyā, and offered his services as charioteer and an accomplished cook under the name of Vāhuka. Damayantī sent out Brahmans to trace her long lost husband.

She sent information to Ṛtuparṇa that Damayantī will once more hold svayamvara; but as the ceremony would take place the day after at sunrise, Nala, acting as his charioteer passed the distance of 500 miles from Ayodhyā to Kuṇḍina in a single day. On the way the king and his charioteer taught each other the secret of the highest skill in dicing and horsemanship respectively. Kali now left his body. The King of Oudh kept his silence as he did not hear anything about the svayamvara. Damayantī examined Vāhuka through her maid and was satisfied of his identity by the flavour of a dish prepared by him. Nala then regained his true form, and was received in royal audience by Bhīma. Nala made his way to his own kingdom, played again with Puṣkara and recovered his throne. He excused his brother and sent him to his state with presents. He brought back his queen and their children and reigned in peace for a long time. The story of Nala and Damayantī is an episode of the Mahābhārata. It has been translated into Latin by Bopp and into English verse by Dean Milman.

His works :—

I. "नलपाकशास्त्रम् Nalapākaçāstra, attributed to king *Nala*, who is said in the well-known story (from the Ma. Bh.) to have been skilled in the *Sūpaçāstra*, etc.

(10, 119) Gr. II. 30. first 2 II. broken ; c. 1700.

Begins :

ekaikanaishadhaḥ prāpya kadācit kalinā vrataḥ ।
ṛituparṇasya nagarīṁ rājānam idam abravīt ॥

N. maddeçaṃ saṃparityajya bāhakākhyo ha mārutaḥ ।
..............................vāhane rājan nāsti matsamaḥ ॥
arthajñāneshu cai'vā haṃ drashtavyo vai puṇyeshu ca ।
annasaṃskāram api ca jāname (mi) piçitasya ca ॥
bhaxyakho...tathālehyaṃ co'shṭyaṃ peyam prayog ataḥ ।
bhedaṃ rasānāṃ shaṇṇāṃ ca çuddhasamkarabhedataḥ ॥

About 420 *gr*.

The king begs for instruction, frightened by the long list of calamities *Nala* mentions as the result of not knowing the properties of articles of diet, and the result is four *prakaraṇa.* This MS. professes to be complete; I have, however, seen (at Madras) a much larger and different work on this subject, also attributed to *Nala.* The receipts here are some of them very curious, and, as red pepper is not mentioned, the book must have been written before the arrival of the Portuguese. Now there is not a single dish made without it."

Burnell, Tanjore Cat, p. 73.

NAKULA AND SAHADEVA.

Nakula and Sahadeva were the twin sons of Mādrī, a sister of the king of Madra, and second wife of Pāṇḍu, but mythologically they were the sons of Aśvins, or more especially of Nāsatya and Dasra respectively. They were the fourth and the youngest of the Pāṇḍu princes. "Nakula was taught the art of training and managing horses by Drona, and when he entered the services of the king Virata he was master of the horse. He had a son name Niramrita by his wife Karenu-mati, a princess of Chedi." Sahadeva learned the Science of Astronomy from Droṇa, and "he was also well acquainted with the management of cattle." He had a son named Suhotra by his wife Vijayā.

That both Nakula and Sahadeva were proficient in the art of curing diseases, we learn from the Mahābhārāta, Ādiparva :—

"Diseases are cured by reciting the names of Nakula and Sahadeva."

In the Birāṭ Parva, Ch. III, Nakula declares himself well-versed in the science of management and treatment of horses; and Sahadeva speaks of his scientific knowledge about the cows. *See also* Ch. XI and XII.

युधिष्ठिर उवाच ॥—

किं त्वं नकुल कुर्व्वाणस्तत्र तात चरिष्यसि ।

कर्म्म तत त्वं समाचक्ष्य राज्ये तस्य महीपतेः ।

सुकुमारश्च शूरश्च दर्शनीयः सुखोचितः ।

नकुल उवाच ॥—

अश्वबन्धो भविष्यामि विराटनृपतेरहं ।

सर्व्वथाज्ञानसम्पन्नः कुशलः परिरक्षणे ।

ग्रन्थिको नाम नाम्नाऽहं कर्म्मतत् सुप्रियं मम।
कुशलोऽस्म्यश्वशिक्षायां तथैवाश्वचिकित्सने।
प्रियाश्च सततं मेऽश्वाः कुरुराज यथा तव।
ये मामामन्त्रयिष्यन्ति विराटनगरे जनाः।
तेभ्य एवं प्रवक्ष्यामि विहरिष्याम्यहं यथा।
पाण्डवेन ह्यहं तात अश्वेष्वधिकृतः पुरा।
विराटनगरे च्छन्नश्चरिष्यामि महीपते।

युधिष्ठिर उवाच ॥

सहदेव क ' तस्य समीपे विहरिष्यसि।
किं वा त्वं कर्म्म कुर्व्वाणः प्रच्छन्नो विहरिष्यसि।

सहदेव उवाच ॥

गोसङ्ख्याता भविष्यामि विराटस्य महीपतेः।
प्रतिषेद्धा च दोग्धा च सङ्ख्याने कुशलो गवां।
तन्तिपाल इति ख्यातो नाम्नाऽहं विदितस्तथ।
निपुनश्च चरिष्यामि व्येतु ते मानसो ज्वरः।
अहं हि सततं गोषु भवता प्रहितः पुरा।
तत्र मे कौशलं सर्व्वमवबुद्धं विशाम्पते।
लक्षणञ्चरितं चापि गवां यच्चापि मङ्गलं।
तत्सर्व्वं मे सुविदितमन्यच्चापि महीपते।
वृषभानपि जानामि राजन् पूजितलक्षणान्।
येषां मूत्रमुपघ्राय अपि वन्ध्या प्रसूयते।
सोऽहमेवं चरिष्यामि प्रीतिरत्र हि मे सदा।
न च मां वेत्स्यते कश्चित्तोषयिष्ये च पार्थिवं।

इति श्रीमहाभारते विराटपर्व्वणि विराटप्रवेशपर्व्वणि युधिष्ठिरादिमन्त्रणे तृतीयोऽध्यायः ॥

सहदेव उवाच ॥

पञ्चानां पाण्डुपुत्राणां ज्येष्ठो भ्राता युधिष्ठिरः।
तस्याष्टशतसाहस्रा गवां वर्गाः शतं शतं।
अपरे दशसाहस्रा द्विस्तावन्तस्तथा परे।
तेषां गोसङ्ख्य आसं वै तन्तिपालेति मां विदुः।

भूतं भव्यं भविष्यच्च यच्च संख्यागतं गवां ।
न मेऽस्त्यविदितं किञ्चित् समन्ताद्दशयोजनं ।
गुणाः सुविदिता ह्यासन्मम तस्य महात्मनः ।
आसीच्च स मया तुष्टः कुरुराजो युधिष्ठिरः ।
क्षिप्रञ्च गावो बहुला भवन्ति न तासु रोगो भवतीह कश्चन ।
येषां मूत्रमुपघ्राय अपि वन्ध्यां प्रसूयते ।

इति श्रीमहाभारते विराटपर्व्वनि पाण्डवप्रवेशपर्व्वणि दशमोऽध्यायः ।

नकुल उवाच ॥

पञ्चानां पाण्डुपुत्राणां ज्येष्ठो भ्राता युधिष्ठिरः ।
तेनाहमश्वेषु पुरा नियुक्तः शत्रुकर्षण ।
अश्वानां प्रकृतिं वेद्मि विनयञ्चापि सर्व्वशः ।
दुष्टानां प्रतिपत्तिञ्च कृत्स्नञ्चैव चिकित्सितं ।
न कातरं स्यान्मम जातु वाहनं न मेऽस्ति दुष्टा वड़वाः कुता हयाः ।
जनस्तु मामाह स चापि पाण्डो युधिष्ठिरो ग्रन्थिकमेव नामतः ॥

इति श्रीमहाभारते विराटपर्व्वनि पाण्डवप्रवेशपर्व्वनि नकुलप्रवेशे द्वादशोऽध्यायः ॥

अश्वैर्व्विनीतैर्जवनैस्तत्र तत्र समागतैः ।
तोषयामास राजानं नकुलो नृपसत्तमं ।
तस्मै प्रदेयं प्रायच्छत् प्रीतो राजा धनं बहु ।
विनीतान् वृषभान् दृष्ट्वा सहदेवस्य चाभितः ।
धनं ददौ बहुविधं विराटः पुरुषर्षभः ।

इति श्रीमहाभारते विराटपर्व्वनि समयपालनपर्व्वनि जीमूतवधे त्रयोदशोऽध्यायः ।

In Gaya, the Kṛṣṇadvāraka Temple was constructed by Damodarlal Dhokri about a hundred years ago. On a wall of the temple is a stone slab with an inscription composed by Sahadeva, a veterinary surgeon.

Books ascribed to Nakula and Sahadeva:

1. *Vaidyaka Sarvasva*—by Nakula. It is mentioned in the Brahmavaivarta Purāṇa. It is not available now.

2. *Vyādhi-Sindhu-Vimardana:* or "Cure of the Ocean of Diseases"—by Sahadeva. It is also referred to in the Brahmavaivarta Purāṇa and is not available.

3. *Aśvacikitsita :* "Treatment of the Diseases of the Horse": This work is ascribed to Nakula and is still extant. The book is also is called Śālihotra. The book has been edited by Umesh Chandra Gupta Kaviratna and printed in the *Bibliotheca Indica,* with the *Aśva-vaidyaka* of Jayadatta Suri in 1887.

MSS. :—

L. 1646 (*Śālihotra*).

L. 1648.

C. P. P. 43.

Bik. MS. 1399.

I. O.: 2764 (1661 A. D.).

Begins :

येन ज्ञानवता हिमालयतरुच्छायासु विक्रीड़ितम्
यः स्नातो हिमपुष्पवात शिशिरे गङ्गाजले पावने ॥
रेमे यस्तु तुरङ्गयूथजनितैर्नानाविधैर्हेषितैः ।
पायाद्वः स तुरङ्गघोषतनयः श्रीशालिहोत्र मुनिः ॥
जयति च पाण्डुवनाथो धर्मसनाथो युधिष्ठिरोनृपतिः ।
भीमार्ज्जुनसहदेवातदनुच ये वाजिशास्त्र तत्त्वज्ञः ॥
दृष्ट्वा सम्यङ्नकुलः शास्त्रं कृत्स्नं च शालिहोत्रीयम् ।
ब्रूते शास्त्रार्थमन्यच्छास्त्रं कृत्वा समासेन ॥
प्रश्नो जातिवर्णमावर्त्तंदन्ता
लक्षं वेगा वाहनं धातुरसम् ।
कालो नस्यं पिण्डमाजंग्र कषायं
शाल्वां चेष्टां वाजिनामत्र वक्ष्ये ॥

End :

अश्वस्याङ्गे प्रलिपेद्धरिद्रया वरिष्टया मङ्गल्या च ।
सुपविचान् दोषघ्नैर्विभूषयेदलङ्कारैः ॥
इति श्रीनकुलकृतोऽश्वचिकित्सितोश्वशालाविधिराष्टादशोऽध्यायः ॥

Analysis of the contents of the *Aśvacikitsita* :—

Chapters.			Subjects.
I.	प्रश्नौ	...	Questions.
II.	जाति	...	On race.
III.	वर्णवर्णन	...	Description of the colour.
IV.	आवर्त्ताः	...	On whorls of hairs.
V.	दन्ता	...	On teeth.
VI.	अवयव प्रमाणम्	...	On measurement of the parts of the body.
VII.	वेगः	...	On speed.
VIII.	आरोहणम्	...	On mounting a horse.
IX.	वाहनः	...	On the management of horse in the different seasons.
X.	धातुपरीक्षा	...	On the examination of horse.
XI.	ऋतुचर्य्या	...	On management of the horse when running.
XII.	नस्य	...	On snuff.
XIII.	पिण्ड	...	On bolus.
XIV.	घृतविधानम्	...	On medicated butters.
XV.	क्वाथः	...	On decoctions.
XVI.	विषम्	...	On poisons.
XVII.	Wanting	...	
XVIII.	अश्वशालाविधि	...	On Stables.

MĀRKAṆḌEYA.

Mārkaṇḍeya was a Maharṣi or great sage who is the reputed author of the *Mārkaṇḍeya Purāṇa*. He was remarkable for his great age whence he was called "Dīrgha āyuṣ" or "the long lived." He is the son of Mṛkuṇda Muni (For the genealogy of the Bhārgavas, see p. 270.) Hislife was calculated to last for twelve years only. His parents were very sorry for it, but Mārkaṇḍeya determined to prolong his life by means of austerities and meditation, यथा चाहं चिरायु स्यात् तथा कुर्य्यामहं तपः. He went to forest, worshipped Hari and was absorbed in meditation. At the appointed time of his death, the servants of Yama, the King of Death, came to take away his life, but were driven away by the messengers of Viṣṇu. On another account Viṣṇu advised him to seek protection from Śiva whose servants drove away the messengers of the King of Death. He is said to have lived for a long time: सप्तकल्पान्तजीवन: "living for seven Kalpas."—Nārasimha Purāṇa, ch. vii.

He is mentioned to be one of the sages who learned the science of medicine from Bharadvāja in *Caraka Samhitā*, I. i

In the *Bower MS.*, he is said to have attained such a long life by the use of the Amrita oil. The sage Cyavana is also described to have regained his youth by the use of the same oil. For the original formula in Sanskrit, the reader is referred to Vol. I, pp. 155-66. The English version is copied from *Bower MS.*, pp. 106-07, and is given below.

(287-312 a) The two truth-speaking Aśvins, the divine physicians, honoured by the Dêvas, have declared the following excellent health-promoting oil, (288) which relieves all diseases, is fit for a king and is as good as ambrosia. It is known by the name of Amṛita (or 'ambrosia'), and is an oil able to make men strong. (289) At the time of Pushya, after having said prayers, performed purificatory rites, and asked the Brâhmans' blessing in a few words, take out the liquorice-roots grown in a favourable place. (290) Of the fresh juice of these roots take four pâtra, and add four pala each of *the following drugs*: Prapauṇḍarîka, Amṛitâ (*Tinospora cordifolia*), knots of lotus-stalks, Śatâvarî (*Asparagus racemosus*), (291) Śṛingâṭaka (*Tropa bispinsosa*), emblic myrobalan, Udumbara (*Ficus glomerata*), Kaśêruka (*Scirpus Kysoor*), the bark of each of the (five) trees with a milky sap, (292) roots of kuśa (*Poa cynosuroides*), Kâsa (*Saccharum spontaneum*) and Ikshu (*Saccharum officinalum*), also of Śara (*Saccharum Sara*) and Vîraṇa (*Andropogon muricatus*), also roots of Gundrâ (*Panicum uliginosum*), of Naḍikâ and of the lotus. (293) Vadarî (*Zizyphus Jujuba*), Vidârî (*Ipomoea digitata*), Vetasa (*Calamus Rotang*), Aḍhurûshaka (*Adhatoda vasica*), Nim, Sâlmalî (*Bombax malabaricum*), dates, cocoanut, Priyangu (*Aglaia Roxburghiana*), (294) Paṭôla (*Trichosanthes dioica*), Kuṭaja (*Holarrhena Antidysenterica*), raisins, leaf-stalk of the lotus, sandal, Kakubha (*Terminalia Arjuna*), Aśvakarṇa (*Shorea robusta*), Lâmajjaka (*Andropogon laniger*), and plumbago-root, (295) also other astringent, sweet or cooling drugs, as many as may be obtainable. Boil all these in two droṇa of water, (296) and when *the whole* is reduced to one-eighth *of the original quantity*, boil in it pastes made of fine powder of one pala each of the following drugs: Balâ (*Sida cordifolia*), Nâgabalâ (*Sida spinosa*), Jîvâ (*Dendrobium multicaule*), cowhage, Kasêruka (*Scirpus Kysoor*), (297) Nata (*Tabernæmontana coronaria*), juice of sugar-cane, Sṛikkâ (*Trigonella corniculata*), small cardamoms and cinnamon-bark, Jîvaka, Ṛishabhaka, Mêdâ, Madhuka (*Bassia latifolia*), and blue lotus (298), the colour producing saffron, aloe wood, and cinnamon-leaves, Vidârî (*Ipomoea digitata*), Kshîrakakôlî, Vîrâ (*Uraria lagopodioides*) and Śârivâ (*Ichnocarpus fruitescens*), (299) Śatâvarî (*Asparagus racemosus*), Priyangu (*Aglaia Roxburghiana*), Guḍûchî (*Tinospora cordifolia*), filaments of the lotus, Lâmajjaka (*Andropogon laniger*), red and white sandal, and fruits of Râjâdana (*Mimusops hexandra*), (300) pearl, coral, conch-shell, moon-stone, sapphire, crystal, silver, gold, and other gems and pearls, (301) liquorice, madder, and Aṁśumatî (*Desmodium gangeticum*). Boil *the whole* slowly over a gentle fire (302) with four Pâtra of (sweet) oil and eight times as much of milk, adding also tamarind-juice and vinegar of rice one half as much as the milk. (303) This boiling should be repeated a hundred or even a thousand times; and when it is thoroughly done, it may be known by this sign, (304) that on the approach of the proper time the oil stiffens by *exposure to* the rays of the sun. After asking the Brahmans' blessing, performing purificatory rites and saying prayers, (305) this Amṛita (or 'ambrosial') oil, highly esteemed by the Dêvas, may be administered *to the patient*, in the form of an injection per anum or per urethrum, or as a draught, or an errhine, or a liniment. (306) It serves the purpose of relieving diseases and imparting strength to the organs of sense. For those who suffer from morbid heat and thirst it makes an excellent and beneficial liniment. (307) It promotes the growth of hair in the old and that of the body in the young; it produces loveliness and grace in women; and also *ensures* numerous offspring, (308) for, by the use of this ambrosial oil, women are predisposed to conception. It cures the eighty nervous diseases, and also those due to *derangement of* the blood or the bile (309) or the phlegm or all the humours concurrently. By its use as an errhine or a liniment the eyes become as sharp as those of an eagle. (310) It keeps off calamities, averts ill fortune, and promotes prosperity.

By the use of this oil the Maharshi Chyavana regained (311) his youth, and was delivered from decrepitude and disease; and the blessed Maharshi Mârkaṇḍêya, who was desirous of a long life, (312a) obtained his desire by the regular use of this oil.

Bower MS., pp. 106-7.

This formula is a phenomenally long one, consisting of no less than eighty-three ingredients, actually named, besides others not named, but permitted (*footnote*, p. 106). The famous Antidotum Mithridatium, or Galene, or Theriaca which consisted of seventy five ingredients, found a place in all the editions of the London Pharmacopœia from 1618 to 1746. Strangely the Egyptian antidote was handed down to us under the name of Ambrosia or Amṛta.

His works:

1. *Mārkaṇḍeya Purāṇa*: "That Purāṇa in which, commencing with the story of the birds that were acquainted with right and wrong, everything is narrated fully by Mārkaṇḍeya as it was explained by holy sages in reply to the question of the Muni, is called Mārkandeya, containing 9,000 verses." Its leading feature is narrative, and it presents an uninterrupted succession of legends." The legend of Hariścandra and Devimāhātmya occur in it. In the *Mahābhārata* Mārkaṇḍeya extolled the charity and devotion

of Śivi, son of Uśīnara, in the story of the pigeon, to protect whom the king gave up his body to the falcon to eat. This Purāṇa has been published in the *Bibliotheca Indica,* and translated by the Rev. Professor K M. Banerjee.

2. *Nāḍīparīkṣā* or "Examination of Pulse." It is ascribed to Mārkaṇḍeya. "It is deposited in some private libraries at Ahmedabad, Bombay. The copy is not available" (Ghosh). Mārkaṇḍeya is quoted as an authority on Pulse in the Nāḍiśastra Saṁgraha, a large MS in G.O.M.L. The last sloka gives the names of 8 sages: Kāśyapa, Kauśika, Vyāsa, Vasiṣṭha, Kumbhasambhava, Parāśara, Bharadvāja and Mārkaṇḍeya from whose works this Saṁgraha was completed.

ĀŚVALĀYANA

He was the celebrated author of *Śrauta Sūtra* and *Gṛhya Sūtra*, and other works on ritual. He is known as the founder of a Śākhā of *Ṛgveda*. Śākhā is a different recension of the text taught by particular schools and teachers and traditionally handed down to posterity. The *Sūtras* have been published by Stenzler, and also in the *Bibliotheca Indica*.

He was a pupil of Śaunaka Muni. His name appears in the list of sages who were desirous to learn Āyurveda as narrated in the *Caraka Saṁhitā* I. i.

Lassen supposes Āśvalāyana to have lived about 350 B.C.

ŚĀṆDILYA

He was a descendant of Saṇdila and the progenitor of the Sāṇdilya family of Brahmans. He was the author of *Bhakti Sūtra* and expounder of the cult of Bhakti or Faith as a religious doctrine. He is said to have written on Law and on Bhāgavat heresy which is opposed to pure Vedantic doctrine of Śaṅkara and regards the individual spirit as at any time distinct from the Supreme Spirit, though it is ultimately absorbed into the latter, The bhakti doctrine makes faith and not works or knowledge the condition of salvation. He seems to be a celebrated writer of antiquity. He was connected with the *Chāndogya Upaniṣada* where he says that the conditioned individual spirit is identical with Brahma :

" Having all actions, having all desires, having all odours, having all tastes, pervading over all this, without speech, without confusion ;—this my self within the heart, is that *Brahma*. I shall attain It, on departing from this world. Verily, one who has this faith, has no uncertainties. Thus said Śāṇdilya,—yea Śāṇdilya."—*Chāndogya Upaniṣada*, Chapter III. xiv. Gangānath Jha's Trans.

He is the author of the *Sāṇdilya Sūtra* and a treatise on law. The *Śāṇdilya Sūtras* or Aphorisms have been published in the *Bibliotheca Indica*. Cowell has shown in the Preface to the work that the extant *Śāṇdilya Sūtras* are modern. (The *Aphorisms of Śāṇdilya*, Trans. by E. B. Cowell, 1878.)

SANKHYA—KAPILA

Kapila is the reputed founder of the Sāṅkhya system of philosophy. Vitatha was his father (*Harivaṁśa*). He is sometimes identified with Viṣṇu, sometimes with Sun and also with Agni. He destroyed the hundred thousand sons of King Sagara with a glance from his fiery eyes (*Rāmāyaṇa*). The legend of Kapila is as follow:

Bāhu was King of Ayodhyā. He was defeated by the Haihayas and took refuge in a forest with his wives. Sagara was his son. Sagara's mother was given a poison by one of his step-mothers to prevent her delivery, and her pregnancy lasted for seven years. Bāhu died. Sagara was born and recovered his paternal throne. He became a paramount sovereign as soon as he obtained Āgneyāstra or fire-weapon from Aubhra. He had two wives: Sumati, the daughter of Kaśyapa, and Keśini, the daughter of the king of Vidarbha. Keśini bore him a son, Asamañja, and Sumati became the mother of sixty thousand sons. Asamañja was a cruel prince and was abandoned by his father. Sagara celebrated the Aśvamedha ceremony or the Sacrifice of a Horse as an emblem of his suzerainty. The horse was being protected by his sons,—but somehow the animal was carried to Pātāla, where the sage Kapila was absorbed in meditation. His sons dug their way to Pātāla, found the horse and considering Kapila to be a thief, insulted him. He once stared at them in anger and the sixty thousand sons were reduced to ashes. Aṁśumat, son of Asamañja, discovered their remains and appeased the wrath of Kapila. The sage granted that Bhagīratha, the grandson of Aṁśumat, would bring down the river Ganges from heaven. The sacred water would wash away their ashes and thus rendered sinless, the son's would ascend to heaven.

Colebrooke says : "A different philosophical system, partly heterodox, partly conformable to the established Hindu creed, is Sāṅkhya ; of which also, as of the preceding, there are two schools ; one usually known by that name, the other commonly termed Yoga." Kapila's system is usually known as the Sāṅkhya. The name was due to the analytical nature of the system. The Yoga system is attributed to Patañjala. The eldest of all systematic philosophies is the dualistic Sāṅkhya. A theistic form of the atheistic Sāṅkhya is called Purānic Sāṅkhya, and Patañjali's system of Yoga with its offshoot, the Pancarātra cult, is thoroughly theistic. The doctrine of Buddha is said to resemble Sāṅkhyan philosophy, but the Sāṅkhyan spirit has, as pointed out by Muller and Oldenberg, nothing corresponding to it in Buddha's system.

"The Sāṅkhya-Sūtras in their existing forms are decidedly later than all these (systems). In reality they are a spurious composition of the 15th century at the earliest and were unknown not only to Śaṅkara and Vāchaspati but also to Madhava, the author of Sarvadarsana Sangraha. It is not clear, therefore, what Sāṅkhya work Badarāyana had in his mind when he repudiated that doctrine."

"The Sāṅkhya system was really taught by Kapila to Āsuri. Āsuri taught it to Panchaśikha who is most probably the author of the original Sāṅkhya-Sūtra. The work of Panchaśikha named Shashtitantra has been admirably abridged by Iśvara Krishna in his 70 *āryās*...... Iśvara Krishna as annotated by Vāchaspati is the ultimate authority on the Sāṅkhya." (Rāmāvatār Śarmā, Sreegopal Basu Mallik Fellowship Lectures, 1907-1908, p. 9).

The name of Kapila occurs in the list of sages, given in the *Caraka Saṁhitā*, who wanted to learn medical science. His name also occurs in the list of sages who are described to be proficient in the science of the healing art in the *Devīpurāṇa*.

The Sāṅkhya system of philosophy as founded by Kapila is atheistical and derives its name from its numeral or discriminative tendencies.

Translation.—Alberuni translated Kapila's work in Arabic. It has been translated in European languages and also into Indian vernaculars. Dr. Ballantyne translated a part of the aphorisms of Kapila in the *Bibliotheca Indica* and in Trubner's Oriental series. (*Sāṅkhya Aphorisms* of Kapila, edited and annotated by Ballantyne, 1885.)

DEVALA

Devala is a Vedic Ṛṣi to whom some hymns are ascribed. He was the son of Asita Muni and became in after life Aṣṭāvakra by the curse of Rambhā. There are several sages of this name: one was the author of a law book, another was an astronomer and a third, the grandfather of Pānini, the famous grammarian.

Devala was present in the meeting of the sages as narrated in the *Caraka Saṁhitā*.

DHAUMYA

He is the younger brother of Devala. In the Mahābhārata he is mentioned as the family priest of the Pāṇḍavas, whom he advised to live in disguise in the court of Virāṭ for one year. Dhaumya is known as the author of a work on law. There are several others of the same name.

The name of Dhaumya occurs in the list of sages who met at the hermitage of Ātreya in his Himalayan retreat as mentioned in the *Caraka Saṁhitā*.

KAUNDIṆYA

Kaundiṇya is known to us as an ancient sage and grammarian. He offended Śiva, but was saved from the god's wrath by Vishnu ; he was hence called Vishnu-Gupta 'saved by Vishnu.' In some editions of *Caraka Saṁhitā* the name is spelt as Kauṇḍilya, but we know of no sage who bore that name. In the edition of Kavirāja Jogindranath Sen, who has tried to collate the text and get the most suitable readings, we find the name of the sage as Kauṇḍiṇya and we accept this reading.

AŚMARATHYA

He was one of the six disciples of Vādarāyaṇa. Aśmarathya was one of the sages who were present at the conclave of physicians mentioned in the *Caraka Saṁhitā* I. i. Aśmarathya was one of the interpreters of the important Upaniṣadic texts. Ātreya is another name in the same field of study. His name also appears as Aśvarathya in some editions of the text of the *Caraka Saṁhitā*.

ŚARKĀRAKṢA

We know nothing of Sarkārakṣa except that he had a son Jāna by name. Jāna Śārkarākṣa is mentioned in the *Chāndogya Upaniṣad*, Ch. V, Khanda XI, p. 67. He was one of the sages who was present in the congress of Ṛṣis as narrated in the *Caraka Saṁhitā*, I. i.

VĀRKṢĪ

Nothing is known of Vārkṣī as a Muni. In the *Mahābhārata* mention is made of Vārkṣī who was a daughter of a sage. She was a virtuous woman, and wife of ten husbands.

Kaikeśeya, Lokākṣa, Paiṅgi, Vaijavāpi, Maimatāyani, Abhijit, and other sages are similarly mentioned to have been present at the meeting, referred to in the *Caraka Saṁhita*, but we know nothing about them.

KĀTYĀYANA

A celebrated author of Ancient India. He wrote his *Vārttikas* or supplementary rules and annotations to complete and correct Pānini's grammar and is known as Varttika-kāra or 'annotator.' He is considered to be identical with Vararuci. He is said to be an incarnation of Puṣpadanta, a demi-god (*Kathāsaritsāgara*). He is also the author of a *Dharma śāstra*, a *Śrauta-sutra* and *Yajurveda Pratiśākhya*.

The age of Kātyāyana has been variously estimated by scholars. Max Muller places him in the second half of the 4th century; Goldstucker in the first half of the 2nd century, and Weber, 25 B.C.

GĀLAVA

Gālava was a pupil of Visvāmitra whom, as related in the *Mahābhārata*. he repeatedly requested to name what presents would satisfy him. His master was annoyed and demanded 800 white horses, each one of which must have one black ear. Gālava went to Garuḍa who took him to Yayāti Rājā who could not satisfy his demand. The king gave to the sage his daughter Mādhavī. Gālava gave her in marriage to Haryāśva, king of Ayodhyā, Divodāsa, king of Kāśi and Uśīnara, king of Bhoja in succession. On the birth of a son to each, they each gave him 200 horses of that peculiar description. Mādhavī still remained a virgin and was presented with the horses to Viśvāmitra who had a son by her Aṣṭaka by name. Aṣṭaka became the owner of the horses and Mādhavī went to her father. Viśvāmitra and Gālava retired to the forest. Ṛcīka first obtained those horses from Varuṇa (*Mahābhārata*).

In the *Harivaṁśa*, Gālava was the son of Viśvāmitra who offered him for sale, having him bound with a cord. Prince Satyavrata gave him liberty.

Pānini mentions Gālava an old grammarian. A teacher of White Yajurveda was also named Gālava.

For the legend of Gālava, and the birth Dhanvantarī see pp. 312-15.

VAIKHAṆASA AND VĀLAKHILYA MUNIS

The Vālakhilyas are mental sons of Brahmā. They are "pigmy sages no bigger than a joint of the thumb, chaste, pious, resplendent as the rays of the sun." So described by the Viṣṇu Purāṇa, which says that they were brought forth by Samanti (humility), wife of Kratu, and were 60,000 in number. They are able to fly swifter than birds The Ṛig-veda says that they sprang from the hairs of Prajapati (Brahmā). They are the guards of the chariot of the sun. They are also called Kharwas. Wilson says they are not improbably connected with the character of Daumling, Thaumlin, Tamlane, Tom-a-lyn or Tom Thumb." (Dowson, *Classical Mythology*, p. 333.)

The term Vālakhilyas is also applied to eleven apocryphal hymns interpolated in the Ṛgveda.

In the *Vṛhat Rāmāyaṇa, Citrakutamāhātmya*, Ch. I, the Vālakhilya Munis are mentioned with Agniveśa and other sages:

विधिना निर्म्मिता पूर्व्वं वेदी परमपावनी ।
अग्निवेश्यादिमुनयो वालाखिल्यादयः स्थिताः ॥

The Vaikhānasa Munis are those sages who adopt Vānaprastha or forest life, the third stage in the life of a Brāhman. They and the Vālakhilya Munis by the regular use of Brāhma-rasāyanavaleha ब्राह्मरसायनावलेह became long-lived. The formula occurs in *Gada Nigraha*, Vol. I, pp. 161-63 :—

पञ्चानां पञ्चमूलानां भागान्दशपलोन्मितान् ।
हरीतकीसहस्रं च त्रिगुणामलकं नवम् ॥

बिदारिगन्धां बृहतीं पृश्निपर्णीं निदिग्धिकाम् ।
विद्याद्विदारिगन्धाद्यं श्वदंष्ट्रापञ्चमं गणम् ॥
बिल्वोऽग्निमन्थः श्योनाकः काश्मर्यः पाटलिस्तथा ।
पुनर्नवा शूर्पपर्ण्यौ बला चैरण्ड एव च ॥
जीवकर्षभकौ वीरा जीवन्ती सशतावरी ।
शरेक्षुदर्भकाशानां शालीनां मूलमेव च ॥
एतेषां पञ्चमूलानां पञ्चानामुपकल्पयेत् ।
भागान्यथोक्तान् तत्सर्वं साध्यं दशगुणेऽम्भसि ॥
दशभागावशेषं तु पूतं तं ग्राहयेद्रसम् ।
हरीतकीश्च ताः सर्वाः सर्वाश्चामलकानि च ॥
तानि सर्वाण्यनस्थीनि फलान्यापोथ्य कूर्चकैः ।
विनीय तस्मिन्निर्यूहे चूर्णानीमानि दापयेत् ॥
मण्डूकपर्ण्याः पिप्पल्याः शङ्खपुष्प्याः प्लवस्य च ।
मुस्तानां सविडङ्गानां चन्दनागुरुणोस्तथा ॥
मधुकस्य हरिद्रायाः वचायाः कनकस्य च ।
भागान् पञ्चपलान्कृत्वा सूक्ष्मैलायास्त्वचस्तथा ॥
सितोपलासहस्रं च चूर्णितं तुलयाधिकम् ।
तैलं स्याद्द्व्याढकं तत्र तथा चौषि च सर्पिषः ।
साध्यं ताम्रमये पात्रे तत्सर्वं मृदुनाऽग्निना ।
ज्ञात्वा लेह्यमदग्धं च शीतं क्षौद्रेण संसृजेत् ॥
क्षौद्रप्रमाणं स्नेहार्धं तत्सर्वं घृतभाजने ।
तिष्ठेत्संमूर्च्छितं तस्य मात्रां काले प्रयोजयेत् ॥
या नोपरुन्ध्यादाहारमेवं मात्रा तु सा स्मृत
षष्टिकः पयसा चात्र जीर्णे भोजनमिष्यते ॥
<u>वैखानसा वालिखिल्यास्तथा चान्ये तपोधनाः</u> ।
रसायनमिदं प्राश्य बभूवुरमितायुषः ॥
मुक्त्वा जीर्णं वपुश्चाग्र्यमवापुस्तरुणं वयः ।
वीततन्द्रा-क्लम-श्वासा निरातङ्काः समाहिताः ॥
मेधास्मृतिबलोपेताश्चिरकालं तपोधनाः ।
ब्राह्मं तपो ब्रह्मचर्यं चेरुश्चात्यन्तनिष्ठया ॥

आयुष्काम: प्रयुञ्जानो ब्राह्मं हीदं रसायनम् ।
दीर्घमायुर्बलं चाग्र्यं कामांश्चेष्टान्समश्नुते ॥

Gada Nigraha, Vol. I, pp. 165-6.

KAPIṢṬHALA.

Kapiṣṭhala is the name of a sage who was present at the meeting of the Rṣis as narrated in the *Caraka Saṁhitā* I. i. In some editions of the book the name occurs as Kapiñjala, and sometimes as Kapidhvaja. But in Sen's edition (1920) we find Kapiṣṭhala which seems to be the correct reading. His disciples were Kapiṣṭhalas "The adherents of the *Yajurveda* split up into several schools, which gradually spread over other parts of India, the Kaṭhas, with their sub-division Kapiṣṭhalas, being in the time of the Greeks, located in the Panjab, and later in Kashmir also. The Kaṭhas are now to be found in Kashmir only, while the Kapiṣṭhalas have entirely disappeared. Of the *Kapiṣṭhala-Kaṭha Saṁhitā* only somewhat corrupt fragments have hitherto come to light and it is very doubtful whether sufficient manuscript material will ever be discovered to render an edition of this text possible."—Macdonnel : *History of Sanskrit Literature*, pp 173-74.

BHĀRGABHA.

The descendants of the sage Bhṛgu are known as the Bhārgabhas. The Bhārgabha is said to have been present in the meeting of the sages as narrated in the *Caraka Saṁhitā*. Now, who is this Bhārgabha? The prominent figures in the race of Bhṛgu are Cyavana, Śaunaka, Jamadagni and Paraśu-Rāma. But the term Bhārgabha is applied specially to Jāmadagna Paraśu-Rām. He was a Brāhmaṇa. The sage Jamadagni was his father, and Renukā, daughter of the royal race of the Kuśikas was his mother. He is regarded as the sixth *Avatāra* of Viṣnu by the Hindus. His exploits have been described before in p. 297. His wrath against the Kṣattriyas was checked by his defeat in his battle with Bhīṣma, the famous warrior of the Kuru race. Bhīṣma and Karṇa learnt the science of archery from him. He cursed Karṇa for concealment of the story of his birth. After the extirpation of the regal race he gave the earth to Kaśyapa and returned to the Mahendra mountain where Arjuna visited him and received instruction in the use of arms (*Mahābhārata*). In the *Rāmāyaṇa* he is said to have suffered defeat in the hands of Rāma, when Paraśu-Rāma obstructed his way to Oudh after his marriage with Sītā, and he lost his celestial seat as a consequence. Jāmadagna was a disciple of Śiva who gave him the invincible Paraśu or axe as his weapon. He is said to have brought Brāhmans into Malabar.

Bhārgava was versed in the science of medicine. He is described to have learned the science in the *Caraka Saṁhitā*, and he is quoted as an authority in the *Hasti-Āyurveda* by Pālakāpya.

End of Volume II.